Vitamin C: From Bench to Bedside

Vitamin C: From Bench to Bedside

Editors
Anitra Carr
Jens Lykkesfeldt

MDPI • Basel • Beijing • Wuhan • Barcelona • Belgrade • Manchester • Tokyo • Cluj • Tianjin

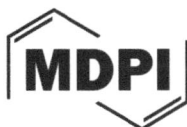

Editors
Anitra Carr
Pathology and Biomedical Science
University of Otago
Christchurch
New Zealand

Jens Lykkesfeldt
Faculty of Health Medical Sciences
University of Copenhagen
Copenhagen
Denmark

Editorial Office
MDPI
St. Alban-Anlage 66
4052 Basel, Switzerland

This is a reprint of articles from the Special Issue published online in the open access journal *Nutrients* (ISSN 2072-6643) (available at: www.mdpi.com/journal/nutrients/special_issues/Vitamin_C_Insights).

For citation purposes, cite each article independently as indicated on the article page online and as indicated below:

LastName, A.A.; LastName, B.B.; LastName, C.C. Article Title. *Journal Name* **Year**, *Volume Number*, Page Range.

ISBN 978-3-0365-1285-3 (Hbk)
ISBN 978-3-0365-1284-6 (PDF)

© 2021 by the authors. Articles in this book are Open Access and distributed under the Creative Commons Attribution (CC BY) license, which allows users to download, copy and build upon published articles, as long as the author and publisher are properly credited, which ensures maximum dissemination and a wider impact of our publications.

The book as a whole is distributed by MDPI under the terms and conditions of the Creative Commons license CC BY-NC-ND.

Contents

About the Editors vii

Preface to "Vitamin C: From Bench to Bedside" ix

Anitra C. Carr and Jens Lykkesfeldt
Vitamin C: From Bench to Bedside
Reprinted from: *Nutrients* **2021**, *13*, 1102, doi:10.3390/nu13041102 1

Jens Lykkesfeldt and Pernille Tveden-Nyborg
The Pharmacokinetics of Vitamin C
Reprinted from: *Nutrients* **2019**, *11*, 2412, doi:10.3390/nu11102412 5

Juliet M. Pullar, Susannah Dunham, Gabi U. Dachs, Margreet C. M. Vissers and Anitra C. Carr
Erythrocyte Ascorbate Is a Potential Indicator of Steady-State Plasma Ascorbate Concentrations in Healthy Non-Fasting Individuals
Reprinted from: *Nutrients* **2020**, *12*, 418, doi:10.3390/nu12020418 25

Mikee Liugan and Anitra C. Carr
Vitamin C and Neutrophil Function: Findings from Randomized Controlled Trials
Reprinted from: *Nutrients* **2019**, *11*, 2102, doi:10.3390/nu11092102 33

Stephanie M. Bozonet and Anitra C. Carr
The Role of Physiological Vitamin C Concentrations on Key Functions of Neutrophils Isolated from Healthy Individuals
Reprinted from: *Nutrients* **2019**, *11*, 1363, doi:10.3390/nu11061363 49

Stephen J. McCall, Allan B. Clark, Robert N. Luben, Nicholas J. Wareham, Kay-Tee Khaw and Phyo Kyaw Myint
Plasma Vitamin C Levels: Risk Factors for Deficiency and Association with Self-Reported Functional Health in the European Prospective Investigation into Cancer-Norfolk
Reprinted from: *Nutrients* **2019**, *11*, 1552, doi:10.3390/nu11071552 63

Liping Gan, Vladimir Camarena, Sushmita Mustafi and Gaofeng Wang
Vitamin C Inhibits Triple-Negative Breast Cancer Metastasis by Affecting the Expression of YAP1 and Synaptopodin 2
Reprinted from: *Nutrients* **2019**, *11*, 2997, doi:10.3390/nu11122997 77

Anitra C. Carr, Emma Spencer, Andrew Das, Natalie Meijer, Carolyn Lauren, Sean MacPherson and Stephen T. Chambers
Patients Undergoing Myeloablative Chemotherapy and Hematopoietic Stem Cell Transplantation Exhibit Depleted Vitamin C Status in Association with Febrile Neutropenia
Reprinted from: *Nutrients* **2020**, *12*, 1879, doi:10.3390/nu12061879 89

Rebecca White, Maria Nonis, John F. Pearson, Eleanor Burgess, Helen R. Morrin, Juliet M. Pullar, Emma Spencer, Margreet C. M. Vissers, Bridget A. Robinson and Gabi U. Dachs
Low Vitamin C Status in Patients with Cancer Is Associated with Patient and Tumor Characteristics
Reprinted from: *Nutrients* **2020**, *12*, 2338, doi:10.3390/nu12082338 99

Sher Ali Khan, Sandipan Bhattacharjee, Muhammad Owais Abdul Ghani, Rachel Walden and Qin M. Chen
Vitamin C for Cardiac Protection during Percutaneous Coronary Intervention: A Systematic Review of Randomized Controlled Trials
Reprinted from: *Nutrients* **2020**, *12*, 2199, doi:10.3390/nu12082199 113

Kuo-Chuan Hung, Yao-Tsung Lin, Kee-Hsin Chen, Li-Kai Wang, Jen-Yin Chen, Ying-Jen Chang, Shao-Chun Wu, Min-Hsien Chiang and Cheuk-Kwan Sun
The Effect of Perioperative Vitamin C on Postoperative Analgesic Consumption: A Meta-Analysis of Randomized Controlled Trials
Reprinted from: *Nutrients* **2020**, *12*, 3109, doi:10.3390/nu12103109 133

Anitra C. Carr, Emma Spencer, Liane Dixon and Stephen T. Chambers
Patients with Community Acquired Pneumonia Exhibit Depleted Vitamin C Status and Elevated Oxidative Stress
Reprinted from: *Nutrients* **2020**, *12*, 1318, doi:10.3390/nu12051318 151

David C. Consoli, Jordan J. Jesse, Kelly R. Klimo, Adriana A. Tienda, Nathan D. Putz, Julie A. Bastarache and Fiona E. Harrison
A Cecal Slurry Mouse Model of Sepsis Leads to Acute Consumption of Vitamin C in the Brain
Reprinted from: *Nutrients* **2020**, *12*, 911, doi:10.3390/nu12040911 161

Won-Young Kim, Jae-Woo Jung, Jae Chol Choi, Jong Wook Shin and Jae Yeol Kim
Subphenotypes in Patients with Septic Shock Receiving Vitamin C, Hydrocortisone, and Thiamine: A Retrospective Cohort Analysis
Reprinted from: *Nutrients* **2019**, *11*, 2976, doi:10.3390/nu11122976 173

Anitra C. Carr and Sam Rowe
The Emerging Role of Vitamin C in the Prevention and Treatment of COVID-19
Reprinted from: *Nutrients* **2020**, *12*, 3286, doi:10.3390/nu12113286 187

About the Editors

Anitra Carr

Associate professor Anitra Carr is the director of the Nutrition in Medicine Research Group at the University of Otago, Christchurch, NZ. Dr. Carr is considered an international 'key opinion leader' on the role of vitamin C in human health and disease. Following a PhD in biochemistry, Dr. Carr was awarded an American Heart Association Fellowship to research vitamin C in cardiovascular disease at the Linus Pauling Institute, Oregon State University, USA. Whilst there, she produced a number of high-impact publications, one of which was used by the US Food and Nutrition Board, Institute of Medicine, as a basis for their increase in the recommended dietary intake for vitamin C. Dr. Carr was recently awarded a Health Research Council of NZ Fellowship and is currently carrying out translational 'bench to bedside' research into the role of vitamin C in the prevention and treatment of severe infection, specifically pneumonia and sepsis, and chronic diseases such as cancer and diabetes.

Jens Lykkesfeldt

Dr. Lykkesfeldt earned his MSc degree in organic chemistry in 1989, his PhD degree in biochemistry in 1992, and later his DSc degree in medicine in 2005 for his thesis on the effect of smoking on vitamin C status. He spent two 3-year postdocs at the University of Copenhagen and UC Berkeley, respectively, the latter with Professor Bruce N. Ames. In 1998, he became principal investigator and associate professor at the University of Copenhagen, Denmark. He was appointed professor and chair of pharmacology and toxicology in 2008 at the Faculty of Health and Medical Sciences, University of Copenhagen, which is his current position. Dr. Lykkesfeldt's research interests include the roles of oxidative stress and antioxidants, in particular that of vitamin C, in early development, chronic diseases, and aging, and he has published >100 articles on vitamin C alone. In 2008, he received the Catherine Pasquiere award from the Society for Free Radical Research, Europe, for his work on vitamin C.

Preface to "Vitamin C: From Bench to Bedside"

Vitamin C (ascorbic acid) is a normal liver metabolite in most animals, with humans being a notable exception due to random genetic mutations that have occurred during our evolution. As such, it has become a vitamin (vital to life), with requirements increasing significantly during various illnesses, particularly severe infections. Recent international clinical trials are highlighting the potential for intravenous vitamin C administration to improve clinical outcomes for patients, particularly those with severe respiratory illness, sepsis, and some cancers. Furthermore, there has been an upsurge in new discoveries and new mechanistic insights, particularly around epigenetic regulation by vitamin C, that are providing rationales for future targeted clinical trials. Although its role in scurvy has been recognized for close to a century, it appears that we still have much to learn about this small carbohydrate molecule. Well-designed observational and interventional studies that consider the baseline status and unique pharmacokinetics of vitamin C are needed moving forward to help address the current gaps in our knowledge. Underpinning mechanistic research will also further our ability to inform good clinical practice.

Anitra Carr, Jens Lykkesfeldt
Editors

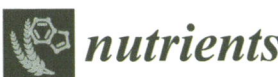

Editorial

Vitamin C: From Bench to Bedside

Anitra C. Carr [1,*] and Jens Lykkesfeldt [2]

1. Nutrition in Medicine Research Group, Department of Pathology & Biomedical Science, University of Otago, Christchurch 8011, New Zealand
2. Faculty of Health & Medical Sciences, University of Copenhagen, 1870 Frederiksberg, Denmark; jopl@sund.ku.dk
* Correspondence: anitra.carr@otago.ac.nz; Tel.: +64-3364-0649

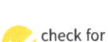

Citation: Carr, A.C.; Lykkesfeldt, J. Vitamin C: From Bench to Bedside. *Nutrients* **2021**, *13*, 1102. https://doi.org/10.3390/nu13041102

Received: 19 March 2021
Accepted: 24 March 2021
Published: 27 March 2021

Publisher's Note: MDPI stays neutral with regard to jurisdictional claims in published maps and institutional affiliations.

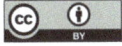

Copyright: © 2021 by the authors. Licensee MDPI, Basel, Switzerland. This article is an open access article distributed under the terms and conditions of the Creative Commons Attribution (CC BY) license (https://creativecommons.org/licenses/by/4.0/).

Vitamin C (ascorbic acid) is a normal liver metabolite in most animals, with humans being a notable exception due to random genetic mutations that have occurred during our evolution. As such, it has become a vitamin (vital to life), with requirements increasing significantly during various illnesses, particularly severe infections. Recent international clinical trials are highlighting the potential for intravenous vitamin C administration to improve clinical outcomes for patients, particularly those with severe respiratory illness and sepsis and some cancers. Furthermore, there has been an upsurge in new discoveries and new mechanistic insights, particularly around epigenetic regulation by vitamin C, that are providing rationales for future targeted clinical trials.

To facilitate the translation of leading-edge research into clinical practice, we held the second "Vitamin C Symposium" in 2019 with the theme of "Vitamin C for Cancer and Infection: From Bench to Bedside" [1]. The speakers were internationally renowned biomedical and clinical researchers and doctors with expertise in the fields of infection and cancer. The symposium was designed as an educational event targeted primarily at doctors and nurses and provided Continuing Professional Development through the Royal New Zealand College of General Practitioners (RNZCGP) and the College of Intensive Care Medicine of Australia and New Zealand (CICM). The content of the symposium comprised translational "bench to bedside" research, from laboratory-based experiments aimed at understanding the underlying mechanisms involved to clinical trials endeavoring to determine the efficacy of vitamin C in various infectious states and cancer types. This symposium was the inspiration for the Nutrients Special Issue "Vitamin C: from Bench to Bedside".

In this Special Issue, we have collected 15 original research papers and comprehensive review articles spanning laboratory-based research, observational studies and intervention trials. These cover the following key research themes: pharmacokinetics, immune function, epidemiology, cancer research, surgical outcomes, and infection research, specifically pneumonia, sepsis, and COVID-19.

Pharmacokinetics: Lykkesfeldt and colleague wrote a comprehensive review highlighting the complex pharmacokinetics of oral and intravenous vitamin C [2], an issue that is often overlooked in the design and interpretation of clinical studies. Research carried out by Pullar and colleagues has indicated that due to the unique kinetics of vitamin C uptake into erythrocytes, these cells could potentially be used as an indicator of vitamin C status in nonfasting individuals [3], thereby overcoming the issue of plasma vitamin C fluctuations in response to recent dietary intake.

Immune function: Carr and colleagues investigated the role of vitamin C in neutrophil function, including a systematic review of randomized controlled trials carried out in different population groups and patient cohorts [4]. The neutrophil functions assessed included chemotaxis, phagocytosis, oxidative burst activity, enzyme activity, and apoptosis. Additional laboratory-based research showed that enhanced uptake of ascorbate by human neutrophils can affect key functions, including chemotaxis and neutrophil extracellular trap (NET) formation [5].

Epidemiology: Dr Myint and colleagues interrogated the large European Prospective Investigation into Cancer-Norfolk (EPIC-Norfolk) database to determine demographic and lifestyle risk factors for vitamin C deficiency and associations with functional health [6]. They found that vitamin C deficiency was associated with older age, being male, lower physical activity, smoking, being more socially deprived and a lower educational attainment. Those in the lowest quartile of vitamin C were also more likely to score in the lowest decile of physical function, bodily pain, general health, and vitality.

Cancer research: Dr Wang and colleagues have identified key molecular targets of vitamin C activity in triple-negative breast cancer metastasis in cell culture and a xenograft model [7], indicating that vitamin C can potentially inhibit metastasis by modulating the expression of SYNPO2 and YAP1. Observational research by Carr and colleagues has indicated that patients undergoing chemotherapy in association with stem cell transplantation exhibit depleted vitamin C status in association with febrile neutropenia [8]. Further observational research by Dachs and colleagues indicated that low vitamin C status in patients with cancer is associated with both patient and tumor characteristics [9].

Surgical outcomes: A systematic review on the effects of vitamin C administration on outcomes of Percutaneous Coronary Intervention (PCI) has indicated that intravenous infusion of vitamin C before PCI may serve as an effective method for cardioprotection against reperfusion injury [10]. A meta-analysis on the effects of perioperative vitamin C administration on postoperative analgesia consumption indicated a lower pain score and a lower morphine consumption in those receiving intravenous vitamin C, but not oral vitamin C [11].

Pneumonia and sepsis: Observational research by Carr and colleagues has indicated that hospitalized patients with community-acquired pneumonia exhibit both depleted vitamin C status and elevated markers of oxidative stress [12]. Pneumonia is a major driver for the development of sepsis. Harrison and colleagues reported enhanced synthesis of vitamin C in mice following a septic insult [13], but despite this, there was still a decrease in vitamin C levels in the brain, as well as upregulation of key inflammatory cytokines (IL-6, IL-1β, TNFα) and chemokines (CXCL1, KC/Gro). Kim et al. retrospectively identified specific subphenotypes in patients with septic shock that may respond differently to treatment with vitamin C, hydrocortisone and thiamine combination therapy [14]. They indicated that clinical outcomes might be better for patients with the hyperinflammatory subphenotype.

Sepsis and COVID-19: Dr Fowler and colleagues wrote a comprehensive review on the emerging role of vitamin C as a treatment for sepsis [15], which covers the pleiotropic functions of vitamin C in sepsis and acute respiratory distress syndrome (ARDS) and includes a discussion of their recent CITRIS-ALI trial which showed decreased mortality in sepsis-induced acute lung injury (ALI) following administration of intravenous vitamin C. As highlighted in the accompanying Editorial [16], this review is particular pertinent in light of the global SARS-CoV-2 pandemic as pneumonia and sepsis are major complications of severe Coronavirus Disease-2019 (COVID-19). Of note, preliminary observational and interventional studies are indicating a potential role for vitamin C in the prevention and treatment of COVID-19 [16].

Collectively, this Special Issue displays the diverse areas of health and disease in which vitamin C plays important roles and the continuing efforts of researchers to unravel the underlying mechanisms of its biological functions. Although its role in scurvy has been recognized for close to a century, it appears that we still have much to learn about this small carbohydrate molecule. Well-designed observational and interventional studies that consider the baseline status and unique pharmacokinetics of vitamin C are needed moving forward to help address the current gaps in our knowledge. Underpinning mechanistic research will also further our ability to inform good clinical practice. We look forward to future discoveries of the roles of vitamin C in human health and disease.

Author Contributions: Conceptualization and writing—original draft preparation, A.C.C.; writing—review and editing, J.L. All authors have read and agreed to the published version of the manuscript.

Funding: This research received no external funding.

Institutional Review Board Statement: Not applicable.

Informed Consent Statement: Not applicable.

Data Availability Statement: Not applicable.

Conflicts of Interest: The authors declare no conflict of interest.

References

1. Carr, A.C. Vitamin C symposium 2019—Vitamin C for cancer and infection: From bench to bedside. *Proceedings* **2019**, *5*, 3. [CrossRef]
2. Lykkesfeldt, J.; Tveden-Nyborg, P. The pharmacokinetics of Vitamin C. *Nutrients* **2019**, *11*, 2412. [CrossRef] [PubMed]
3. Pullar, J.; Dunham, S.; Dachs, G.; Vissers, M.; Carr, A.C. Erythrocyte ascorbate is a potential indicator of steady-state plasma ascorbate concentrations in healthy non-fasting individuals. *Nutrients* **2020**, *12*, 418. [CrossRef] [PubMed]
4. Liugan, M.; Carr, A.C. Vitamin C and neutrophil function: Findings from randomized controlled trials. *Nutrients* **2019**, *11*, 2102. [CrossRef] [PubMed]
5. Bozonet, S.M.; Carr, A.C. The role of physiological Vitamin C concentrations on key functions of neutrophils isolated from healthy individuals. *Nutrients* **2019**, *11*, 1363. [CrossRef] [PubMed]
6. McCall, S.J.; Clark, A.B.; Luben, R.N.; Wareham, N.J.; Khaw, K.T.; Myint, P.K. Plasma Vitamin C levels: Risk factors for deficiency and association with self-reported functional health in the European Prospective Investigation into Cancer-Norfolk. *Nutrients* **2019**, *11*, 1552. [CrossRef] [PubMed]
7. Gan, L.; Camarena, V.; Mustafi, S.; Wang, G. Vitamin C inhibits triple-negative breast cancer metastasis by affecting the expression of YAP1 and Synaptopodin 2. *Nutrients* **2019**, *11*, 2997. [CrossRef] [PubMed]
8. Carr, A.C.; Spencer, E.; Das, A.; Meijer, N.; Lauren, C.; MacPherson, S.; Chambers, S.T. Patients undergoing myeloablative chemotherapy and hematopoietic stem cell transplantation exhibit depleted Vitamin C status in association with febrile neutropenia. *Nutrients* **2020**, *12*, 1879. [CrossRef] [PubMed]
9. White, R.; Nonis, M.; Pearson, J.F.; Burgess, E.; Morrin, H.R.; Pullar, J.M.; Spencer, E.; Vissers, M.C.M.; Robinson, B.A.; Dachs, G.U. Low Vitamin C status in patients with cancer is associated with patient and tumor characteristics. *Nutrients* **2020**, *12*, 2338. [CrossRef] [PubMed]
10. Khan, S.A.; Bhattacharjee, S.; Ghani, M.O.A.; Walden, R.; Chen, Q.M. Vitamin C for cardiac protection during percutaneous coronary intervention: A systematic review of randomized controlled trials. *Nutrients* **2020**, *12*, 2199. [CrossRef] [PubMed]
11. Hung, K.C.; Lin, Y.T.; Chen, K.H.; Wang, L.K.; Chen, J.Y.; Chang, Y.J.; Wu, S.C.; Chiang, M.H.; Sun, C.K. The effect of perioperative Vitamin C on postoperative analgesic consumption: A meta-analysis of randomized controlled trials. *Nutrients* **2020**, *12*, 3109. [CrossRef] [PubMed]
12. Carr, A.C.; Spencer, E.; Dixon, L.; Chambers, S.T. Patients with community acquired pneumonia exhibit depleted Vitamin C status and elevated oxidative stress. *Nutrients* **2020**, *12*, 1318. [CrossRef] [PubMed]
13. Consoli, D.C.; Jesse, J.J.; Klimo, K.R.; Tienda, A.A.; Putz, N.D.; Bastarache, J.A.; Harrison, F.E. A cecal slurry mouse model of sepsis leads to acute consumption of Vitamin C in the brain. *Nutrients* **2020**, *12*, 911. [CrossRef] [PubMed]
14. Kim, W.Y.; Jung, J.W.; Choi, J.C.; Shin, J.W.; Kim, J.Y. Subphenotypes in patients with septic shock receiving Vitamin C, hydrocortisone, and thiamine: A retrospective cohort analysis. *Nutrients* **2019**, *11*, 2976. [CrossRef] [PubMed]
15. Kashiouris, M.G.; L'Heureux, M.; Cable, C.A.; Fisher, B.J.; Leichtle, S.W.; Fowler, A.A. The emerging role of Vitamin C as a treatment for sepsis. *Nutrients* **2020**, *12*, 292. [CrossRef] [PubMed]
16. Carr, A.C.; Rowe, S. The emerging role of Vitamin C in the prevention and treatment of COVID-19. *Nutrients* **2020**, *12*, 3286. [CrossRef] [PubMed]

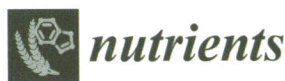

Review

The Pharmacokinetics of Vitamin C

Jens Lykkesfeldt * and Pernille Tveden-Nyborg

Faculty of Health and Medical Sciences, Department of Veterinary and Animal Sciences,
University of Copenhagen, DK-1870 Frederiksberg C, Denmark; ptn@sund.ku.dk
* Correspondence: jopl@sund.ku.dk; Tel.: +45-3533-3163

Received: 17 September 2019; Accepted: 8 October 2019; Published: 9 October 2019

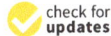

Abstract: The pharmacokinetics of vitamin C (vitC) is indeed complex. Regulated primarily by a family of saturable sodium dependent vitC transporters (SVCTs), the absorption and elimination are highly dose-dependent. Moreover, the tissue specific expression levels and subtypes of these SVCTs result in a compartmentalized distribution pattern with a diverse range of organ concentrations of vitC at homeostasis ranging from about 0.2 mM in the muscle and heart, and up to 10 mM in the brain and adrenal gland. The homeostasis of vitC is influenced by several factors, including genetic polymorphisms and environmental and lifestyle factors such as smoking and diet, as well as diseases. Going from physiological to pharmacological doses, vitC pharmacokinetics change from zero to first order, rendering the precise calculation of dosing regimens in, for example, cancer and sepsis treatment possible. Unfortunately, the complex pharmacokinetics of vitC has often been overlooked in the design of intervention studies, giving rise to misinterpretations and erroneous conclusions. The present review outlines the diverse aspects of vitC pharmacokinetics and examines how they affect vitC homeostasis under a variety of conditions.

Keywords: vitamin C; pharmacokinetics; homeostasis; human disease

1. Introduction

Humans rely solely on dietary intake for the maintenance of the body pool of vitamin C (vitC). In contrast to the vast majority of vertebrates, in which L-gulonolactone oxidase catalyzes the final step in the biosynthesis of ascorbic acid, evolutionarily conserved deletions have made the corresponding gene inactive in primates, flying mammals, guinea pigs, and some bird and fish species, thereby disabling its formation [1]. This evolutionary event may in fact have resulted in an adaptational process where our ability to prevent vitC deficiency has been improved by various measures changing the pharmacokinetics, including more efficient absorption, recycling, and renal reuptake of vitC compared to vitC synthesizing species [2,3].

The absorption, distribution, metabolism, and excretion of vitC in humans is highly complex and unlike that of most low molecular weight compounds. The majority of intestinal uptake, tissue distribution, and renal reuptake is handled by the sodium-dependent vitC transporter (SVCT) family of proteins [4] that cotransports sodium ions and ascorbate (ASC) across membranes with the ability to generate considerable concentration gradients [5,6]. It is the differential expression, substrate affinity, and concentration dependency of the SVCTs between organs that gives rise to the unique compartmentalization and nonlinear pharmacokinetics of vitC at physiological levels [7].

The hydrophilic nature of ASC and the likely resulting absence of passive diffusion across biological membranes has puzzled pharmacologists. However, two decades ago, active transport of vitC was found to be essential for life, when Sotiriou et al. showed that SVCT2 knockout mice die immediately after birth from respiratory failure with severe brain hemorrhage [8]. Acknowledging the role of SVCTs in vitC homeostasis has naturally sparked an interest in possible differences in SVCT activity between individuals and potential impact on vitC status. Thus, a number of polymorphisms have been identified, and these may affect the pharmacokinetics of vitC significantly. Although not investigated in clinical studies yet, pharmacokinetic modelling has suggested that several of the identified SVCT alleles result in a lower plasma steady state level and consequently completely altered homeostasis [9] with the lowest saturation level leading to permanent vitC deficiency, i.e., a plasma concentration < 23 µM [10,11].

In contrast to the physiological concentrations achievable by oral ingestion, pharmacological concentrations, i.e., millimolar plasma concentrations, can be reached by parenteral administration, mostly intravenous infusion [12]. Interestingly, the pharmacokinetics of vitC appears to change from zero to first order following high-dose infusion displaying a constant and dose-independent half-life [13].

A final factor contributing to the complexity of vitC pharmacology is its metabolism. Low molecular weight drugs and xenobiotics are normally metabolized by a combination of phase I and II enzymes leading to oxidized and conjugated metabolites with increased water solubility and enhanced clearance. VitC takes part in numerous physiological reactions as an electron donor [14]. Acting both as a specific cofactor or antioxidant, ASC is oxidized to the ascorbyl radical, which subsequently may undergo dismutation to form ASC and dehydroascorbic acid (DHA) [15]. Although DHA has a half-life of only a few minutes [16], it is normally reduced back to ASC by enzymatic means, an intracellular process that is both efficient and quantitative in healthy individuals. However, it has been shown that the recycling process may be inadequate during disease and among smokers, for example, resulting in an increased turnover of vitC [17,18]. Thus, increased intake of vitC may be necessary to achieve homeostasis in high-risk individuals.

The present review outlines the pharmacokinetics of vitC under various conditions and discusses how it affects the vitC status.

2. Pharmacokinetics of Vitamin C

Pharmacokinetics constitutes the description of absorption, distribution, metabolism, and excretion of drugs. Pharmacokinetics is based on a number of theoretical models, all of which have a set of assumptions that need to be fulfilled for their validity. Compared to a typical orally administered low molecular weight drug, vitC differs in multiple ways with respect to pharmacokinetic properties [19]. Unfortunately, lack of proper attention to particularly the nonlinearity of vitC pharmacokinetics has led to misinterpretation of a major part of the clinical literature as reviewed elsewhere [11,19,20]. In the following, the kinetics of vitC is explored in more detail.

2.1. Oral Route of Administration

Oral ingestion of food or supplements is the primary route of administration for vitC. VitC is ubiquitous in nature and particularly fruits and vegetables contain relatively large amounts of ASC [21]. For healthy individuals, it is possible to get sufficient amounts of vitC through the diet provided it contains high amounts of vitC-rich sources [22,23]. However, in many diseases and in people with very poor vitC status including smokers, for example, the dietary intake may be insufficient to provide adequate amounts of vitC [19,24,25].

2.1.1. Absorption

VitC exists primarily in two forms in vivo, ASC (reduced form) and DHA (oxidized form), of which the former is by far the predominant [26]. Due to the efficient intracellular recycling of DHA to ASC by most cell types, the total available vitC capacity is considered the combined pool of ASC and DHA [27]. With regard to vitC, three potential modes of membrane transport exist: passive diffusion, facilitated diffusion, and active transport [6].

For most low molecular weight drugs, simple diffusion is the primary means of membrane transport. However, vitC is predominantly represented by its anionic form (>99.9%) at neutral pH and is highly water-soluble. As such, it will only be able to diffuse across the plasma membrane at a relatively slow rate even in the presence of a considerable concentration gradient. However, in the milieu of the stomach (pH 1) or small intestine (pH 5), the proportion of unionized ascorbic acid increases to 99.9% and 15%, respectively, and under these local conditions, passive diffusion could perhaps play a more significant role in vitC uptake. Studies in individuals with normal vitC status have reported similar times to maximal plasma concentration following oral administration of ascorbic and erythorbic acid, respectively [28,29], even though erythorbic acid, an isoform of ASC with low vitC activity, is poorly transported by epithelial SVCT1 [30]. However, it remains undisclosed if passive diffusion of ASC contributes significantly to its absorption from these compartments.

Facilitated diffusion across membranes occurs through carrier proteins but like passive diffusion, it depends on an electrochemical gradient. DHA has been shown to compete with glucose for transport through several glucose transporters [31,32]. While only present in negligible amounts in the blood of healthy individuals [17,33], intestinal concentrations are presumably much higher, most likely due to the absence of intracellular recycling and relatively higher concentration in foodstuffs. This may explain the repeated finding of similar bioavailability of ASC and DHA as vitC sources [2,34–36]. Moreover, this could explain the observation of equal absorption rates of ascorbic and erythorbic acid from the intestine as dehydroerythorbic acid would be expected to pass through glucose transporters. DHA uptake is expectedly inhibited by excess glucose, while the maximal rates of uptake for ASC and DHA are similar when glucose is absent [37].

Finally, concentration gradient-independent active transport plays a significant role in vitC absorption. As early as the 1970s, it was observed that the bioavailability of ASC is highly dose-dependent [38]. Increasing oral doses were shown to lead to decreasing absorption fractions and it was concluded by several authors that intestinal ASC absorption is subject to saturable active transport [38,39]. Malo and Wilson discovered that DHA and ASC are taken up by separate mechanisms in the intestine and that uptake of ASC is sodium-dependent [37]. This coincided with the discovery and characterization of the SVCT family of transporters by Tsukaguchi et al. [4]. They subsequently showed that the intestine contains the low affinity/high capacity active transporter SVCT1 [30]. Thus, ASC is efficiently transported across the apical membrane of the intestinal epithelial cells via active transport but its release into the blood stream is less well understood. As intracellular vitC is effectively kept reduced, facilitating further uptake of DHA, efflux to the blood through glucose transporters is unlikely to provide a significant contribution. As mentioned above, the intracellular pH of 7.0 renders the anionic ASC predominant (99.9%) and given its hydrophilic nature, passive efflux of ascorbic acid via simple diffusion will be relatively slow. However, as the cellular release of vitC to the blood stream is vital for the absorption process and must occur to a high extend considering the rapid uptake of vitC (plasma Tmax of about 3 h [29]), it strongly implies the existence of yet undiscovered channels or transporters facilitating vitC efflux. It has been proposed that ASC efflux may occur through volume-sensitive anion channels in the basolateral membranes of epithelial cells [6]. In the brain, however, studies in human microvascular pericytes have shown that volume-sensitive anion channels are apparently not involved in the ASC efflux from these cells and may therefore not represent a general mechanism of basal ASC efflux [40]. A schematic overview of intestinal vitC absorption is shown in Figure 1.

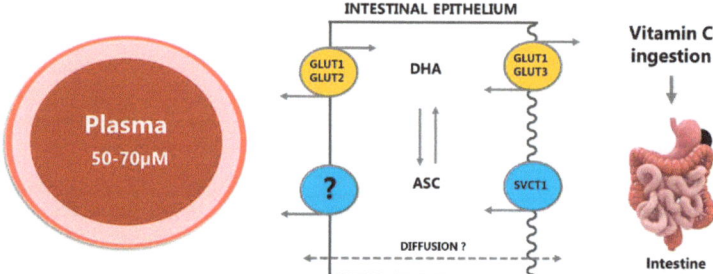

Figure 1. Ingested vitamin C (vitC) is absorbed across the intestinal epithelium primarily by membrane transporters in the apical brush border membrane, either as ascorbate (ASC) by sodium-coupled active transport via the SVCT1 transporter or as dehydroascorbic acid (DHA) through facilitated diffusion via GLUT1 or GLUT3 transporters. Once inside the cell, DHA is efficiently converted to ASC or transported to the blood stream by GLUT1 and GLUT2 in the basolateral membrane, hereby maintaining a low intracellular concentration and facilitating further DHA uptake. ASC is conveyed to plasma by diffusion, possibly also by facilitated diffusion through volume-sensitive anion channels or by yet unidentified active transporters; the precise efflux mechanisms remain unknown. Modified from [5].

2.1.2. Distribution

The distribution of vitC is highly compartmentalized (Figure 2). Simple diffusion is unlikely to play a major role in vitC transport across membranes, at least in the further distribution from the blood stream. From a theoretical point of view, ASC plasma steady state concentrations would be 2.5-fold higher than in tissue as calculated by a dissociation-determined equilibrium. In reality, intracellular concentrations of ASC range from about 0.5 to 10 mM compared to the mere 50–80 µM in the plasma of healthy individuals [7], confirming a many-fold preference for tissue. Although the glucose transporters (GLUTs 1–4 and 8) capable of facilitating diffusion of DHA are widely represented throughout the body [31,32,41–43], the negligible amount of oxidized vitC present in plasma of healthy individuals precludes that GLUT mediated transport per se is of major importance in the diverse distribution of vitC. One apparent exception is erythrocytes that do not contain SVCTs but are only able to take up vitC through facilitated diffusion [44–46]. Human erythrocytes are able to recycle DHA to ASC and maintain an intracellular vitC concentration similar to that of plasma [18]. It has been estimated that the erythrocytes alone are capable of reducing the total amount of vitC present in blood approximately once every 3 min [47,48]. Consequently, the recycling capacity of the erythrocytes may constitute a substantial antioxidant reserve in vivo. Recent investigations actually suggest that ASC is necessary for the structural integrity of the erythrocytes and that intracellular erythrocyte ASC is essential to maintain ASC plasma concentrations in vivo [49,50]. However, collectively speaking and considering the quantitative importance of mechanisms, ASC is primarily distributed via active transport.

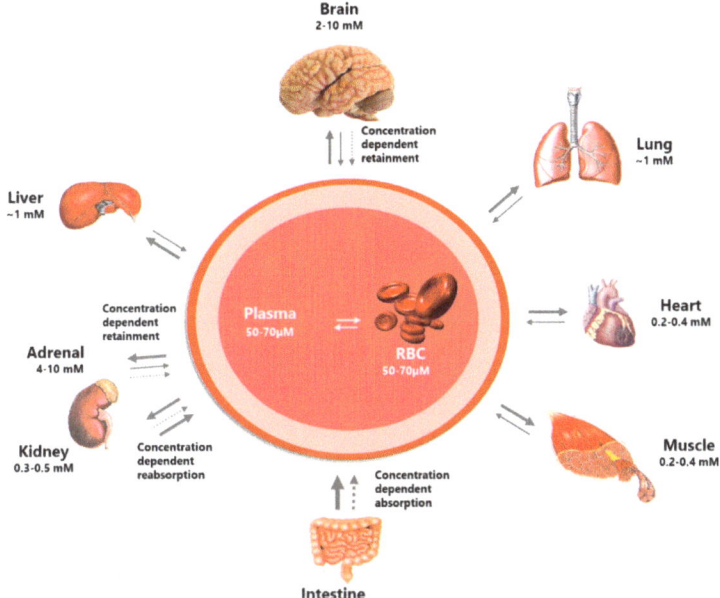

Figure 2. The figure illustrates the highly differential distribution of vitC in the body. Several organs have concentration-dependent mechanisms for the retention of vitC, maintaining high levels during times of inadequate supply at the expense of other organs. Particularly protected is the brain. In addition, the concentration-dependent absorption and re-absorption mechanisms contribute to the homeostatic control of the vitC in the body. Modified from [5].

In contrast to epithelial ASC uptake and reuptake mediated by the high capacity/low affinity SVCT1 (Vmax of about 15 pmol/min/cell and Km of about 65–252 µM [5,30,51]), distribution from the blood stream to the various tissues is mainly governed by the slightly larger SVCT2 [52]. SVCT2 is a low capacity/high affinity transporter of vitC (Vmax of about 1 pmol/min/cell and Km of about 8–69 µM [5,30,51]) and is widely expressed in all organs [4]. The respective transport capacities and affinities for vitC fit well with the accepted notion that SVCT1 mediates the systemic vitC homeostasis, while SVCT2 secures local demands [53]. This is particularly evident for the brain, which upholds one of the highest concentrations of vitC in the body [7,54]. Transport of vitC into the brain is believed to take place through SVCT2s located in the choroid plexus [55], although it has been suggested that other yet undiscovered mechanisms may also be involved [56,57]. However, the pivotal role of SVCT2 in the brain remains undisputed as supported by convincing studies in *Slc23a2* knockout mice that display severe brain hemorrhage and high perinatal mortality [8].

Apart from its remarkably high steady state concentration, the brain also distinguishes itself by being exceptional in the retention of vitC during states of deficiency [54,58–64]. This retention occurs at the expense of the other organs and has been proposed to be essential for the maintenance of proper brain function [63,65,66] (Figure 3). Also, during repletion, the brain, as well as the adrenal glands, has a remarkable affinity for ASC, and detailed in vivo studies in guinea pigs, which, like humans, are unable to synthesize vitC, have revealed that these tissues in particular are the fastest to re-establish homeostasis [7].

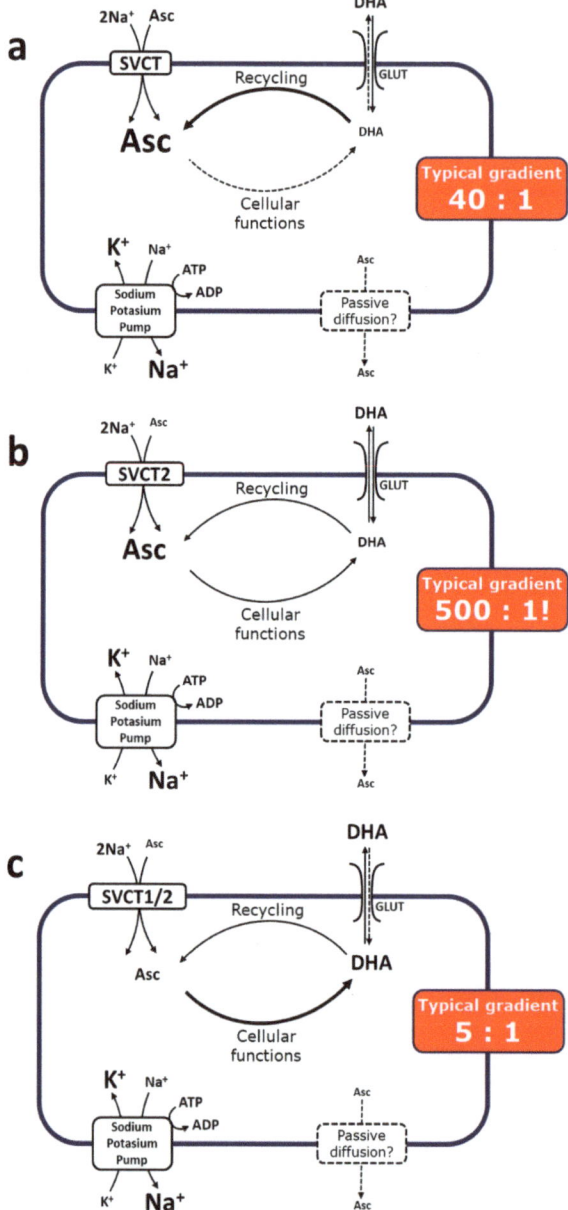

Figure 3. Tissue accumulation of vitC depends on both local and systemic conditions. The ratios are based on data obtained from guinea pigs that like human cannot synthesize vitC [7]. (**a**): During sufficiency, tissues accumulate vitC primarily through the sodium-dependent vitC transporters (SVCTs) perhaps with a small contribution from influx of DHA, which is rapidly converted to ASC. (**b**): During deficiency, prioritized retainment of vitC occurs in, for example the brain, at the expense of other tissues (**c**): where increased oxidative stress may result in elevated DHA concentrations, limited recycling capacity and poor tissue accumulation through DHA influx.

The mechanism(s) underlying the highly differential steady state concentrations of vitC in various tissues remains largely unknown. The potential existence of multiple tissue-specific isoforms of the SVCT2 has not been confirmed, leading to the assumption that the individual SVCT2 expression level of the cells of the tissues may define organ steady state levels of vitC subject to plasma availability. This implies that tissue and cell type composition are mainly responsible. However, in the brain of guinea pigs, for example, substantial differences in vitC steady state levels have been observed between the individual regions, with the highest concentrations being found in the cerebellum, which also appears to saturate first [7]. This does not directly coincide with cerebellum being the most neuron-rich brain region, although neurons contain the highest concentrations of vitC of the brains cells. Moreover, regional SVCT2-abundance has mostly been investigated through RNA expression levels leaving little information on the possible influence of, e.g., post-translational modifications, activation, and/or relocation of the functional protein to the cell membrane.

2.1.3. Metabolism

In contrast to plants, where a number of ASC derivatives and analogues, including several glucosides, have been identified, only ASC exists in mammals [67]. The metabolism of ASC is intimately linked to its antioxidant function. Through its enediol structure (Figure 4) that is highly resonance stabilized and influenced by the acidity of the molecule, ASC serves as an efficient electron donor in biological reactions. In supplying reducing equivalents as either a cofactor or free radical quencher, ASC itself is oxidized to the comparatively stable radical intermediate, ascorbyl free radical, two molecules of which may be disproportionate at a physiological pH to one molecule of ASC and one of DHA [21,68]. As mentioned earlier, DHA is efficiently reduced intracellularly by a number of cell types, thereby preserving the ASC pool. Turnover of vitC is therefore particularly linked to the catabolism of DHA which occurs through hydrolysis to 2,3-diketogulonic acid and decarboxylation to L-xylonate and L-lyxonate, both of which can enter the pentose phosphate pathway for further degradation (Figure 4) [69].

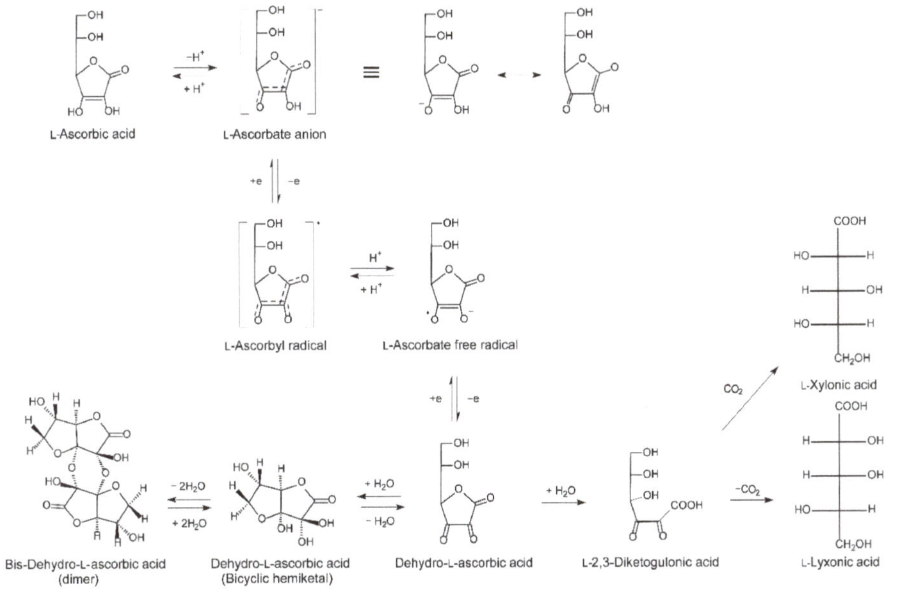

Figure 4. Schematic outline of vitC metabolism. Modified from [21].

2.1.4. Excretion and Reuptake

As a highly hydrophilic low molecular weight compound, ASC would be expected to be efficiently excreted through the kidneys. Indeed, ASC is quantitatively filtered through glomerulus by means of the hydrostatic pressure gradient and concentrated in the pre-urine subsequently to the resorption of water (Figure 5). Here, the pH drops to about five, resulting in an increased proportion of unionized ascorbic acid to that of ASC. The ascorbic acid increase from <0.01% in plasma to about 15% in the pre-urine, representing a concentration gradient of 1500:1, would for most molecules result in substantial passive reabsorption but does apparently not occur for ascorbic acid presumably due to its low lipid solubility. Instead, reuptake of ASC in the proximal renal tubules is controlled by saturable active transport through SVCT1. However, for individuals with saturated plasma levels, excretion of surplus vitC is quantitative [70,71].

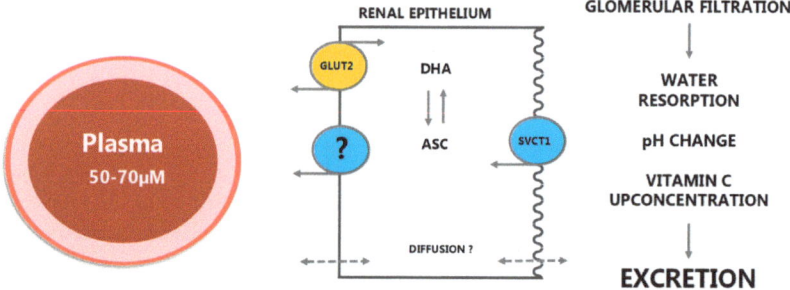

Figure 5. In the kidney, vitC is efficiently filtered by glomerulus to the renal tubule lumen. Reabsorption under vitC deficient conditions is primarily achieved by SVCT1 transporters in the apical membrane although diffusion from the luminal surface may also contribute to the overall uptake. As in the intestinal epithelium, ASC is presumably released to the blood stream through diffusion but the extent and mechanisms of this are not known in detail. GLUT2 transporters are located in the basolateral membrane enabling transport of DHA to plasma. Under saturated conditions, vitC is quantitatively excreted. Modified from [5].

The importance of SVCT1 for intestinal vitC uptake and, in particular, for renal reuptake has been illustrated by Corpe et al. who showed that *Slc23a1-/-* mice display an 18-fold increased excretion of ASC, lower body pool and vitC homeostasis, and increased mortality [32]. They also modelled the effect of known human polymorphisms in the SVCT1 on the plasma saturation level and came to the astonishing conclusion that the most severely affected SNP (A772G rs35817838) would result in a maximal plasma concentration of less than 20 µM [32], i.e., a potential life-long state of vitC deficiency regardless of intake. The renal reuptake of ASC is highly concentration-dependent. Levine and coworkers have shown in detail that the renal excretion coefficient of ASC ranges from 0 to 1 depending on the individual's vitC status, i.e., corresponding to quantitative reuptake in individuals with poor vitC status and quantitative excretion in individuals with saturated status [70,71]. The fact that the excretion ratio is about 1 for intakes higher than about 500 mg/day in healthy individuals supports that passive reabsorption of vitC does not play a significant role in the kidneys.

2.1.5. Steady State Homeostasis of Vitamin C Following Oral Administration/Intake

Most low molecular weight drug pharmacokinetics can be modelled by first order kinetics within their therapeutic range, i.e., a doubling of the dose results in a doubling of the steady state plasma concentration. However, the dominant role of the saturable active transport mechanisms in the absorption, distribution, and excretion of ASC results in nonlinear dose-dependent pharmacokinetics. With increasing vitC intake, the plasma steady state concentration reaches a maximal level of about 70–80 µM [70,71]. From the available literature, it appears that a daily intake of about 200–400 mg of vitC ensures saturation of the blood in healthy individuals [20]. During periods of altered distribution due to temporary physiological needs such as pregnancy or increased turnover during disease or smoking, higher intakes are needed to maintain sufficient levels.

It may be possible to exceed the homeostatic saturation level of 70–80 µM by several fold through multiple daily gram doses of vitC. At supraphysiological levels, vitC gradually adheres to first order kinetics as discussed under intravenous administration. Hence, it is possible to estimate that, for example, a dose of 2 g of vitC given three times a day is likely to result in a steady state plasma concentration of about 250 µM (calculations based to data from ref [13]). However, the possible health benefits from such supraphysiological levels have yet to be documented.

2.1.6. Effect of Dosing Forms and Formulations

Several attempts have been made to bypass the maximum steady state plasma concentration of about 70–80 µM achievable through oral administration. A slow release formulation would theoretically extend the uptake period resulting in a prolonged and thus increased accumulated uptake thereby increasing the overall exposure. However, Viscovich et al. did not find any significant differences in exposure or other pharmacokinetic variables between plain and slow release vitC supplements given to smokers, neither at study start nor after 4 weeks of supplementation [29]. Another approach to increase the maximum achievable plasma concentration through oral administration has been liposomes. The pharmacokinetic properties of a bolus of four grams of liposome-encapsulated vitC were compared to those of plain vitC and placebo in eleven volunteers in a crossover trial [72]. The authors found a 35% increase in exposure (AUC0–4hours) with a plasma C_{max} of about 200 µM after 3 h. Unfortunately, plasma concentrations were not measured beyond the 4 h time point. In an attempt to show a potential biological significance of increased plasma vitC status, the participants were subjected to a 20-min partial ischemia induced by a blood pressure cuff at 200 mm Hg. However, no beneficial effect on ischemia-reperfusion-induced oxidative stress was observed on lipid peroxidation over that of the non-encapsulated dose of vitC [72]. Regardless, this technology has shown some promise and continues to be explored in anticancer therapy, where chemotherapeutics can be delivered together with vitC for a potentially synergistic effect [73]. In another sophisticated approach, the particular ability of the brain to take up vitC has been used by linking ASC to the surface of liposomes containing chemotherapeutics thereby making a brain-specific drug delivery system by using the endogenous vitC transport mechanisms [74].

2.2. Intravenous Route of Administration

Intravenous administration of drugs generally produces a predictable plasma concentration by avoiding absorption limitations, resulting in 100% bioavailability. For vitC specifically, intravenous administration bypasses the saturable absorption mechanisms. This virtually removes the upper limit of the maximum achievable plasma concentration. Parenteral administration of vitC is typically handled by intravenous infusion. This approach results in a predictable plasma steady state concentration that will remain constant until infusion is discontinued. For vitC, a linear relationship between dose and C_{max} can be observed for doses up to about 70 g/m^2 in humans as complied from clinical pharmacokinetic studies, resulting in a plasma concentration of about 50 mM (Figure 6, calculations based on [13,75]). For higher doses, the linearity seems to disappear and resembles a level of saturation. However, more data are needed to establish if 50 mM constitutes an upper steady state vitC concentration in plasma.

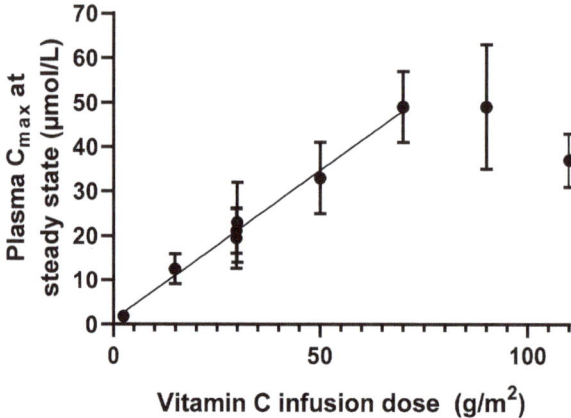

Figure 6. Relationship between infusion dose of vitC and plasma C_{max} in cancer patients as compiled from [13,75]. The data suggests that a linear relationship between dose and C_{max} exists for doses between 1 and 70 g/m^2 ($p < 0.001$, $r^2 > 0.99$), while higher doses results do not translate into higher plasma C_{max}.

2.2.1. Distribution

As for all compounds in circulation, the distribution of vitC following infusion depends at least initially on the vascularization of the various tissues. Whereas the millimolar plasma concentrations do not seem to affect normal tissue distribution beyond saturation, particular interest has been devoted the poorly vascularized tumors as ASC has shown to be cytotoxic to cancer cells but not normal cells at high concentrations in in vitro and in vivo studies, possibly through a pro-oxidant function [76–78]. Campell et al. [79] measured ASC concentrations in tumor tissue following high-dose vitC administration in a mouse model and found that daily injections were necessary to delay tumor growth and suppress the transcription factor hypoxia-inducible factor 1. Interestingly, it was also found that elimination was significantly delayed in tumor compared to normal tissue [79], which may help in preserving the effect of ASC in tumors between infusions. In an attempt to mimic tissue diffusion rates and availability in both normal and tumor tissue, Kuiper and coworkers [80] used a multicell-layered, three-dimensional pharmacokinetic model to measure ASC diffusion and transport parameters through dense tissue in vitro. They were able to simulate diffusion under a number of conditions, including tumors, and concluded that supraphysiological concentrations of ASC, achievable only by intravenous infusion, are necessary for effective delivery of ASC into poorly vascularized tumors [80]. Using these data, it was recently rationalized that normal body saturation obtained by adequate oral dosing will be able to diffuse to cover the distance between vessels in normal well-perfused tissue, and thus provide sufficient vitC for the entire body. In contrast, this diffusion distance is insufficient to increase the vitC content of tumors with poor vascularization, which requires above millimolar concentrations plasma concentrations for effective vitC diffusion [81]. Other than that, very little is known about the organ and tissue homeostasis following intravenous infusion of high-dose vitC.

2.2.2. Metabolism and Excretion

In normal tissue, metabolism of ASC has not been shown to deviate from the general pattern illustrated in Figure 4. However, in poorly vascularized tumor tissues, high-dose vitC combined with the hypoxic tumor environment has been proposed to promote the formation of cytotoxic levels of hydrogen peroxide, thus providing a putative mode of action and a potential role of ASC in cancer treatment [26,82,83].

Following high-dose intravenous administration of vitC, the dose-dependency of the elimination phase, as evident at levels below saturation as described above, is surpassed [84]. VitC is quickly eliminated through glomerular filtration with no significant reuptake. This renders the half-life constant and the elimination kinetics first order [13]. Several pharmacokinetic studies of high-dose vitC have calculated a constant elimination half-life of about 2 h following the discontinuation of intravenous infusion [13,75,85]. This suggests that the millimolar plasma concentrations achieved by intravenous infusion are normalized to physiological levels in about 16 h. In this perspective, the observation that tumor tissue may maintain an elevated level for as much as 48 h is interesting [79], and may be mediated by increased stability in the hypoxic tumor environment, but most likely also by the delayed clearance due to poor vascularization.

3. Factors Affecting Vitamin C Homeostasis and Requirements

As described in detail in the above, vitC homeostasis is tightly controlled in healthy individuals giving rise to a complex relationship between the steady state levels of the various bodily organs and tissues. This interrelationship depends primarily on the availability of vitC in the diet and the specific "configurations" and expression levels of SVCTs of the tissues. However, a number of other factors may interfere with the body's attempt control the vitC homeostasis, and some major contributors are discussed below.

3.1. Influence of Polymorphisms

With the acknowledgement of the importance of SVCTs for regulation of vitC homeostasis and the evolution of genomic sequencing techniques, it has become clear that a large number of polymorphisms exist that influence the steady state level of vitC. This has been reviewed in detail elsewhere [3], but little is known about the potential clinical impact of these. A Mendelian randomization study in 83,256 individuals from the Copenhagen General Population Study used a genetic variant rs33972313 in Slc23a1 resulting in higher than average vitC status to test if improved vitC status is associated with low risk of ischemic heart disease and all-cause mortality [86]. The authors found that high intake of fruits and vegetables was associated with low risk of ischemic heart disease and all-cause mortality. Effect sizes were comparable for vitC, albeit not significantly. As mentioned earlier, modelling studies have proposed that the functionally poorest SVCT allele identified so far (A772G, rs35817838) results in a plasma saturation level of only one fourth of that of the background population corresponding to a condition of life-long vitC deficiency [9]. It would indeed be interesting to test how this allele compares for morbidity and mortality.

3.2. Smoking

Smoking is a major source of oxidants and estimates have suggested that every puff of a cigarette equals the inhalation of about 1014 tar phase radicals and 1015 gas phase radicals [87]. Not surprisingly, this draws a major toll on the antioxidant defense of the body as demonstrated by a persistent association between tobacco smoke and poor antioxidant status in general, and poor vitC status in particular [17,25]. Active smoking typically depletes the vitC pool by 25–50% compared to never-smokers [88], while environmental tobacco smoke exposure results in a drop of about half that size [89,90]. The direct cause of the smoking-induced vitC depletion has been investigated, and smoking cessation has been shown to immediately restore about half of the vitC depletion observed as a result of smoking [91]. This immediate albeit partial recovery has pointed towards an oxidative stress mediated depletion of vitC caused by smoking. Moreover, both oxidative stress and ASC recycling are induced by smoking regardless of antioxidant intake [18,92]. However, the lack of full recovery suggests that other factors also contribute to the lower vitC status among smokers. Studies have suggested that the difference in vitC status between smokers and nonsmokers is not related to altered pharmacokinetics of vitC [28,29]. However, as smokers in general have a lower intake of fruits and vegetables and a larger intake of fat compared to nonsmokers [93], this may account for the difference in vitC levels observed between ex-smokers and never-smokers [19]. Indeed, an analysis of the Second National Health and Nutrition Examination Survey (NHANES II) confirmed that the vitC intake of smokers is significantly lower than that of nonsmokers, but also that the increased risk of poor vitC status was independent of this lower intake [94].

Various attempts have been made to estimate the amount of vitC needed to compensate for tobacco smoking. Schectman et al. analyzed the NHANES II data, comparing daily intake vs. serum concentrations of vitC among 4182 smokers and 7020 non-smokers. They estimated by regression analysis that smokers would need an additional 130 mg/day to overcome the adverse effect of smoking on vitC status [95]. In a separate analysis, it was concluded that smokers need an intake > 200 mg/day to lower the risk of vitC deficiency to that of nonsmokers [96]. These results were later indirectly supported by Lykkesfeldt et al. using a different approach. Measuring the steady state oxidation ratio of vitC in smokers and nonsmokers, it was shown that in particular smokers with poor vitC status had an increased steady state oxidation of their vitC pool compared to nonsmokers [17]. The authors concluded that smokers need at least 200 mg vitC per day to compensate for the effect of smoking on the oxidation of vitC [17]. These data stand in contrast to previous data by Kallner et al., who used ^{14}C-labelled ASC to estimate the turnover of vitC in smokers [97]. Seventeen male smoking volunteers between 21 and 69 years of age and weighing between 55 and 110 kg received doses from 30 to 180 mg/day and were instructed to ingest a diet completely devoid of vitC. Urinary excretion of radioactivity was used to estimate the vitC pharmacokinetics using a three-compartment model. Based on these data, Kallner et al. concluded that smokers needed only about 35 mg more than nonsmokers per day to compensate for their habit [97]. This recommendation was later adopted by the Institute of Medicine in their dietary reference intakes [22]. However, several problems are associated with the latter study. Namely, radioactivity rather than ASC per se was quantified as a surrogate for vitC excretion. Moreover, only 17 individuals with considerable variation in age and body composition were included in the study. Finally, these studies were carried out prior to the identification of the SVCTs and their importance for the nonlinear pharmacokinetics of vitC at physiological levels. In fact, such a dose-concentration relationship formally rules out the use of compartment as well as noncompartment kinetic modelling, as the fundamental assumption of a terminal first order elimination phase is not fulfilled. Thus, it appears likely that the turnover in smokers may be underestimated by Kallner et al.

3.3. Pregnancy

Several preclinical studies have illustrated the importance of vitC in early development, in particular that of the brain and cognition [60,63,98–100]. In humans, studies have shown that poor maternal vitC status results in increased fetal oxidative stress, impaired implantation and increased risk of complications including preeclampsia [101,102]. It is not clear to what extent vitC supplementation may ameliorate this risk. The few controlled studies that have been carried out have produced mixed results [103–106], but unfortunately, none of them have considered vitC status in the recruitment or group allocation process and they are therefore of limited value.

During pregnancy, the human fetus relies completely on an adequate maternal vitC intake and transplacental transport of vitC. Experimental evidence suggests that this transport is primarily governed by SVCT2 and thus constitutes the primary means of fetal vitC supply [60]. Expectedly, maternal vitC status has been shown to gradually decline from the 1st to 3rd trimester, a change not only explainable by the increased volume of distribution but rather by the selective accumulation across the placenta [107]. Fetal and postnatal steady state concentrations exceed those of the mother, and both during pregnancy and lactation, most authorities recommend an increased intake ranging from 10 to 35 additional mg vitC/day to compensate for this increased draw on maternal resources [22].

3.4. Disease

A plethora of disease conditions, including infectious diseases, cancer, cardiovascular disease, stroke, diabetes, and sepsis, have been associated with poor vitC status (reviewed in [19,20]).

Considerable epidemiological evidence has shown vitC deficiency to negatively affect independent risk factors of, for example, cardiovascular disease development [14]. However, causal linkage between disease etiology and vitC status remains scarce, except for that of scurvy [108]. The decreased vitC status in disease is often explained by a combination of a sometimes massively increased turnover due to oxidative stress and inflammation and a decreased dietary intake of vitC associated with the disease [81,109].

An obvious display of increased vitC turnover in critical illness is that large doses are often needed to replete the individual to the level of a healthy control. These doses exceed those necessary to saturate a healthy individual by many-fold [110]. One current example is sepsis patients where systemic inflammation and oxidative stress presumably increases the expenditure of vitC [111,112]. Recently published data on critically ill patients ($n = 44$, both septic and nonseptic patients) show that actual plasma vitC concentrations are on average 60% lower than the values predicted from patient vitC intake during hospitalization (either enteral or parenterally administered nutrition) [110]. Although several causes of the apparent vitC depletion are likely, e.g., interactions with administered care and therapeutics potentially affecting vitC bioavailabilty, the data suggest significant alterations in the pharmacokinetics of vitC in this group of patients, reflected by the discrepancy in the almost linear course of the plasma concentration curve opposed to the predicted increase over time. Whether reestablishing normal vitC status in critically ill patients has a significant clinical impact on disease prognosis remains to be established, but promising results are emerging [113,114] and controlled trials are under way. A very recent meta-analysis suggests that vitC therapy significantly shortens the stay of patients in the intensive care unit [115].

In diabetes, reduced levels of plasma vitC is reported in both insulin demanding and noninsulin demanding diabetic patients [116–119]. A prospective evaluation of older adults in the National Institutes of Health-American Association of Retired Persons (NIH-AARP) Diet and Health Study cohort, indicate that the use of vitC supplementation may reduce the risk of diabetes, supporting further investigations and controlled trials to identify a putative relationship between vitC levels and diabetes [120]. Supplementation with vitC (500 mg/day) increased insulin sensitivity and the expression of the SVCT2 transporter in skeletal muscle in type 2 diabetic patients [121], supporting findings that an intake of high-dose ascorbic acid (above 1 mg/day) exerted a beneficial effect on maintaining blood sugar homeostasis and decreasing insulin resistance in type 2 diabetic patients [119]. In a randomized controlled cross-over study of type 2 diabetes patients, an intake of 500 mg vitC twice daily for four months significantly improved glucose homeostasis as well as decreased blood pressure compared to placebo treated controls, linking vitC supplement to improved blood-sugar balance and cardiovascular function [122]. Positive effects of vitC on vascular hallmarks linked to diabetes have previously been indicated; in young diabetes type 1 patients, poor vitC status was linked to increases in the arterial vascular wall, indicating a putatively increased risk of atherosclerotic disease in these patients [123]. In type 2 diabetic patients with coronary artery disease, a high-dose supplementation (2 mg/day) for 4 weeks reduced circulating markers of thrombosis, supporting a beneficial role of vitC on the vascular system [124]. Collectively, the above evidence suggests that a higher metabolic turnover of vitC in diabetes can be counter-balanced by supplementation. However, if it also improves the long-term prognosis remains to be evaluated.

4. Concluding Remarks

The pharmacokinetics of vitC is complex, dose-dependent, and compartmentalized at physiological levels, while independent of dose and first order at pharmacological levels. The lack of this fundamental knowledge has left deep traces of design flaws, misconceptions, misinterpretations, and erroneous conclusions in the scientific literature. Unfortunately, these inherited problems continue to hamper our ability to properly evaluate the role of vitC in human health and its potential relevance in disease prevention and treatment. So far, the overtly exaggerated optimistic view that enough vitC can cure everything has been battling the dismissive negligence of refusal to re-examine the literature based on new evidence. The balance between these two extremes needs to be identified in order to realize the potential of vitC in both health and disease for the future.

Author Contributions: J.L. drafted the manuscript, which was subsequently critically revised by P.T.-N.

Funding: This paper received no external funding.

Conflicts of Interest: The authors declare no conflict of interest.

References

1. Yang, H. Conserved or lost: Molecular evolution of the key gene GULO in vertebrate vitamin C biosynthesis. *Biochem. Genet.* **2013**, *51*, 413–425. [CrossRef] [PubMed]
2. Frikke-Schmidt, H.; Tveden-Nyborg, P.; Lykkesfeldt, J. L-dehydroascorbic acid can substitute l-ascorbic acid as dietary vitamin C source in guinea pigs. *Redox Biol.* **2016**, *7*, 8–13. [CrossRef] [PubMed]
3. Michels, A.J.; Hagen, T.M.; Frei, B. Human genetic variation influences vitamin C homeostasis by altering vitamin C transport and antioxidant enzyme function. *Annu. Rev. Nutr.* **2013**, *33*, 45–70. [CrossRef]
4. Tsukaguchi, H.; Tokui, T.; Mackenzie, B.; Berger, U.V.; Chen, X.Z.; Wang, Y.; Brubaker, R.F.; Hediger, M.A. A family of mammalian Na^+-dependent L-ascorbic acid transporters. *Nature* **1999**, *399*, 70–75. [CrossRef]
5. Lindblad, M.; Tveden-Nyborg, P.; Lykkesfeldt, J. Regulation of vitamin C homeostasis during deficiency. *Nutrients* **2013**, *5*, 2860–2879. [CrossRef] [PubMed]
6. Wilson, J.X. Regulation of vitamin C transport. *Annu. Rev. Nutr.* **2005**, *25*, 105–125. [CrossRef]
7. Hasselholt, S.; Tveden-Nyborg, P.; Lykkesfeldt, J. Distribution of vitamin C is tissue specific with early saturation of the brain and adrenal glands following differential oral dose regimens in guinea pigs. *Br. J. Nutr.* **2015**, *113*, 1539–1549. [CrossRef]
8. Sotiriou, S.; Gispert, S.; Cheng, J.; Wang, Y.; Chen, A.; Hoogstraten-Miller, S.; Miller, G.F.; Kwon, O.; Levine, M.; Guttentag, S.H.; et al. Ascorbic-acid transporter Slc23a1 is essential for vitamin C transport into the brain and for perinatal survival. *Nat. Med.* **2002**, *8*, 514–517. [CrossRef]
9. Corpe, C.P.; Tu, H.; Eck, P.; Wang, J.; Faulhaber-Walter, R.; Schnermann, J.; Margolis, S.; Padayatty, S.; Sun, H.; Wang, Y.; et al. Vitamin C transporter Slc23a1 links renal reabsorption, vitamin C tissue accumulation, and perinatal survival in mice. *J. Clin. Investig.* **2010**, *120*, 1069–1083. [CrossRef]
10. Smith, J.L.; Hodges, R.E. Serum levels of vitamin C in relation to dietary and supplemental intake of vitamin C in smokers and nonsmokers. *Ann. N. Y. Acad. Sci.* **1987**, *498*, 144–152. [CrossRef]
11. Lykkesfeldt, J.; Poulsen, H.E. Is vitamin C supplementation beneficial? Lessons learned from randomised controlled trials. *Br. J. Nutr.* **2010**, *103*, 1251–1259. [CrossRef] [PubMed]
12. Chen, Q.; Espey, M.G.; Krishna, M.C.; Mitchell, J.B.; Corpe, C.P.; Buettner, G.R.; Shacter, E.; Levine, M. Pharmacologic ascorbic acid concentrations selectively kill cancer cells: Action as a pro-drug to deliver hydrogen peroxide to tissues. *Proc. Natl. Acad. Sci. USA* **2005**, *102*, 13604–13609. [CrossRef] [PubMed]
13. Nielsen, T.K.; Hojgaard, M.; Andersen, J.T.; Poulsen, H.E.; Lykkesfeldt, J.; Mikines, K.J. Elimination of ascorbic acid after high-dose infusion in prostate cancer patients: A pharmacokinetic evaluation. *Basic Clin. Pharmacol. Toxicol.* **2015**, *116*, 343–348. [CrossRef] [PubMed]
14. Carr, A.; Frei, B. Does vitamin C act as a pro-oxidant under physiological conditions? *FASEB J.* **1999**, *13*, 1007–1024. [CrossRef] [PubMed]
15. Buettner, G.R. The pecking order of free radicals and antioxidants: Lipid peroxidation, alpha-tocopherol, and ascorbate. *Arch. Biochem. Biophys.* **1993**, *300*, 535–543. [CrossRef] [PubMed]
16. Bode, A.M.; Cunningham, L.; Rose, R.C. Spontaneous decay of oxidized ascorbic acid (dehydro-L-ascorbic acid) evaluated by high-pressure liquid chromatography. *Clin. Chem.* **1990**, *36*, 1807–1809. [PubMed]
17. Lykkesfeldt, J.; Loft, S.; Nielsen, J.B.; Poulsen, H.E. Ascorbic acid and dehydroascorbic acid as biomarkers of oxidative stress caused by smoking. *Am. J. Clin. Nutr.* **1997**, *65*, 959–963. [CrossRef] [PubMed]
18. Lykkesfeldt, J.; Viscovich, M.; Poulsen, H.E. Ascorbic acid recycling in human erythrocytes is induced by smoking in vivo. *Free Radic. Biol. Med.* **2003**, *35*, 1439–1447. [CrossRef] [PubMed]
19. Tveden-Nyborg, P.; Lykkesfeldt, J. Does vitamin C deficiency increase lifestyle-associated vascular disease progression? Evidence based on experimental and clinical studies. *Antiox. Redox Signal.* **2013**, *19*, 2084–2104. [CrossRef] [PubMed]

20. Frei, B.; Birlouez-Aragon, I.; Lykkesfeldt, J. Authors' perspective: What is the optimum intake of vitamin C in humans? *Crit. Rev. Food Sci. Nutr.* **2012**, *52*, 815–829. [CrossRef]
21. Frikke-Schmidt, H.; Tveden-Nyborg, P.; Lykkesfeldt, J. Vitamin C in human nutrition. In *Vitamins in the Prevention of Human Disease*; Herrmann, W., Obeid, R., Eds.; De Gruyter: Berlin, Germany, 2011; pp. 323–347.
22. Food and Nutrition Board Staff; Panel on Dietary Antioxidants; Institute of Medicine Staff. *Dietary Reference Intakes for Vitamin C, Vitamin E, Selenium and Carotenoids: A Report of the Panel on Dietary Antioxidants and Related Compounds, Subcommitties on Upper Reference Levels of Nutrients and of the Interpretation and Use of Dietary Reference Intakes, and the Standing Committee on the Scientific Evaluation of Dietary Reference Intakes, Food and Nutrition Board, Institute of Medicine*; National Academy Press: Washington, DC, USA, 2000.
23. Carr, A.C.; Bozonet, S.M.; Pullar, J.M.; Simcock, J.W.; Vissers, M.C. A randomized steady-state bioavailability study of synthetic versus natural (kiwifruit-derived) vitamin C. *Nutrients* **2013**, *5*, 3684–3695. [CrossRef] [PubMed]
24. Dachs, G.U.; Munn, D.G.; Carr, A.C.; Vissers, M.C.; Robinson, B.A. Consumption of vitamin C is below recommended daily intake in many cancer patients and healthy volunteers in Christchurch. *N. Z. Med. J.* **2014**, *127*, 73–76. [PubMed]
25. Lykkesfeldt, J.; Christen, S.; Wallock, L.M.; Chang, H.H.; Jacob, R.A.; Ames, B.N. Ascorbate is depleted by smoking and repleted by moderate supplementation: A study in male smokers and nonsmokers with matched dietary antioxidant intakes. *Am. J. Clin. Nutr.* **2000**, *71*, 530–536. [CrossRef] [PubMed]
26. Du, J.; Cullen, J.J.; Buettner, G.R. Ascorbic acid: Chemistry, biology and the treatment of cancer. *Biochim. Biophys. Acta* **2012**, *1826*, 443–457. [CrossRef] [PubMed]
27. May, J.; Asard, H. Ascorbate recycling. In *Vitamin C*; Asard, H., May, J.M., Smirnoff, N., Eds.; BIOS Scientific Publishers Ltd.: Oxford, UK, 2004; pp. 189–202.
28. Lykkesfeldt, J.; Bolbjerg, M.L.; Poulsen, H.E. Effect of smoking on erythorbic acid pharmacokinetics. *Br. J. Nutr.* **2003**, *89*, 667–671. [CrossRef] [PubMed]
29. Viscovich, M.; Lykkesfeldt, J.; Poulsen, H.E. Vitamin C pharmacokinetics of plain and slow release formulations in smokers. *Clin. Nutr.* **2004**, *23*, 1043–1050. [CrossRef] [PubMed]
30. Wang, Y.; Mackenzie, B.; Tsukaguchi, H.; Weremowicz, S.; Morton, C.C.; Hediger, M.A. Human vitamin C (L-ascorbic acid) transporter SVCT1. *Biochem. Biophys. Res. Commun.* **2000**, *267*, 488–494. [CrossRef] [PubMed]
31. Vera, J.C.; Rivas, C.I.; Fischbarg, J.; Golde, D.W. Mammalian facilitative hexose transporters mediate the transport of dehydroascorbic acid. *Nature* **1993**, *364*, 79–82. [CrossRef]
32. Corpe, C.P.; Eck, P.; Wang, J.; Al-Hasani, H.; Levine, M. Intestinal dehydroascorbic acid (DHA) transport mediated by the facilitative sugar transporters, GLUT2 and GLUT8. *J. Biol. Chem.* **2013**, *288*, 9092–9101. [CrossRef] [PubMed]
33. Lykkesfeldt, J. Ascorbate and dehydroascorbic acid as reliable biomarkers of oxidative stress: Analytical reproducibility and long-term stability of plasma samples subjected to acidic deproteinization. *Cancer Epidemiol. Prev. Biomark.* **2007**, *16*, 2513–2516. [CrossRef]
34. Todhunter, E.N.; Mc, M.T.; Ehmke, D.A. Utilization of dehydroascorbic acid by human subjects. *J. Nutr.* **1950**, *42*, 297–308. [CrossRef] [PubMed]
35. Linkswiler, H. The effect of the Ingestion of ascorbic acid and dehydroascorbic acid upon the blood levels of these two components in human subjects. *J. Nutr.* **1958**, *64*, 43–54. [CrossRef]
36. Sabry, J.H.; Fisher, K.H.; Dodds, M.L. Human utilization of dehydroascorbic acid. *J. Nutr.* **1958**, *64*, 457–466. [CrossRef] [PubMed]
37. Malo, C.; Wilson, J.X. Glucose modulates vitamin C transport in adult human small intestinal brush border membrane vesicles. *J. Nutr.* **2000**, *130*, 63–69. [CrossRef] [PubMed]
38. Kubler, W.; Gehler, J. Kinetics of intestinal absorption of ascorbic acid. Calculation of non-dosage-dependent absorption processes. *Int. Z. Vitaminforsch.* **1970**, *40*, 442–453. [PubMed]
39. Mayersohn, M. Ascorbic acid absorption in man—Pharmacokinetic implications. *Eur. J. Pharmacol.* **1972**, *19*, 140–142. [CrossRef]
40. May, J.M.; Qu, Z.C. Ascorbic acid efflux from human brain microvascular pericytes: Role of re-uptake. *Biofactors* **2015**, *41*, 330–338. [CrossRef]

41. Rumsey, S.C.; Daruwala, R.; Al-Hasani, H.; Zarnowski, M.J.; Simpson, I.A.; Levine, M. Dehydroascorbic acid transport by GLUT4 in Xenopus oocytes and isolated rat adipocytes. *J. Biol. Chem.* **2000**, *275*, 28246–28253. [CrossRef]
42. Rumsey, S.C.; Kwon, O.; Xu, G.W.; Burant, C.F.; Simpson, I.; Levine, M. Glucose transporter isoforms GLUT1 and GLUT3 transport dehydroascorbic acid. *J. Biol. Chem.* **1997**, *272*, 18982–18989. [CrossRef]
43. Mardones, L.; Ormazabal, V.; Romo, X.; Jana, C.; Binder, P.; Pena, E.; Vergara, M.; Zuniga, F.A. The glucose transporter-2 (GLUT2) is a low affinity dehydroascorbic acid transporter. *Biochem. Biophys. Res. Commun.* **2011**, *410*, 7–12. [CrossRef]
44. May, J.M.; Qu, Z.; Morrow, J.D. Mechanisms of ascorbic acid recycling in human erythrocytes. *Biochim. Biophys. Acta* **2001**, *1528*, 159–166. [CrossRef]
45. Mendiratta, S.; Qu, Z.C.; May, J.M. Enzyme-dependent ascorbate recycling in human erythrocytes: Role of thioredoxin reductase. *Free Radic. Biol. Med.* **1998**, *25*, 221–228. [CrossRef]
46. Mendiratta, S.; Qu, Z.C.; May, J.M. Erythrocyte ascorbate recycling: Antioxidant effects in blood. *Free Radic. Biol. Med.* **1998**, *24*, 789–797. [CrossRef]
47. Lykkesfeldt, J. Increased oxidative damage in vitamin C deficiency is accompanied by induction of ascorbic acid recycling capacity in young but not mature guinea pigs. *Free Radic. Res.* **2002**, *36*, 567–574. [CrossRef] [PubMed]
48. May, J.M.; Qu, Z.C.; Whitesell, R.R. Ascorbic acid recycling enhances the antioxidant reserve of human erythrocytes. *Biochemistry* **1995**, *34*, 12721–12728. [CrossRef] [PubMed]
49. Tu, H.; Li, H.; Wang, Y.; Niyyati, M.; Wang, Y.; Leshin, J.; Levine, M. Low Red Blood Cell Vitamin C Concentrations Induce Red Blood Cell Fragility: A Link to Diabetes Via Glucose, Glucose Transporters, and Dehydroascorbic Acid. *EBioMedicine* **2015**, *2*, 1735–1750. [CrossRef] [PubMed]
50. Tu, H.; Wang, Y.; Li, H.; Brinster, L.R.; Levine, M. Chemical Transport Knockout for Oxidized Vitamin C, Dehydroascorbic Acid, Reveals Its Functions in vivo. *EBioMedicine* **2017**, *23*, 125–135. [CrossRef] [PubMed]
51. Daruwala, R.; Song, J.; Koh, W.S.; Rumsey, S.C.; Levine, M. Cloning and functional characterization of the human sodium-dependent vitamin C transporters hSVCT1 and hSVCT2. *FEBS Lett.* **1999**, *460*, 480–484. [CrossRef]
52. Savini, I.; Rossi, A.; Pierro, C.; Avigliano, L.; Catani, M.V. SVCT1 and SVCT2: Key proteins for vitamin C uptake. *Amino Acids* **2008**, *34*, 347–355. [CrossRef]
53. Eck, P.; Kwon, O.; Chen, S.; Mian, O.; Levine, M. The human sodium-dependent ascorbic acid transporters SLC23A1 and SLC23A2 do not mediate ascorbic acid release in the proximal renal epithelial cell. *Physiol. Rep.* **2013**, *1*, e00136. [CrossRef]
54. Lykkesfeldt, J.; Trueba, G.P.; Poulsen, H.E.; Christen, S. Vitamin C deficiency in weanling guinea pigs: Differential expression of oxidative stress and DNA repair in liver and brain. *Br. J. Nutr.* **2007**, *98*, 1116–1119. [CrossRef] [PubMed]
55. Harrison, F.E.; May, J.M. Vitamin C function in the brain: Vital role of the ascorbate transporter SVCT2. *Free Radic. Biol. Med.* **2009**, *46*, 719–730. [CrossRef] [PubMed]
56. Meredith, M.E.; Harrison, F.E.; May, J.M. Differential regulation of the ascorbic acid transporter SVCT2 during development and in response to ascorbic acid depletion. *Biochem. Biophys. Res. Commun.* **2011**, *414*, 737–742. [CrossRef] [PubMed]
57. Sogaard, D.; Lindblad, M.M.; Paidi, M.D.; Hasselholt, S.; Lykkesfeldt, J.; Tveden-Nyborg, P. In vivo vitamin C deficiency in guinea pigs increases ascorbate transporters in liver but not kidney and brain. *Nutr. Res.* **2014**, *34*, 639–645. [CrossRef] [PubMed]
58. Frikke-Schmidt, H.; Tveden-Nyborg, P.; Birck, M.M.; Lykkesfeldt, J. High dietary fat and cholesterol exacerbates chronic vitamin C deficiency in guinea pigs. *Br. J. Nutr.* **2011**, *105*, 54–61. [CrossRef] [PubMed]
59. Paidi, M.D.; Schjoldager, J.G.; Lykkesfeldt, J.; Tveden-Nyborg, P. Prenatal vitamin C deficiency results in differential levels of oxidative stress during late gestation in foetal guinea pig brains. *Redox Biol.* **2014**, *2*, 361–367. [CrossRef] [PubMed]
60. Schjoldager, J.G.; Paidi, M.D.; Lindblad, M.M.; Birck, M.M.; Kjaergaard, A.B.; Dantzer, V.; Lykkesfeldt, J.; Tveden-Nyborg, P. Maternal vitamin C deficiency during pregnancy results in transient fetal and placental growth retardation in guinea pigs. *Eur. J. Nutr.* **2015**, *54*, 667–676. [CrossRef] [PubMed]

61. Schjoldager, J.G.; Tveden-Nyborg, P.; Lykkesfeldt, J. Prolonged maternal vitamin C deficiency overrides preferential fetal ascorbate transport but does not influence perinatal survival in guinea pigs. *Br. J. Nutr.* **2013**, *110*, 1573–1579. [CrossRef] [PubMed]
62. Tveden-Nyborg, P.; Hasselholt, S.; Miyashita, N.; Moos, T.; Poulsen, H.E.; Lykkesfeldt, J. Chronic vitamin C deficiency does not accelerate oxidative stress in ageing brains of guinea pigs. *Basic Clin. Pharmacol. Toxicol.* **2012**, *110*, 524–529. [CrossRef]
63. Tveden-Nyborg, P.; Johansen, L.K.; Raida, Z.; Villumsen, C.K.; Larsen, J.O.; Lykkesfeldt, J. Vitamin C deficiency in early postnatal life impairs spatial memory and reduces the number of hippocampal neurons in guinea pigs. *Am. J. Clin. Nutr.* **2009**, *90*, 540–546. [CrossRef]
64. Tveden-Nyborg, P.; Lykkesfeldt, J. Does vitamin C deficiency result in impaired brain development in infants? *Redox Rep.* **2009**, *14*, 2–6. [CrossRef] [PubMed]
65. Tveden-Nyborg, P.; Vogt, L.; Schjoldager, J.G.; Jeannet, N.; Hasselholt, S.; Paidi, M.D.; Christen, S.; Lykkesfeldt, J. Maternal vitamin C deficiency during pregnancy persistently impairs hippocampal neurogenesis in offspring of guinea pigs. *PLoS ONE* **2012**, *7*, e48488. [CrossRef] [PubMed]
66. May, J.M. Vitamin C transport and its role in the central nervous system. In *Water Soluble Vitamins*; Springer: Dordrecht, The Netherlands, 2012; pp. 85–103.
67. Smirnoff, N. Ascorbic acid metabolism and functions: A comparison of plants and mammals. *Free Radic. Biol. Med.* **2018**, *122*, 116–129. [CrossRef] [PubMed]
68. Buettner, G.R.; Schafer, F.Q. Ascorbate as an antioxidant. In *Vitamin C: Its Functions and Biochemistry in Animals and Plants*; Asard, H., May, J.M., Smirnoff, N., Eds.; BIOS Scientific Publishers Limited: Oxford, UK, 2004; pp. 173–188.
69. Banhegyi, G.; Braun, L.; Csala, M.; Puskas, F.; Mandl, J. Ascorbate metabolism and its regulation in animals. *Free Radic. Biol. Med.* **1997**, *23*, 793–803. [CrossRef]
70. Levine, M.; Conry-Cantilena, C.; Wang, Y.; Welch, R.W.; Washko, P.W.; Dhariwal, K.R.; Park, J.B.; Lazarev, A.; Graumlich, J.F.; King, J.; et al. Vitamin C pharmacokinetics in healthy volunteers: Evidence for a recommended dietary allowance. *Proc. Natl. Acad. Sci. USA* **1996**, *93*, 3704–3709. [CrossRef] [PubMed]
71. Levine, M.; Wang, Y.; Padayatty, S.J.; Morrow, J. A new recommended dietary allowance of vitamin C for healthy young women. *Proc. Natl. Acad. Sci. USA* **2001**, *98*, 9842–9846. [CrossRef] [PubMed]
72. Davis, J.L.; Paris, H.L.; Beals, J.W.; Binns, S.E.; Giordano, G.R.; Scalzo, R.L.; Schweder, M.M.; Blair, E.; Bell, C. Liposomal-encapsulated Ascorbic Acid: Influence on Vitamin C Bioavailability and Capacity to Protect Against Ischemia-Reperfusion Injury. *Nutr. Metab. Insights* **2016**, *9*, 25–30. [CrossRef] [PubMed]
73. Miura, Y.; Fuchigami, Y.; Hagimori, M.; Sato, H.; Ogawa, K.; Munakata, C.; Wada, M.; Maruyama, K.; Kawakami, S. Evaluation of the targeted delivery of 5-fluorouracil and ascorbic acid into the brain with ultrasound-responsive nanobubbles. *J. Drug Target.* **2018**, *26*, 684–691. [CrossRef]
74. Peng, Y.; Zhao, Y.; Chen, Y.; Yang, Z.; Zhang, L.; Xiao, W.; Yang, J.; Guo, L.; Wu, Y. Dual-targeting for brain-specific liposomes drug delivery system: Synthesis and preliminary evaluation. *Bioorg. Med. Chem.* **2018**, *26*, 4677–4686. [CrossRef]
75. Stephenson, C.M.; Levin, R.D.; Spector, T.; Lis, C.G. Phase I clinical trial to evaluate the safety, tolerability, and pharmacokinetics of high-dose intravenous ascorbic acid in patients with advanced cancer. *Cancer Chemother. Pharmacol.* **2013**, *72*, 139–146. [CrossRef]
76. Chen, P.; Yu, J.; Chalmers, B.; Drisko, J.; Yang, J.; Li, B.; Chen, Q. Pharmacological ascorbate induces cytotoxicity in prostate cancer cells through ATP depletion and induction of autophagy. *Anticancer Drugs* **2012**, *23*, 437–444. [CrossRef]
77. Chen, Q.; Espey, M.G.; Sun, A.Y.; Pooput, C.; Kirk, K.L.; Krishna, M.C.; Khosh, D.B.; Drisko, J.; Levine, M. Pharmacologic doses of ascorbate act as a prooxidant and decrease growth of aggressive tumor xenografts in mice. *Proc. Natl. Acad. Sci. USA* **2008**, *105*, 11105–11109. [CrossRef]
78. Chen, Q.; Espey, M.G.; Sun, A.Y.; Lee, J.H.; Krishna, M.C.; Shacter, E.; Choyke, P.L.; Pooput, C.; Kirk, K.L.; Buettner, G.R.; et al. Ascorbate in pharmacologic concentrations selectively generates ascorbate radical and hydrogen peroxide in extracellular fluid in vivo. *Proc. Natl. Acad. Sci. USA* **2007**, *104*, 8749–8754. [CrossRef]
79. Campbell, E.J.; Vissers, M.C.M.; Wohlrab, C.; Hicks, K.O.; Strother, R.M.; Bozonet, S.M.; Robinson, B.A.; Dachs, G.U. Pharmacokinetic and anti-cancer properties of high dose ascorbate in solid tumours of ascorbate-dependent mice. *Free Radic. Biol. Med.* **2016**, *99*, 451–462. [CrossRef]

80. Kuiper, C.; Vissers, M.C.; Hicks, K.O. Pharmacokinetic modeling of ascorbate diffusion through normal and tumor tissue. *Free Radic. Biol. Med.* **2014**, *77*, 340–352. [CrossRef]
81. Vissers, M.C.M.; Das, A.B. Potential Mechanisms of Action for Vitamin C in Cancer: Reviewing the Evidence. *Front. Physiol.* **2018**, *9*, 809. [CrossRef]
82. Schoenfeld, J.D.; Alexander, M.S.; Waldron, T.J.; Sibenaller, Z.A.; Spitz, D.R.; Buettner, G.R.; Allen, B.G.; Cullen, J.J. Pharmacological Ascorbate as a Means of Sensitizing Cancer Cells to Radio-Chemotherapy While Protecting Normal Tissue. *Semin. Radiat. Oncol.* **2019**, *29*, 25–32. [CrossRef]
83. Doskey, C.M.; Buranasudja, V.; Wagner, B.A.; Wilkes, J.G.; Du, J.; Cullen, J.J.; Buettner, G.R. Tumor cells have decreased ability to metabolize H2O2: Implications for pharmacological ascorbate in cancer therapy. *Redox Biol.* **2016**, *10*, 274–284. [CrossRef]
84. Padayatty, S.J.; Sun, H.; Wang, Y.; Riordan, H.D.; Hewitt, S.M.; Katz, A.; Wesley, R.A.; Levine, M. Vitamin C pharmacokinetics: Implications for oral and intravenous use. *Ann. Intern. Med.* **2004**, *140*, 533–537. [CrossRef]
85. Ou, J.; Zhu, X.; Lu, Y.; Zhao, C.; Zhang, H.; Wang, X.; Gui, X.; Wang, J.; Zhang, X.; Zhang, T.; et al. The safety and pharmacokinetics of high dose intravenous ascorbic acid synergy with modulated electrohyperthermia in Chinese patients with stage III-IV non-small cell lung cancer. *Eur. J. Pharm. Sci.* **2017**, *109*, 412–418. [CrossRef]
86. Kobylecki, C.J.; Afzal, S.; Davey Smith, G.; Nordestgaard, B.G. Genetically high plasma vitamin C, intake of fruit and vegetables, and risk of ischemic heart disease and all-cause mortality: A Mendelian randomization study. *Am. J. Clin. Nutr.* **2015**, *101*, 1135–1143. [CrossRef]
87. Pryor, W.A.; Stone, K. Oxidants in cigarette smoke. Radicals, hydrogen peroxide, peroxynitrate, and peroxynitrite. *Ann. N. Y. Acad. Sci.* **1993**, *686*, 12–27. [CrossRef]
88. Lykkesfeldt, J. Smoking depletes vitamin C: Should smokers be recommended to take supplements? In *Cigarette Smoke and Oxidative Stress*; Halliwell, B., Poulsen, H.E., Eds.; Springer: Heidelberg, Berlin, 2006; pp. 237–260.
89. Preston, A.M.; Rodriguez, C.; Rivera, C.E. Plasma ascorbate in a population of children: Influence of age, gender, vitamin C intake, BMI and smoke exposure. *P. R. Health Sci. J.* **2006**, *25*, 137–142.
90. Preston, A.M.; Rodriguez, C.; Rivera, C.E.; Sahai, H. Influence of environmental tobacco smoke on vitamin C status in children. *Am. J. Clin. Nutr.* **2003**, *77*, 167–172. [CrossRef]
91. Lykkesfeldt, J.; Prieme, H.; Loft, S.; Poulsen, H.E. Effect of smoking cessation on plasma ascorbic acid concentration. *BMJ* **1996**, *313*, 91. [CrossRef]
92. Lykkesfeldt, J.; Viscovich, M.; Poulsen, H.E. Plasma malondialdehyde is induced by smoking: A study with balanced antioxidant profiles. *Br. J. Nutr.* **2004**, *92*, 203–206. [CrossRef]
93. Canoy, D.; Wareham, N.; Welch, A.; Bingham, S.; Luben, R.; Day, N.; Khaw, K.T. Plasma ascorbic acid concentrations and fat distribution in 19,068 British men and women in the European Prospective Investigation into Cancer and Nutrition Norfolk cohort study. *Am. J. Clin. Nutr.* **2005**, *82*, 1203–1209. [CrossRef]
94. Schectman, G. Estimating ascorbic acid requirements for cigarette smokers. *Ann. N. Y. Acad. Sci.* **1993**, *686*, 335–345. [CrossRef]
95. Schectman, G.; Byrd, J.C.; Gruchow, H.W. The influence of smoking on vitamin C status in adults. *Am. J. Public Health* **1989**, *79*, 158–162. [CrossRef]
96. Schectman, G.; Byrd, J.C.; Hoffmann, R. Ascorbic acid requirements for smokers: Analysis of a population survey. *Am. J. Clin. Nutr.* **1991**, *53*, 1466–1470. [CrossRef]
97. Kallner, A.B.; Hartmann, D.; Hornig, D.H. On the requirements of ascorbic acid in man: Steady-state turnover and body pool in smokers. *Am. J. Clin. Nutr.* **1981**, *34*, 1347–1355. [CrossRef]
98. Hansen, S.N.; Schou-Pedersen, A.M.V.; Lykkesfeldt, J.; Tveden-Nyborg, P. Spatial Memory Dysfunction Induced by Vitamin C Deficiency Is Associated with Changes in Monoaminergic Neurotransmitters and Aberrant Synapse Formation. *Antioxidants* **2018**, *7*, 82. [CrossRef]
99. Hansen, S.N.; Tveden-Nyborg, P.; Lykkesfeldt, J. Does vitamin C deficiency affect cognitive development and function? *Nutrients* **2014**, *6*, 3818–3846. [CrossRef]
100. Harrison, F.E.; Meredith, M.E.; Dawes, S.M.; Saskowski, J.L.; May, J.M. Low ascorbic acid and increased oxidative stress in gulo (-/-) mice during development. *Brain Res.* **2010**, *1349*, 143–152. [CrossRef]
101. Jauniaux, E.; Poston, L.; Burton, G.J. Placental-related diseases of pregnancy: Involvement of oxidative stress and implications in human evolution. *Hum. Reprod. Update* **2006**, *12*, 747–755. [CrossRef]

102. Juhl, B.; Lauszus, F.F.; Lykkesfeldt, J. Poor Vitamin C Status Late in Pregnancy Is Associated with Increased Risk of Complications in Type 1 Diabetic Women: A Cross-Sectional Study. *Nutrients* **2017**, *9*, 186. [CrossRef]
103. Chappell, L.C.; Seed, P.T.; Kelly, F.J.; Briley, A.; Hunt, B.J.; Charnock-Jones, D.S.; Mallet, A.; Poston, L. Vitamin C and E supplementation in women at risk of preeclampsia is associated with changes in indices of oxidative stress and placental function. *Am. J. Obstet. Gynecol.* **2002**, *187*, 777–784. [CrossRef]
104. Beazley, D.; Ahokas, R.; Livingston, J.; Griggs, M.; Sibai, B.M. Vitamin C and E supplementation in women at high risk for preeclampsia: A double-blind, placebo-controlled trial. *Am. J. Obstet. Gynecol.* **2005**, *192*, 520–521. [CrossRef]
105. Villar, J.; Purwar, M.; Merialdi, M.; Zavaleta, N.; Thi Nhu Ngoc, N.; Anthony, J.; De Greeff, A.; Poston, L.; Shennan, A.; WHO Vitamin C and Vitamin E trial group. World Health Organisation multicentre randomised trial of supplementation with vitamins C and E among pregnant women at high risk for pre-eclampsia in populations of low nutritional status from developing countries. *BJOG* **2009**, *116*, 780–788. [CrossRef]
106. Chappell, L.C.; Seed, P.T.; Briley, A.L.; Kelly, F.J.; Lee, R.; Hunt, B.J.; Parmar, K.; Bewley, S.J.; Shennan, A.H.; Steer, P.J.; et al. Effect of antioxidants on the occurrence of pre-eclampsia in women at increased risk: A randomised trial. *Lancet* **1999**, *354*, 810–816. [CrossRef]
107. Juhl, B.; Lauszus, F.F.; Lykkesfeldt, J. Is Diabetes Associated with Lower Vitamin C Status in Pregnant Women? A Prospective Study. *Int. J. Vitam. Nutr. Res.* **2016**, *86*, 184–189. [CrossRef]
108. Frikke-Schmidt, H.; Lykkesfeldt, J. Role of marginal vitamin C deficiency in atherogenesis: In vivo models and clinical studies. *Basic Clin. Pharmacol. Toxicol.* **2009**, *104*, 419–433. [CrossRef]
109. Traber, M.G.; Buettner, G.R.; Bruno, R.S. The relationship between vitamin C status, the gut-liver axis, and metabolic syndrome. *Redox Biol.* **2019**, *21*, 101091. [CrossRef]
110. Carr, A.C.; Rosengrave, P.C.; Bayer, S.; Chambers, S.; Mehrtens, J.; Shaw, G.M. Hypovitaminosis C and vitamin C deficiency in critically ill patients despite recommended enteral and parenteral intakes. *Crit. Care* **2017**, *21*, 300. [CrossRef]
111. Marik, P.E. Vitamin C for the treatment of sepsis: The scientific rationale. *Pharmacol. Ther.* **2018**, *189*, 63–70. [CrossRef]
112. Carr, A.C.; Shaw, G.M.; Fowler, A.A.; Natarajan, R. Ascorbate-dependent vasopressor synthesis: A rationale for vitamin C administration in severe sepsis and septic shock? *Crit. Care* **2015**, *19*, 418. [CrossRef]
113. Fowler, A.A., 3rd; Syed, A.A.; Knowlson, S.; Sculthorpe, R.; Farthing, D.; DeWilde, C.; Farthing, C.A.; Larus, T.L.; Martin, E.; Brophy, D.F.; et al. Phase I safety trial of intravenous ascorbic acid in patients with severe sepsis. *J. Transl. Med.* **2014**, *12*, 32. [CrossRef]
114. Marik, P.E.; Khangoora, V.; Rivera, R.; Hooper, M.H.; Catravas, J. Hydrocortisone, Vitamin C, and Thiamine for the Treatment of Severe Sepsis and Septic Shock: A Retrospective Before-After Study. *Chest* **2017**, *151*, 1229–1238. [CrossRef]
115. Hill, A.; Clasen, K.C.; Wendt, S.; Majoros, A.G.; Stoppe, C.; Adhikari, N.K.J.; Heyland, D.K.; Benstoem, C. Effects of Vitamin C on Organ Function in Cardiac Surgery Patients: A Systematic Review and Meta-Analysis. *Nutrients* **2019**, *11*, 2103. [CrossRef]
116. Maxwell, S.R.; Thomason, H.; Sandler, D.; Leguen, C.; Baxter, M.A.; Thorpe, G.H.; Jones, A.F.; Barnett, A. HAntioxidant status in patients with uncomplicated insulin-dependent and non-insulin-dependent diabetes mellitus. *Eur. J. Clin. Investig.* **1997**, *27*, 484–490. [CrossRef]
117. Stankova, L.; Riddle, M.; Larned, J.; Burry, K.; Menashe, D.; Hart, J.; Bigley, R. Plasma ascorbate concentrations and blood cell dehydroascorbate transport in patients with diabetes mellitus. *Metabolism* **1984**, *33*, 347–353. [CrossRef]
118. Feskens, E.J.; Virtanen, S.M.; Rasanen, L.; Tuomilehto, J.; Stengard, J.; Pekkanen, J.; Nissinen, A.; Kromhout, D. Dietary factors determining diabetes and impaired glucose tolerance. A 20-year follow-up of the Finnish and Dutch cohorts of the Seven Countries Study. *Diabetes Care* **1995**, *18*, 1104–1112.
119. Paolisso, G.; Balbi, V.; Volpe, C.; Varricchio, G.; Gambardella, A.; Saccomanno, F.; Ammendola, S.; Varricchio, M.; D'Onofrio, F. Metabolic benefits deriving from chronic vitamin C supplementation in aged non-insulin dependent diabetics. *J. Am. Coll. Nutr.* **1995**, *14*, 387–392. [CrossRef]
120. Song, Y.; Xu, Q.; Park, Y.; Hollenbeck, A.; Schatzkin, A.; Chen, H. Multivitamins, individual vitamin and mineral supplements, and risk of diabetes among older U.S. adults. *Diabetes Care* **2011**, *34*, 108–114. [CrossRef]

121. Mason, S.A.; Baptista, R.; Della Gatta, P.A.; Yousif, A.; Russell, A.P.; Wadley, G.D. High-dose vitamin C supplementation increases skeletal muscle vitamin C concentration and SVCT2 transporter expression but does not alter redox status in healthy males. *Free Radic. Biol. Med.* **2014**, *77*, 130–138. [CrossRef]
122. Mason, S.A.; Rasmussen, B.; van Loon, L.J.C.; Salmon, J.; Wadley, G.D. Ascorbic acid supplementation improves postprandial glycaemic control and blood pressure in individuals with type 2 diabetes: Findings of a randomized cross-over trial. *Diabetes Obes. Metab.* **2019**, *21*, 674–682. [CrossRef]
123. Odermarsky, M.; Lykkesfeldt, J.; Liuba, P. Poor vitamin C status is associated with increased carotid intima-media thickness, decreased microvascular function, and delayed myocardial repolarization in young patients with type 1 diabetes. *Am. J. Clin. Nutr.* **2009**, *90*, 447–452. [CrossRef]
124. Tousoulis, D.; Antoniades, C.; Tountas, C.; Bosinakou, E.; Kotsopoulou, M.; Toutouzas, P.; Stefanadis, C. Vitamin C affects thrombosis/fibrinolysis system and reactive hyperemia in patients with type 2 diabetes and coronary artery disease. *Diabetes Care* **2003**, *26*, 2749–2753. [CrossRef]

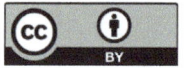 © 2019 by the authors. Licensee MDPI, Basel, Switzerland. This article is an open access article distributed under the terms and conditions of the Creative Commons Attribution (CC BY) license (http://creativecommons.org/licenses/by/4.0/).

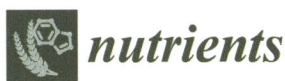

Article

Erythrocyte Ascorbate Is a Potential Indicator of Steady-State Plasma Ascorbate Concentrations in Healthy Non-Fasting Individuals

Juliet M. Pullar [1,*], **Susannah Dunham** [1], **Gabi U. Dachs** [2], **Margreet C. M. Vissers** [1] and **Anitra C. Carr** [3]

[1] Centre for Free Radical Research, Department of Pathology and Biomedical Science, University of Otago, Christchurch, PO Box 4345, 8140 Christchurch, New Zealand; Susannah.Dunham@cdhb.health.nz (S.D.); margreet.vissers@otago.ac.nz (M.C.M.V.)
[2] Mackenzie Cancer Research Group, Department of Pathology and Biomedical Science, University of Otago, Christchurch, PO Box 4345, 8140 Christchurch, New Zealand; gabi.dachs@otago.ac.nz
[3] Nutrition in Medicine Research Group, Department of Pathology and Biomedical Science, University of Otago, Christchurch, PO Box 4345, 8140 Christchurch, New Zealand; anitra.carr@otago.ac.nz
* Correspondence: juliet.pullar@otago.ac.nz; Tel.: +64-3364-1559

Received: 16 January 2020; Accepted: 3 February 2020; Published: 6 February 2020

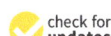

Abstract: Plasma vitamin C concentrations fluctuate in response to recent dietary intake; therefore levels are typically determined in the fasting state. Erythrocyte ascorbate concentrations have been shown to be similar to plasma levels, but little is known about the kinetics of ascorbate accumulation in these cells. In this study, we investigated ascorbate uptake into erythrocytes after dietary supplementation with vitamin C and compared it to changes in plasma ascorbate concentrations. Seven individuals with baseline fasting plasma vitamin C concentrations ≥ 50 µmol/L were depleted of vitamin C-containing foods and drinks for one week, and then supplemented with 250 mg vitamin C/day in addition to resuming their normal diet. Fasting or steady-state plasma ascorbate concentrations declined to almost half of their baseline concentration over the week of vitamin C depletion, and then returned to saturation within two days of beginning supplementation. Erythrocyte ascorbate concentrations exhibited a very similar profile to plasma levels, with values ~76% of plasma, and a strong linear correlation ($r = 0.89$, $p < 0.0001$). Using a pharmacokinetic study design in six individuals with baseline fasting plasma vitamin C concentrations ≥50 µmol/L, we also showed that, unlike plasma, which peaked between 2 and 4 h following ingestion of 200 mg of vitamin C, erythrocyte ascorbate concentrations did not change in the six hours after supplementation. The data from these two intervention studies indicate that erythrocyte ascorbate concentration provides a stable measure of steady-state plasma ascorbate status and could be used to monitor ascorbate status in healthy non-fasting individuals.

Keywords: vitamin C; ascorbate; plasma; erythrocyte; steady-state; pharmacokinetic; dehydroascorbic acid

---

1. Introduction

Humans, unlike most other animals, have lost the ability to synthesise vitamin C (ascorbate) due to evolutionary conserved mutations in the gene encoding L-gulonolactone oxidase, which catalyses the final step in the biosynthetic pathway [1]. A diet severely lacking in vitamin C can result in the deficiency disease scurvy, which is characterised by the breakdown of connective tissue, causing localised bruising and bleeding, and ultimately leading to death [2,3]. Although scurvy is now rarely seen, the inadequate dietary intake of vitamin C is thought to be much more common and hypovitaminosis C (plasma ascorbate concentrations < 23 µmol/L) has been described in up to 15% of individuals [4,5]. These levels are associated with early symptoms of scurvy, such as fatigue and depression [6].

After ingestion, vitamin C is absorbed via the small intestine, released into the bloodstream and distributed to the tissues [7]. Accumulation into cells occurs via the sodium-dependent vitamin C transporters SVCT1 and SVCT2, which actively transport the vitamin against a concentration gradient to reach millimolar concentrations inside the cells [8,9]. It is well recognised that the SVCTs are vital for ascorbate distribution in the body [10,11]. Cells can also transport the oxidised form of vitamin C, dehydroascorbic acid (DHA) using the facilitative glucose transporters (GLUTs) in competition with glucose [12,13]. Once inside the cells, DHA is reduced to ascorbate [9,14]. GLUT-mediated DHA transport seems to be critical for ascorbate uptake into the erythrocytes. Mature erythrocytes do not contain SVCT proteins [15,16] and are thought to be reliant on the GLUTs, particularly GLUT1, for obtaining ascorbate from circulation [13,17,18]. Previous studies have shown that the ascorbate concentration in erythrocytes is similar to that of plasma [19–21], indicating that these cells do not concentrate ascorbate against the plasma concentration gradient.

Vitamin C status is typically determined by measuring the plasma concentrations of the vitamin [5,14]. However, the accuracy of this measurement is dependent on the use of fasting blood samples, as plasma vitamin C levels can fluctuate depending on recent dietary intake [15]. Providing fasting samples can be clinically challenging and inconvenient, and can also be difficult to incorporate into some study design scenarios. Thus, an accurate measurement of the vitamin C status in non-fasting individuals would be a useful tool. Given the observation that erythrocyte ascorbate levels are similar to plasma levels [19–21], we hypothesised that the intracellular erythrocyte ascorbate concentration may be a useful indicator of the steady-state plasma ascorbate concentration. In this study, we used both steady-state and short-term pharmacokinetic study designs to determine the kinetics of ascorbate uptake into erythrocytes and the relationship between erythrocyte levels and plasma ascorbate status.

2. Materials and Methods

2.1. Steady-State Study

Ethical approval was obtained from the New Zealand Southern Health and Disability Ethics Committee URA/06/12/083/AM02. Seven healthy participants were recruited from the University of Otago, Christchurch, with all participants providing written informed consent. Participants were eligible if they were non-smokers and had fasting plasma ascorbate concentrations of ≥50 µmol/L. The study design is shown in Figure 1. At recruitment, participants were asked to refrain from eating and drinking vitamin C-containing food for one week and were provided with an extensive list of foods to avoid, as well as a list of those that lacked vitamin C. After one week, participants resumed their normal diet and were given a 250 mg vitamin C tablet daily (Tishcon Corp., Westbury, NY, USA). Plasma and erythrocyte ascorbate concentrations were assessed at day 1 and every 2–3 days throughout the study period. All blood samples were obtained via venous puncture after an overnight fast, which included sampling prior to the ingestion of the daily vitamin C supplement in the second week of the study.

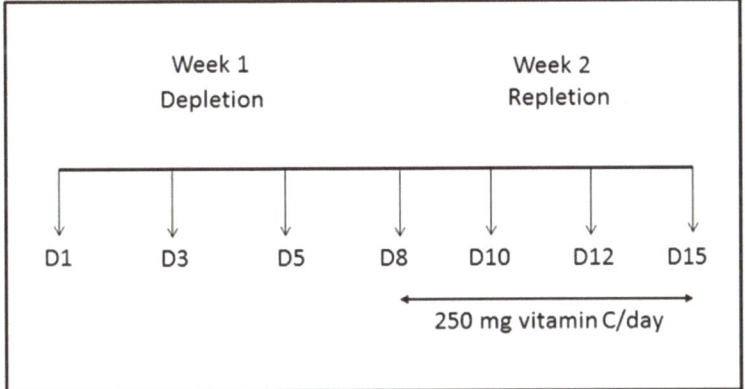

Figure 1. Steady-state study design. Participants were depleted of vitamin C-containing foods and beverages for one week and then supplemented with 250 mg of vitamin C per day for another week, in addition to returning to their normal diet. Fasting blood samples were obtained at the days indicated and analysed for plasma and erythrocyte ascorbate (D1 is day 1, etc.).

2.2. Pharmacokinetic Study

Ethical approval was obtained from the University of Otago Ethics Committee (H14/123) to conduct a short-term pharmacokinetic study, comparing the uptake of ascorbate into plasma and erythrocytes following dietary intake. Six healthy volunteers with fasting plasma ascorbate concentrations of ≥50 μmol/L were recruited from the University of Otago, Christchurch. Participants with healthy vitamin C levels (≥50 μmol/L) were chosen to avoid the possible preferential uptake of ascorbate by the tissues in individuals with a low vitamin C status, which could confound the comparison between plasma and erythrocyte ascorbate. All participants provided written informed consent. Following an overnight fast, a blood sample was obtained and the participants were supplemented with 200 mg of vitamin C tablets (Tishcon Corp., Westbury, NY, USA). Blood samples were collected every two hours for the next six hours (four samples in total, including the baseline). Following baseline blood collection, the participants were asked to avoid vitamin C-containing goods for the remaining six hours. The blood samples were processed for plasma and erythrocyte ascorbate analyses at the time of collection.

2.3. Plasma Ascorbate Sample Processing

Blood was collected in K_3-EDTA vacutainer tubes (Becton Dickinson, Auckland, New Zealand), immediately placed on ice, and processed within two hours of collection. All the following procedures were carried out on ice or at 4 °C. The blood was centrifuged at 3200× g for 15 min at 4 °C to separate the cells from the plasma. An aliquot of plasma was removed for ascorbate analysis and was acidified with an equal volume of ice-cold 0.54 mol/L perchloric acid containing 100 μmol/L diethylenetriaminepentaacetic acid (DTPA). The perchloric acid extracts were centrifuged and supernatants stored at −80 °C until HPLC analysis.

2.4. Erythrocyte Ascorbate Sample Processing

An analysis of erythrocyte ascorbate was undertaken using an adaptation of the method of Levine and co-workers [21]. Firstly, the remaining plasma and buffy coat layer were carefully removed from the centrifuged blood and discarded. The packed erythrocytes were washed once with a 10-fold excess of ice-cold PBS containing 500 μmol/L DTPA. Following centrifugation, 150 μL aliquots of packed erythrocytes were stored at −80 °C. On the day of the HPLC analysis, the erythrocytes were rapidly thawed and the cells lysed with the addition of a four times volume of ice-cold milliQ water containing

500 µmol/L DTPA, vortex mixing and incubation on ice for 2 min. A 200 µL aliquot was added to the top of a centrifugal filter unit (Amicon Ultra 0.5 mL, 10K Ultracel®; Millipore) and the lysate was centrifuged at 14,000 × g for 20 min at 4 °C to remove haemoglobin. An equal volume of ice-cold 0.54 mol/L perchloric acid containing 100 µmol/L DTPA was immediately added to the ultrafiltrate and the samples were vortexed and spun. The samples were incubated with tris (2-carboxyethyl) phosphine hydrochloride (TCEP) to reduce any DHA present in the sample, as described previously [22].

2.5. Ascorbate HPLC Analysis

The vitamin C content of the plasma and erythrocyte samples was analysed by reverse-phase HPLC with coulometric electrochemical detection [22]. A standard curve of sodium ascorbate was freshly prepared each day in 77 mmol/L perchloric acid containing 100 µmol/L DTPA. Plasma and erythrocyte ascorbate are expressed as µmol/L.

2.6. Statistical Analyses

Statistical analyses were carried out using GraphPad Prism version 8 (La Jolla, CA, USA). The data are represented as the mean ± SEM, with p values ≤ 0.05 considered significant. Correlations were tested using Pearson's linear correlation and differences between paired data were tested using two-tailed paired t-tests.

3. Results

3.1. Steady-State Study

Seven healthy individuals with plasma vitamin C concentrations of ≥50 µmol/L were depleted via elimination of vitamin C-containing foods and drinks for one week and then supplemented with 250 mg of vitamin C/day for the following week, in addition to resuming their normal diet. Fasting plasma and erythrocyte ascorbate concentrations were measured every two to three days. The mean baseline fasting plasma ascorbate concentration was 82.8 ± 9.0 µmol/L (Figure 2A). Plasma ascorbate levels decreased rapidly upon withdrawal of vitamin C from the diet, reaching 44.1 ± 5.2 µmol/L after 7 days (Figure 2A; ~47% reduction). However, ascorbate concentrations were quickly restored upon the addition of vitamin C to the diet, with the group reaching plasma saturation (≥80 µmol/L) within two days of beginning supplementation.

Similarly, erythrocyte ascorbate concentrations decreased over the week in which vitamin C was removed from the diet, dropping from a starting concentration of 58.3 ± 6.0 µmol/L to 32.0 ± 5.7 µmol/L over the 7 days (Figure 2A; ~45% reduction). When participants were supplemented with vitamin C, a rapid and significant increase in erythrocyte ascorbate was observed. Like the plasma, the erythrocyte ascorbate concentration plateaued within two days of beginning supplementation.

The data show that changes in the steady-state ascorbate concentration of individuals, as evidenced by their fasting plasma ascorbate levels, are also reflected in their erythrocyte ascorbate content. Indeed, a strong positive linear relationship was observed between the two (Figure 2B: Pearson correlation coefficient r of 0.887; $p < 0.0001$). For every 1 µmol/L increase in plasma ascorbate, there was a ~0.76 µmol/L increase in erythrocyte ascorbate (regression line: y = 0.76 x −1), demonstrating a lower ascorbate concentration in the erythrocytes than in plasma. As expected, erythrocytes do not accumulate ascorbate to the millimolar concentrations observed in other cell types.

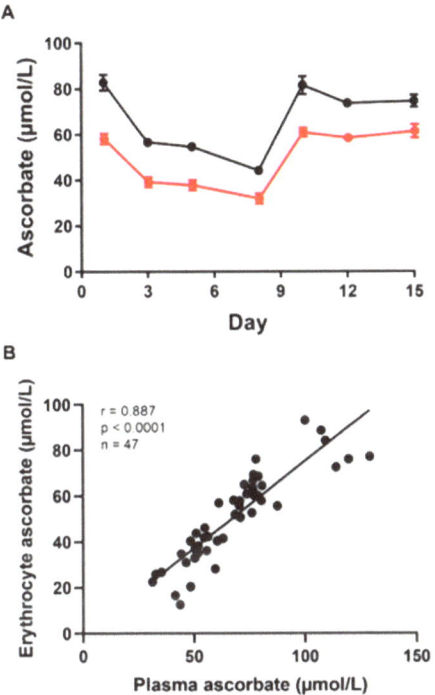

Figure 2. Changes in steady-state ascorbate concentrations during the two-week study. (**A**) Fasting plasma (●) and erythrocyte (●) ascorbate concentrations over time. Each symbol represents the mean ± SEM of 5 to 7 individuals, as not all 7 individuals provided samples on each day of the study. (**B**) Linear correlation of the plasma and erythrocyte ascorbate concentrations (n = 47 points). For Figure A, paired t-tests showed that days 3, 5 and 8 were significantly different to the baseline for both plasma and erythrocytes. For Figure B, a Pearson linear correlation analysis was performed.

3.2. Short-Term Pharmacokinetic Study

To investigate the short-term effects of vitamin C supplementation on erythrocyte ascorbate concentrations, a pharmacokinetic study was conducted in six individuals who had plasma vitamin C concentrations of ≥50 μmol/L. Fasting participants were given 200 mg vitamin C tablets and plasma and erythrocyte ascorbate were monitored over the following 6 h (Figure 3). A statistically significant increase in plasma ascorbate was observed at 2 and 4 h post-supplementation, with levels returning towards baseline at 6 h. In comparison, erythrocyte ascorbate did not significantly differ from baseline for the duration of the time course. A significant difference between plasma and erythrocyte ascorbate was found at two and four hours, but not at six 6 hours ($p < 0.05$). As such, plasma and erythrocyte ascorbate were not linearly correlated ($r = 0.08$, $p = 0.7$). The data indicate that erythrocyte ascorbate concentrations do not show the same rapid increase as occurs in plasma after the ingestion of vitamin C [6,23], suggesting that these levels more accurately reflect steady-state ascorbate levels and may be a useful indicator of their status in non-fasting blood samples.

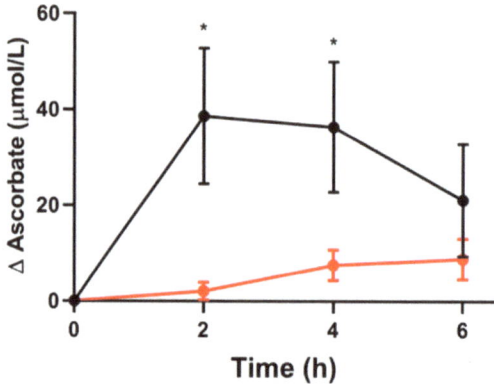

Figure 3. Pharmacokinetic study. The change in plasma (●) and erythrocyte (●) ascorbate following ingestion of 200 mg of vitamin C. The zero time point is fasting, with supplementation occurring immediately after this sample was taken. The data represent the mean ± SEM (n = 6). The baseline ascorbate concentrations were 67.2 ± 8.8 µmol/L and 58.7 ± 4.6 µmol/L for plasma and erythrocytes, respectively. Paired t-tests indicate that erythrocyte ascorbate time points were not significantly different from the baseline, whereas plasma ascorbate was different from the baseline at 2 and 4 h ($p < 0.05$). Furthermore, erythrocyte and plasma ascorbate were significantly different from each other at the time points indicated * ($p < 0.02$).

4. Discussion

Unlike most other cell types, which actively take up ascorbate using the SVCTs, erythrocytes accumulate ascorbate primarily by the passive transport of DHA via the GLUTs [17]. In our study of healthy individuals, we found that the ascorbate content of erythrocytes did not change following dietary intake of the vitamin, despite there being a transient peak observed in the plasma. This indicates that erythrocyte ascorbate does not respond to a transient change in plasma levels and more accurately reflects steady-state plasma ascorbate. This was supported by the observation that changes in the steady-state plasma ascorbate concentration were reflected in the erythrocyte ascorbate concentration. Red cell ascorbate concentrations were ~0.76 of those of plasma, using the gradient of the regression line. These findings suggest that erythrocyte ascorbate content could be used as an indicator of the steady-state plasma ascorbate concentrations in non-fasting individuals, as this measurement does not seem to be subject to transient fluctuations following dietary intake.

It is well known that intracellular erythrocyte ascorbate concentrations are comparable to the plasma concentrations of the vitamin [14,19–21,24]; however, less is known about the short-term uptake kinetics of these cells. A previous study by Williamson and Winterbourn [19] indicated that plasma ascorbate concentrations increased two to three-fold two hours after oral administration of 2 g of vitamin C, whereas the erythrocyte ascorbate increased by only about 20%. Although this was higher than the increase observed in our study, it is likely to reflect the 10-fold higher vitamin C dose used in their study. They also conducted a supplementation study with 1 g of vitamin C/day for 2–3 weeks in 11 individuals and showed increases in both the fasting plasma and erythrocyte ascorbate concentrations. However, the ratio of erythrocyte to plasma ascorbate was ~1.6 in their study [19], which is higher than our measurements. This difference may relate to the colourimetric assay used to measure erythrocyte ascorbate in their study, which may be affected by haemoglobin iron and therefore, may be less accurate than our assay, which overcomes many of the problems associated with measuring erythrocyte ascorbate, notably the high iron content of these cells [21].

There are, however, some limitations to using erythrocyte ascorbate concentration as an indicator of steady-state plasma ascorbate status in non-fasting individuals. The erythrocyte assay is more expensive and time-consuming, with additional handling required over the plasma method [21]. Moreover, the values obtained cannot be used interchangeably with those of plasma. While we have found that erythrocyte ascorbate is about 75% of plasma ascorbate in our healthy cohort, and others have found a similar result [21], whether this ratio would hold for ascorbate concentrations above or below the normal range (~40–120 µmol/L in our study) or in individuals who are unwell and may have higher DHA concentrations due to oxidative stress is not clear. Recent work has also highlighted that erythrocytes from individuals with a severe vitamin C deficiency are fragile and prone to lysis [24], which may have affected the accuracy of our assay in deficient individuals.

5. Conclusions

In this study, we provide valuable data that contribute to the understanding of erythrocyte ascorbate accumulation and pharmacokinetics. These cells are often ignored with regard to vitamin C; however, they represent a substantial pool of ascorbate in the body, making up 40%–50% of blood volume. Further work investigating erythrocyte ascorbate concentrations in acute and chronically ill cohorts, and particularly those who are receiving intravenous vitamin C infusions, is warranted. Such studies would help clarify whether erythrocyte ascorbate could be useful as an indicator of steady-state plasma ascorbate concentrations in non-fasting individuals.

Author Contributions: Conceptualisation, G.U.D. and J.M.P.; methodology, J.M.P., G.U.D., A.C.C. and M.C.M.V.; formal analysis, J.M.P.; investigation, S.D. and J.M.P.; writing—original draft preparation, J.M.P.; writing—review and editing, A.C.C., G.U.D. and M.C.M.V.; visualisation, J.M.P.; supervision, G.U.D., A.C.C., J.M.P. and M.C.M.V.; project administration, S.D. and J.M.P.; funding acquisition, G.U.D. and J.M.P. All authors have read and agreed to the published version of the manuscript.

Funding: This research was funded by the Canterbury Medical Research Foundation, grant number 15/03.

Acknowledgments: We would like to thank the participants of the two studies. AC is the recipient of a Health Research Council of New Zealand Sir Charles Hercus Health Research Fellowship.

Conflicts of Interest: The authors declare no conflict of interest.

References

1. Smirnoff, N. Ascorbic acid metabolism and functions: A comparison of plants and mammals. *Free. Radic. Boil. Med.* **2018**, *122*, 116–129. [CrossRef] [PubMed]
2. Khalife, R.; Grieco, A.; Khamisa, K.; Tinmouh, A.; McCudden, C.; Saidenberg, E. Scurvy, an old story in a new time: The hematologist's experience. *Blood Cells Mol. Dis.* **2019**, *76*, 40–44. [CrossRef] [PubMed]
3. Padayatty, S.J.; Levine, M. Vitamin C: The known and the unknown and Goldilocks. *Oral Dis.* **2016**, *22*, 463–493. [CrossRef] [PubMed]
4. Pearson, J.F.; Pullar, J.M.; Wilson, R.; Spittlehouse, J.K.; Vissers, M.C.M.; Skidmore, P.M.L.; Willis, J.; Cameron, V.A.; Carr, A.C. Vitamin C Status Correlates with Markers of Metabolic and Cognitive Health in 50-Year-Olds: Findings of the CHALICE Cohort Study. *Nutrients* **2017**, *9*, 831. [CrossRef] [PubMed]
5. Schleicher, R.L.; Carroll, M.D.; Ford, E.S.; Lacher, D.A. Serum vitamin C and the prevalence of vitamin C deficiency in the United States: 2003–2004 National Health and Nutrition Examination Survey (NHANES). *Am. J. Clin. Nutr.* **2009**, *90*, 1252–1263. [CrossRef]
6. Levine, M.; Conry-Cantilena, C.; Wang, Y.; Welch, R.W.; Washko, P.W.; Dhariwal, K.R.; Park, J.B.; Lazarev, A.; Graumlich, J.F.; King, J.; et al. Vitamin C pharmacokinetics in healthy volunteers: Evidence for a recommended dietary allowance. *Proc. Natl. Acad. Sci. USA* **1996**, *93*, 3704–3709. [CrossRef]
7. Wilson, J.X. Regulation of Vitamin C Transport. *Annu. Rev. Nutr.* **2005**, *25*, 105–125. [CrossRef]
8. Savini, I.; Rossi, A.; Pierro, C.; Avigliano, L.; Catani, M.V. SVCT1 and SVCT2: Key proteins for vitamin C uptake. *Amino Acids* **2008**, *34*, 347–355. [CrossRef]
9. Du, J.; Cullen, J.J.; Buettner, G.R. Ascorbic acid: Chemistry, biology and the treatment of cancer. *Biochim. Biophys. Acta Bioenerg.* **2012**, *1826*, 443–457. [CrossRef]

10. Sotiriou, S.; Gispert, S.; Cheng, J.; Wang, Y.; Chen, A.; Hoogstraten-Miller, S.; Miller, G.F.; Kwon, O.; Levine, M.; Guttentag, S.H.; et al. Ascorbic-acid transporter Slc23a1 is essential for vitamin C transport into the brain and for perinatal survival. *Nat. Med.* **2002**, *8*, 514–517. [CrossRef]
11. Corpe, C.P.; Tu, H.; Eck, P.; Wang, J.; Faulhaber-Walter, R.; Schnermann, J.; Margolis, S.; Padayatty, S.; Sun, H.; Wang, Y.; et al. Vitamin C transporter Slc23a1 links renal reabsorption, vitamin C tissue accumulation, and perinatal survival in mice. *J. Clin. Investig.* **2010**, *120*, 1069–1083. [CrossRef]
12. Vera, J.C.; Rivas, C.I.; Fischbarg, J.; Golde, D.W. Mammalian facilitative hexose transporters mediate the transport of dehydroascorbic acid. *Nature* **1993**, *364*, 79–82. [CrossRef]
13. Rumsey, S.C.; Kwon, O.; Xu, G.W.; Burant, C.; Simpson, I.; Levine, M. Glucose Transporter Isoforms GLUT1 and GLUT3 Transport Dehydroascorbic Acid. *J. Boil. Chem.* **1997**, *272*, 18982–18989. [CrossRef] [PubMed]
14. Mendiratta, S.; Qu, Z.-C.; May, J.M. Erythrocyte Ascorbate Recycling: Antioxidant Effects in Blood. *Free. Radic. Boil. Med.* **1998**, *24*, 789–797. [CrossRef]
15. May, J.M.; Qu, Z.C.; Qiao, H.; Koury, M.J. Maturational loss of the vitamin C transporter in erythrocytes. *Biochem. Biophys. Res. Commun.* **2007**, *360*, 295–298. [CrossRef] [PubMed]
16. May, J.M. Ascorbate function and metabolism in the human erythrocyte. *Front. Biosci.* **1998**, *3*, d1–d10. [CrossRef]
17. Tu, H.; Wang, Y.; Li, H.; Brinster, L.R.; Levine, M. Chemical Transport Knockout for Oxidized Vitamin C, Dehydroascorbic Acid, Reveals Its Functions in vivo. *EBioMedicine* **2017**, *23*, 125–135. [CrossRef]
18. Sage, J.M.; Carruthers, A. Human erythrocytes transport dehydroascorbic acid and sugars using the same transporter complex. *Am. J. Physiol. Physiol.* **2014**, *306*, C910–C917. [CrossRef]
19. Williamson, D.; Winterbourn, C.C. Effect of oral administration of ascorbate on acetylphenylhydrazine-induced Heinz body formation. *Br. J. Haematol.* **1980**, *46*, 319–321. [CrossRef]
20. Evans, R.M.; Currie, L.; Campbell, A. The distribution of ascorbic acid between various cellular components of blood, in normal individuals, and its relation to the plasma concentration. *Br. J. Nutr.* **1982**, *47*, 473–482. [CrossRef]
21. Li, H.; Tu, H.; Wang, Y.; Levine, M. Vitamin C in mouse and human red blood cells: An HPLC assay. *Anal. Biochem.* **2012**, *426*, 109–117. [CrossRef] [PubMed]
22. Pullar, J.M.; Bayer, S.; Carr, A.C. Appropriate Handling, Processing and Analysis of Blood Samples Is Essential to Avoid Oxidation of Vitamin C to Dehydroascorbic Acid. *Antioxidants* **2018**, *7*, 29. [CrossRef] [PubMed]
23. Levine, M.; Wang, Y.; Padayatty, S.J.; Morrow, J. A new recommended dietary allowance of vitamin C for healthy young women. *Proc. Natl. Acad. Sci. USA* **2001**, *98*, 9842–9846. [CrossRef] [PubMed]
24. Tu, H.; Li, H.; Wang, Y.; Niyyati, M.; Wang, Y.; Leshin, J.; Levine, M. Low Red Blood Cell Vitamin C Concentrations Induce Red Blood Cell Fragility: A Link to Diabetes Via Glucose, Glucose Transporters, and Dehydroascorbic Acid. *EBioMedicine* **2015**, *2*, 1735–1750. [CrossRef]

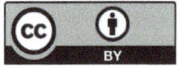

© 2020 by the authors. Licensee MDPI, Basel, Switzerland. This article is an open access article distributed under the terms and conditions of the Creative Commons Attribution (CC BY) license (http://creativecommons.org/licenses/by/4.0/).

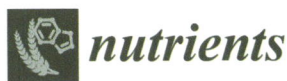

Review

Vitamin C and Neutrophil Function: Findings from Randomized Controlled Trials

Mikee Liugan [1] and Anitra C. Carr [2,*]

[1] Centre for Postgraduate Nursing Studies, University of Otago, Christchurch 8011, New Zealand
[2] Nutrition in Medicine Research Group, Department of Pathology & Biomedical Science, University of Otago, Christchurch 8011, New Zealand
* Correspondence: anitra.carr@otago.ac.nz; Tel.: +64-3364-0649

Received: 16 August 2019; Accepted: 3 September 2019; Published: 4 September 2019

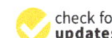

Abstract: Vitamin C is known to support immune function and is accumulated by neutrophils to millimolar intracellular concentrations suggesting an important role for the vitamin in these cells. In this review, the effects of vitamin C, as a mono- or multi-supplement therapy, on neutrophil function were assessed by conducting a systematic review of randomized controlled trials (RCTs). Specifically, trials which assessed neutrophil migration (chemotaxis), phagocytosis, oxidative burst, enzyme activity, or cell death (apoptosis) as primary or secondary outcomes were assessed. A systematic literature search was conducted using the Cochrane Central Register of Controlled Trials, EMBASE, Embase Classic, Joanna Briggs Institute EBP, Ovid MEDLINE®, Ovid MEDLINE® In-Process & Other Non-Indexed Citations, Ovid Nursing Database, CINAHL and PubMed database, which identified 16 eligible RCTs. Quality appraisal of the included studies was carried out using the Cochrane Risk of Bias tool. Three of the studies assessed neutrophil chemotaxis in hospitalised patients or outpatients, two of which showed improved neutrophil function following intravenous vitamin C administration. Ten RCTs assessed neutrophil phagocytosis and/or oxidative burst activity; five were exercise studies, one in smokers, one in myocardial infarction patients and three in healthy volunteers. Two of the multi-supplement studies showed a difference between the intervention and control groups: increased oxidative burst activity in athletes post-exercise and decreased oxidant generation in myocardial infarction patients. Two studies assessed neutrophil enzyme activity; one showed deceased antioxidant enzyme activity in divers and the other showed increased antioxidant enzyme activity in athletes. One final study showed decreased neutrophil apoptosis in septic surgical patients following intravenous vitamin C administration. Overall, 44% of the RCTs assessed in this review showed effects of vitamin C supplementation on neutrophil functions. However, the studies were very heterogeneous, comprising different participant cohorts and different dosing regimens. There were also a number of limitations inherent in the design of many of these RCTs. Future RCTs should incorporate prescreening of potential participants for low vitamin C status or utilize cohorts known to have low vitamin status, such as hospitalized patients, and should also comprise appropriate vitamin C dosing for the cohort under investigation.

Keywords: vitamin C; ascorbic acid; neutrophils; polymorphonuclear leukocytes; migration; chemotaxis; apoptosis; phagocytosis; oxidative burst; systematic review

1. Introduction

Neutrophils are a vital component of the innate immune system, providing a first line of defense against invading pathogens [1]. Following microbial invasion, neutrophils migrate to the site of infection in response to pathogen- and host-derived pro-inflammatory mediators, known as chemotaxis [1]. The neutrophils then proceed to phagocytose, kill and digest the invading pathogens via both oxidative and enzymatic mechanisms [2]. Spent neutrophils subsequently undergo a process of programmed cell death which results in recognition and clearance of the cells by macrophages [3]. Effective clearance of neutrophils from inflammatory loci is vital for resolution of the pro-inflammatory response as release of necrotic cell contents results in tissue damage [4]. Chromatin released from neutrophils, known as neutrophil extracellular traps, comprises both oxidative and proteolytic enzymes, and has been implicated in host tissue damage and various pathologies [5].

Defective neutrophil function is observed in a number of conditions, such as chronic granulomatous disease and Chédiak-Higashi syndrome, which result in recurrent infections [6,7]. Patients with recurrent infections and sepsis can also present with dysfunctional neutrophils, sometimes referred to as immune paralysis due to the inability of the cells to migrate appropriately [8]. It is noteworthy that patients with severe infections and sepsis present with depleted vitamin C status [9,10]. Vitamin C is known to have pleiotropic roles in the immune system, through its antioxidant and enzyme cofactor activities, including potentially supporting neutrophil function [11]. Preclinical studies indicate that neutrophils isolated from scorbutic guinea pigs exhibit attenuated chemotaxis, phagocytosis, oxidant production and microbial killing compared with control animals, and supplementation with vitamin C reversed the dysfunctional activities [12–14]. Vitamin C-deficient gulonolactone oxidase (Gulo) knockout mice exhibit dysfunctional neutrophil cell death and diminished uptake by macrophages [15], and vitamin C supplementation can decrease neutrophil extracellular traps formation in septic Gulo knockout mice [16].

Although mean plasma vitamin C concentrations are typically around 50 µmol/L, neutrophils accumulate millimolar intracellular vitamin C concentrations against a concentration gradient which is thought to indicate an important role for the vitamin in these cells [17]. Thus, the depleted vitamin C status of neutrophils observed during infectious episodes could potentially compromise their function [18]. Numerous non-controlled studies have investigated the effects of vitamin C supplementation on the neutrophil functions of chemotaxis, phagocytosis, oxidant generation and microbial killing and predominantly showed positive effects (reviewed in [11]). A number of these studies included patients with known neutrophil dysfunction e.g., those with chronic granulomatous disease or Chédiak-Higashi syndrome, or individuals with allergic or infectious conditions. Exercise, both single bouts and prolonged training over several weeks, can produce changes in the distribution and function of various cellular and humoral components of the immune system [19]. Studies have reported high susceptibility of athletes to infections, especially upper respiratory tract infections, following heavy and intensive training as well as after marathon and ultramarathon running [20,21]. Thus, the effect of vitamin C supplementation on neutrophil function in athletes is also of interest.

The purpose of this review was to identify RCTs which investigated the effects of vitamin C supplementation on the functions of neutrophils. These included RCTs in athletes, healthy volunteers and patient groups, but excluding participants with existing neutrophilic dysfunction disorders. Studies comprising vitamin C administered as monotherapy or in combination with other micronutrients, such as vitamin E, were included. No restriction was placed on the route of administration (oral or intravenous) or the source of vitamin C (supplemental or food-derived) [22].

2. Methodology

The research question for this review was formulated using the PICO tool which comprises Population, Intervention, Comparison and Outcomes, an approach endorsed by the Cochrane Collaboration [23]. The PICO question was: What are the effects of vitamin C supplementation on neutrophil function, particularly on neutrophil chemotaxis/motility/migration, phagocytosis, oxidative burst, enzyme activity, apoptosis/clearance or necrosis/necrotic cell death in humans?

Preliminary literature searches were conducted using the databases PROSPERO, DARE, NICE, and the Cochrane Database of Systematic Reviews to determine any existing literature available on the topic area, to identify any existing or ongoing reviews of relevance to the topic area to ensure that the topic to be reviewed was novel and that there were no published reviews with the same research question in the current literature. A thorough literature search was then conducted using the Cochrane Central Register of Controlled Trials (May 2018), EMBASE (1980 to June 2018), Embase Classic (1947 to 1979), Joanna Briggs Institute EBP (June 2018), Ovid MEDLINE® In-Process & Other Non-Indexed Citations (June 2018), Ovid MEDLINE® (1946 to Present with Daily Update), Ovid Nursing Database (1946 to May 2018), CINAHL and PubMed databases using the following keywords: (1) vitamin C OR ascorbic acid OR ascorbate OR antiscorbutic factor OR l-ascorbate OR l-ascorbic acid; AND (2) neutrophils OR polymorphonuclear leukocytes OR immune system OR immunity OR immune function OR inflammation; AND (3) migration OR mobility OR chemotaxis OR apoptosis OR phagocytosis OR clearance OR necrosis OR necrotic cell death OR oxidative burst OR neutrophil enzyme activity. No restrictions were placed for the publication date, study location, age of participants, nature of participants, route of administration of vitamin C, and the source of vitamin C (supplemental or food-derived). However, only published RCTs and publications in English were included in this review.

The abstracts and titles of the papers obtained from the literature search were screened to ensure that all the PICO components were covered and also that the inclusion/exclusion criteria were met (Table 1). Studies that did not meet the inclusion/exclusion criteria were rejected. Full-texts of the relevant papers were obtained using the University of Otago library and ResearchGate websites. Each of the full-text articles gathered for analysis were critically appraised for quality and risk of bias using the Cochrane Risk of Bias tool for RCTs [23]. For every criterion, each study was rated either low, unclear or high risk of bias and therefore appraised as good, fair or poor-quality research. The primary outcome measure for this review was the relationship between vitamin C and neutrophil function in humans.

Table 1. Inclusion and exclusion criteria.

Inclusion	Exclusion
Randomized Controlled Trial	
Peer-reviewed publication	
Human Subjects	
Full-text access	
English papers	
Any of the following neutrophil functions as primary or secondary outcomes:	Participants with existing neutrophilic dysfunction disorders
Migration/chemotaxis/motility	Review articles
Phagocytosis	
Oxidative burst	
Enzyme activity	
Apoptosis/clearance	
Necrosis/necrotic cell death	

3. Results

3.1. Literature Search Outcome

The process of selection and screening of studies is illustrated in Figure 1 using the PRISMA flow chart [24]. Screening was based on the predetermined inclusion/exclusion criteria as well as the PICO components. After the screening process, sixteen papers were found to be eligible and were quality appraised for risks of bias using the Cochrane Risk of Bias tool (Figure 2) [23]. Four publications were rated low-quality following the critical appraisal, of which two papers failed to meet allocation concealment and blinding requirements scoring as high-risk for selection bias and performance bias while the other two papers had flawed statistical analysis owing to missing data thus scoring as high-risk for attrition bias and other bias. Due to the limited number of studies available, these four publications were included in the analysis and results, however, the limitations of these papers were highlighted. Thus, sixteen papers were included in the synthesis.

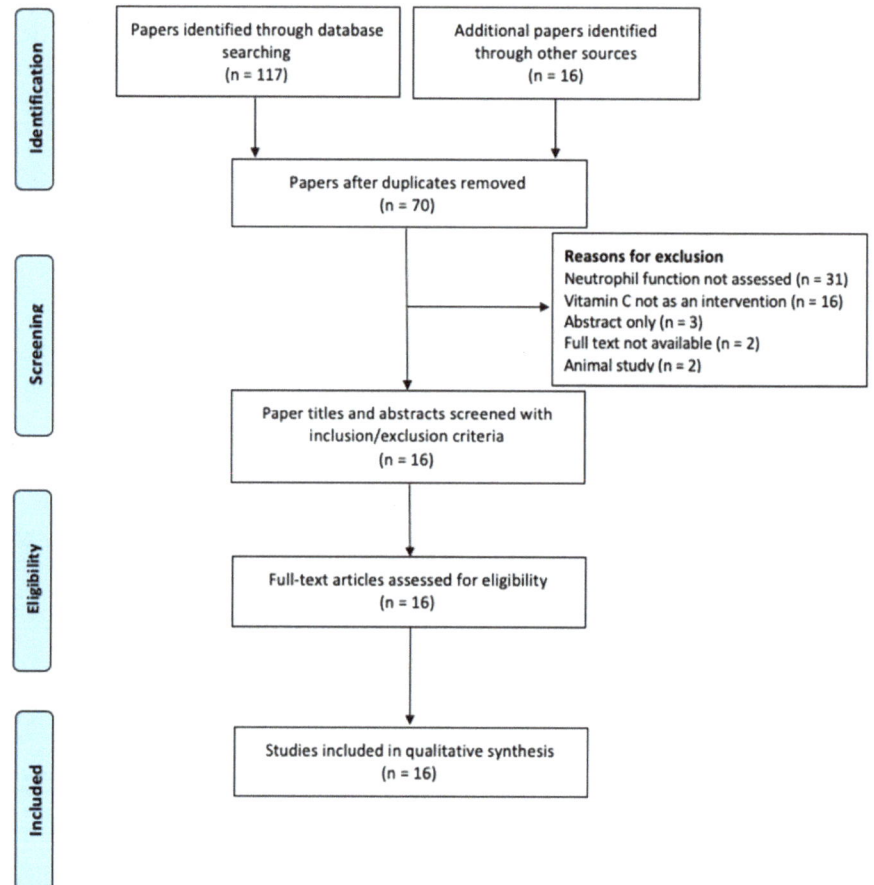

Figure 1. The study selection process presented using the PRISMA flow chart.

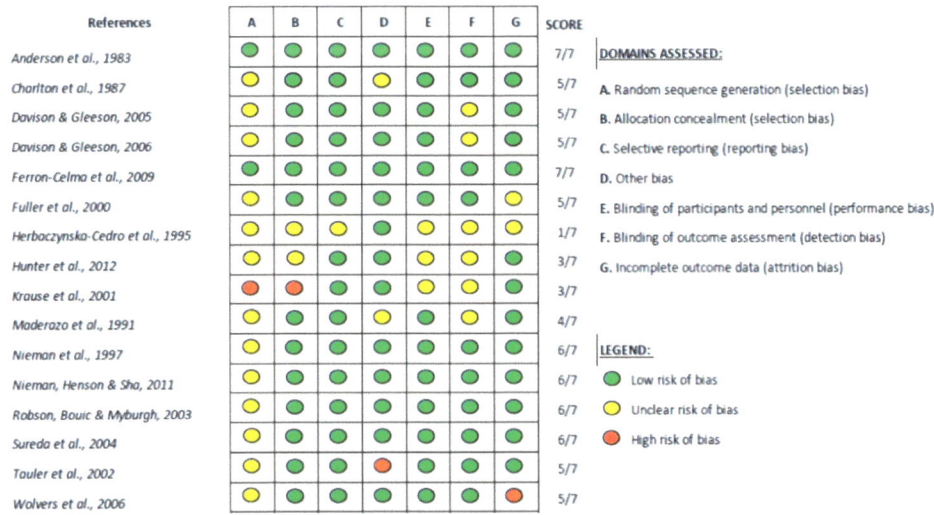

Figure 2. Quality appraisal results of the included studies using the Cochrane Risk of Bias tool.

3.2. Study Characteristics

The 16 studies described were conducted in nine locations. These included Africa ($n = 1$), Austria ($n = 1$), New Zealand ($n = 1$), the Netherlands ($n = 1$), Poland ($n = 1$), Spain ($n = 3$), South Africa ($n = 1$), United States ($n = 4$), and the United Kingdom ($n = 3$). The 16 studies comprised nine that used vitamin C as monotherapy and seven that used combination supplementation. As illustrated in Table 2a and Table 2b (vitamin C only and combination studies, respectively), participants were recruited from a number of different settings including schools, clinics, communities, and surgical departments of hospitals. However, some studies did not specify the trial settings. The time frames of the studies ranged from one day to six-month long trials. The sample size of the studies ranged from six to 131 participants garnering a total number of 497 participants. There was a wide variation in the methodologies used between studies, e.g., the neutrophil assays were either carried out with whole blood or the cells were isolated prior to analysis in buffer or culture media (Table 2a and Table 2b), the intervention was administered at different doses, via different routes of administration (four studies used intravenous vitamin C, with trauma, surgical, and septic cohorts), and the treatment periods also varied dramatically from one day to six months (Table 3a and Table 3b). The included studies also covered a wide range of age groups as illustrated in Table 4. Furthermore, the control measures instigated for potential confounding factors were also variable, e.g., not all studies measured the plasma vitamin C concentrations at baseline, and diet control as well as smoking status were often not taken into consideration or reported (Table 4). Overall, three studies assessed neutrophil chemotaxis (with one also assessing phagocytosis), ten studies assessed neutrophil phagocytosis and/or oxidative burst activity, two studies assessed neutrophil enzyme activity, and one study assessed neutrophil apoptosis.

Table 2a. Characteristics of vitamin C-only supplementation studies.

Reference	Title of Study	Location	Trial Setting	Time Frame of Study	Neutrophil Function Assessed
Anderson et al. (1983) [25]	Ascorbic acid in bronchial asthma	Africa	Hospital Paediatric Respiratory Clinic	6 months	Chemotaxis, phagocytosis (isolated cells)
Charlton et al. (1987) [26]	Neutrophil mobility during anaesthesia in children. A trial for ascorbate premedication.	United Kingdom	Surgical Hospital	1 day	Chemotaxis (isolated cells)
Maderazo et al. (1991) [27]	A randomized trial of replacement antioxidant vitamin therapy for neutrophil locomotory dysfunction in blunt trauma	United States	Hospital	1 week	Chemotaxis (isolated cells)
Davison and Gleeson (2005) [28]	Influence of acute vitamin C and/or carbohydrate ingestion on hormonal, cytokine, and immune responses to prolonged exercise.	United Kingdom	Laboratory	3 weeks	Oxidative burst (whole blood)
Davison and Gleeson (2006) [29]	The effect of 2 weeks vitamin C supplementation on immunoendocrine responses to 2.5 h cycling exercise in man.	United Kingdom	Laboratory	2 weeks	Oxidative burst (whole blood)
Fuller et al. (2000) [30]	The effect of vitamin E and vitamin C supplementation on LDL oxidizability and neutrophil respiratory burst in young smokers	United States (North Carolina)	Community	8 weeks	Oxidative burst (isolated cells)
Krause et al. (2001) [31]	Effect of vitamin C on neutrophil function after high-intensity exercise	Austria	Outdoor Biathlon	1 week	Phagocytosis; oxidative burst (isolated cells and whole blood)
Nieman et al. (1997) [19]	Vitamin C supplementation does not alter the immune response to 2.5 h of running	United States (North Carolina)	Human Performance Laboratory	8 days	Phagocytosis; oxidative burst (whole blood)
Sureda et al. (2004) [32]	Hypoxia/reoxygenation and vitamin C intake influence NO synthesis and antioxidant defences of neutrophils.	Spain	Not specified	1 week	Enzyme activity (isolated cells)
Ferron-Celma et al. (2009) [33]	Effects of vitamin C administration on neutrophil apoptosis in patients after abdominal surgery.	Spain	Digestive Surgery Department	6 days	Apoptosis (isolated cells)

Table 2b. Characteristics of combination supplementation studies.

Reference	Title of Study	Country	Trial Setting	Time Frame of Study	Neutrophil Function Assessed
Herbaczynska-Cedro et al. (1995) [34]	Supplementation with vitamins C and E suppresses leukocyte oxygen free radical production in patients with myocardial infarction	Poland	Hospital	2 weeks	Oxidative burst (isolated cells)
Robson et al. (2003) [35]	Antioxidant supplementation enhances neutrophil oxidative burst in trained runners following prolonged exercise.	South Africa	Laboratory	7 weeks	Oxidative burst (whole blood)
Hunter et al. (2012) [36]	Consumption of gold kiwifruit reduces severity and duration of selected upper respiratory tract infection symptoms and increases plasma vitamin C concentration in healthy older adults	New Zealand	Community	20 weeks	Phagocytosis (whole blood)
Nieman et al. (2011) [37]	Ingestion of micronutrient fortified breakfast cereal has no influence on immune function in healthy children: A randomized controlled trial	United States (North Carolina)	Community	8 weeks	Phagocytosis; oxidative burst (whole blood)
Wolvers et al. (2006) [38]	Effect of a mixture of micronutrients, but not of bovine colostrum concentrate, on immune function parameters in healthy volunteers: a randomized placebo-controlled study.	The Netherlands	Unilever Food and Health Research Institute	12 weeks	Phagocytosis; oxidative burst (whole blood)
Tauler et al. (2002) [39]	Diet supplementation with vitamin E, vitamin C and B-carotene cocktail enhances basal neutrophil antioxidant enzymes in athletes.	Spain	Not specified	12 weeks	Enzyme activity (isolated cells)

Table 3a. The participant characteristics and interventions used, the frequency of intervention and the route of administration for vitamin C-only studies.

References	Participant Characteristics			Intervention and Dose Administered	Frequency of Intervention	Route of Administration
	Number (n)	Mean Age (Years)	Gender (% Women)			
Anderson et al. (1983) [25]	$n = 16$ asthmatic children	9.5	25%	Vitamin C (1000 mg/day) with standard anti-asthma chemoprophylaxis (SAC) OR SAC only	Once daily for six months	Intravenous
Charlton et al. (1987) [26]	$n = 20$ surgical patients	10	-	Vitamin C (10 mg/kg; mean = 363 mg) OR placebo	One-off	Intravenous
Maderazo et al. (1991) [27]	$n = 46$ trauma patients	24	21%	Vitamin C (200 mg/day) OR vitamin E (50 mg/day) OR both OR placebo	Once daily for one week	Intravenous
Davison and Gleeson (2005) [28]	$n = 6$ healthy athletes	25	0%	Vitamin C (3400 mg) OR carbohydrate OR both OR placebo	One-off for each intervention (crossover study)	Oral
Davison and Gleeson (2006) [29]	$n = 9$ healthy athletes	26	0%	Vitamin C (1000 mg/day) OR placebo	Once daily for two weeks	Oral
Fuller et al. (2000) [30]	$n = 30$ healthy smokers	20	73%	Vitamin C (1000 mg/day) OR vitamin E (400 IU/day) OR both OR placebo	Once daily for eight weeks	Oral
Krause et al. (2001) [31]	$n = 10$ healthy adults	29	0%	Vitamin C (2000 mg/day) OR none	Once daily for one week	Oral
Nieman et al. (1997) [19]	$n = 12$ healthy athletes	41	25%	Vitamin C (1000 mg/day) OR placebo	Once daily for eight days	Oral
Sureda et al. (2004) [32]	$n = 7$ healthy divers	-	0%	Vitamin C (1000 mg/day) OR placebo	Once daily for one week	Oral
Ferron-Celma et al. (2009) [33]	$n = 20$ surgical patients	67	45%	Vitamin C (450 mg/day) OR placebo	Once daily for six days post-operative	Intravenous

Table 3b. The participant characteristics and interventions used, the frequency of intervention and the route of administration for combination studies.

References	Participant Characteristics			Intervention and Dose Administered	Frequency of Intervention	Route of Administration
	Number (n)	Mean Age (Years)	Gender (% Women)			
Herbaczynska-Cedro et al. (1995) [34]	n = 45 cardiac patients	59	13%	Vitamins C and E (600 mg/day) OR conventional treatment only	Once daily for two weeks	Oral
Robson et al. (2003) [35]	n = 12 healthy athletes	30	50%	Multivitamin supplement: vitamin C content 60 mg/day AND antioxidant supplement: vitamin C content 900 mg/day OR placebo	Once daily for one week	Oral
Hunter et al. (2012) [36]	n = 32 healthy elderly	71	63%	2 fresh Gold kiwifruit AND 2 freeze dried Gold kiwifruit (comprising total of ~360 mg vitamin C) OR 2 freeze dried bananas	Once daily for four weeks; crossover (8 weeks washout)	Oral
Nieman et al. (2011) [37]	n = 65 healthy children	10	43%	Cereal fortified with micronutrients PLUS: Low: vitamin C content of 0.8 mg/day Medium: vitamin C content of 20 mg/day High: vitamin C content of 100 mg/day	Once daily for two months	Oral
Wolvers et al. (2006) [38]	n = 131 healthy volunteers	57	68%	Micronutrient mix (with vitamin C ~375 mg/day) OR bovine colostrum OR both OR placebo	Once daily for ten weeks	Oral
Tauler et al. (2002) [39]	n = 20 healthy athletes	23	0%	Antioxidant cocktail (vitamin E and β-carotene) PLUS vitamin C 500 mg/day (only in last 15 days) OR placebo	Once daily for three months (only last 15 days for vitamin C)	Oral

Table 4. Measurement of plasma vitamin C concentrations and control of diet and smoking status within studies.

References	Mean Plasma Vitamin C Levels		Diet Control	Smoking Status
	Baseline	Post-Intervention		
Vitamin C-Only Studies				
Anderson et al. (1983) [25]	~61 µmol/L	~137 µmol/L	Not controlled	-
Charlton et al. (1987) [26]	-	-	Not controlled	-
Maderazo et al. (1991) [27]	~51 µmol/L (~25 µmol/L day 1)	~54 µmol/L	Nutrition by mouth or feeding tube as needed (parenteral nutrition excluded until end of study)	-
Davison and Gleeson (2005) [28]	-	-	24-hour food diary of diet prior to exercise trials and maintained during trials	Non-smokers
Davison and Gleeson (2006) [29]	-	-	24-hour food diary prior to exercise trials and maintained during trials	All smokers
Fuller et al. (2000) [30]	-	92 µmol/L	3-day food record completed and maintained usual diet	-
Krause et al. (2001) [31]	39 µmol/L	62 µmol/L	not controlled	-
Nieman et al. (1997) [19]	-	-	7-day food record, carbohydrate intake ~60% of total energy, moderate vitamin C intake (~100 mg/day); refrained from nutrient supplement use	-
Sureda et al. (2004) [32]	30 µmol/L	80 µmol/L	7-day 24-hour recall of dietary intake and maintained during trials (Mediterranean diet)	-
Ferron-Celma et al. (2009) [33]	-	-	Not controlled	-
Combination Studies				
Herbaczynska-Cedro et al. (1995) [34]	38 µmol/L	77 µmol/L	Not controlled	58% smokers
Robson et al. (2003) [35]	~70 µmol/L	~90 µmol/L	Dietary intake recorded a week before exercise trials and maintained	-
Hunter et al. (2012) [36]	-	73 µmol/L	Refrained from consumption of vitamin C supplements, kiwifruit and kiwifruit products	Non-smokers
Nieman et al. (2011) [37]	-	~70 µmol/L	3-day food record pre-study, at 1 month and at 2 months	-
Wolvers et al. (2006) [38]	~37 µmol/L	~94 µmol/L	Maintained Dutch dietary habits	Non-smokers
Tauler et al. (2002) [39]	~57 µmol/L		Not controlled	-

3.3. Outcomes

3.3.1. Neutrophil Chemotaxis

Three of the included RCTs assessed neutrophil migration in response to chemoattractants; two were hospitalized cohorts (surgical premedication and trauma) and one from an outpatient clinic, and all three used intravenous vitamin C [25–27]. Anderson et al. [25] showed that administration of intravenous vitamin C (1000 mg once daily) to asthmatic children was associated with improved neutrophil chemotaxis compared with standard anti-asthma chemoprophylaxis (SAC) treatment alone. Charlton et al. [26] showed that premedication (papaveretum and hyoscine) used prior to surgery caused a decline in neutrophil chemotaxis in children undergoing elective surgical procedures. After the premedication was administered, neutrophil chemotaxis still fell significantly in the vitamin C group (single dose of 10 mg/kg) and was not significantly different to the placebo group. This suggests that vitamin C supplementation before premedication does not protect against depression of neutrophil chemotaxis in children as a result of the premedication given.

Neutrophil chemotaxis following serious blunt trauma was shown to be significantly decreased soon after injury, reaching maximum depression by day two of injury [27]. Plasma vitamin C concentrations also decreased to half initial levels. Neutrophil chemotaxis increased for those treated for a week with both vitamins C and E (200 and 50 mg/day, respectively). For the patients who received either vitamin C or E alone, there was a slightly better response than the placebo group, but this did not reach statistical significance, likely due to the low participant numbers (e.g., only three analysed in the vitamin C group). Thus, the combination of vitamins C and E together gave a better response than either vitamin C or E alone with regard to neutrophil chemotaxis.

3.3.2. Phagocytosis and Oxidative Burst

Five studies investigated the effects of either vitamin C alone or antioxidant combinations on exercise-induced changes in neutrophil oxidative burst activity and/or phagocytosis [19,28,29,31,35]. Nieman et al. [19] showed that exercise caused a significant increase in granulocyte phagocytosis and a decrease in granulocyte oxidative burst post-exercise. The vitamin C group (1 g/day for eight days) did not differ significantly from the placebo group which suggests that vitamin C supplementation had no effect on the exercise-induced changes in granulocyte phagocytosis and oxidative burst activity. Krause et al. [31] reported decreased phagocytosis and bactericidal activity of neutrophils isolated after high-intensity exercise (biathlon), although no change in intracellular reactive oxygen species generation was observed. There were no differences between the vitamin C supplementation (2 g for one week) and the placebo groups in this study.

Davison and Gleeson [28] investigated the influence of acute vitamin C supplementation (3.4 g single dose) and/or carbohydrate ingestion on neutrophil degranulation and oxidative burst activity after a prolonged exercise trial. They found that neutrophil degranulation was significantly decreased in the vitamin C and carbohydrate + vitamin C groups post-exercise but did not differ to the placebo group. In addition, neither vitamin C nor carbohydrate had an effect on the decrease in neutrophil oxidative burst activity post-exercise. Therefore, in this study, vitamin C supplementation had no effect on neutrophil degranulation or oxidative burst activity post-exercise. In a similar study conducted by the same investigators [29], it was reported that both oxidative burst activity and neutrophil degranulation was decreased post-exercise. Vitamin C supplementation (1 g/day for two weeks) was no different to the placebo group and thus did not influence neutrophil oxidative burst or degranulation.

In contrast to the vitamin C-alone supplementation studies, Robson et al. [35] showed that neutrophil oxidative burst was significantly higher in trained runners following prolonged exercise in the antioxidant group (with vitamin C 960 mg/day for one week) compared to the placebo group post-exercise. Thus, antioxidant combinations may provide improved neutrophil function in athletes compared to vitamin C monotherapy.

One study investigated the effects of vitamin C supplementation on neutrophil oxidative burst of smokers [30]. Smoking increases susceptibility to bacterial and viral infections and compromises the anti-microbial functions of neutrophils [40,41]. Furthermore, smoking is associated with lower plasma vitamin C concentrations [42–45]. Fuller et al. [30] supplemented healthy smokers with vitamin C (1 g/day for eight weeks) and/or vitamin E but found no difference in neutrophil superoxide production in any of the treatment groups compared with placebo, despite an increase in plasma vitamin C status (from 39 to 62 µmol/L).

Ischemia/reperfusion injury can also result in increased production of reactive oxygen species, inducing oxidative stress, and is common in disease states such as stroke and myocardial ischemia [46]. In a study of patients with acute myocardial infarction, Herbaczynska et al. [34] found that supplementation with vitamins C and E (600 mg/day) decreased oxygen free radical generation by neutrophils. Thus, the combination of vitamins C and E appeared to exhibit antioxidant functions in these patients.

Two studies investigated the effects of micronutrient supplementation on neutrophil phagocytosis and oxidative burst activities in healthy individuals [37,38]. Wolvers et al. [38] found that the consumption of micronutrient (with ~375 mg/day of vitamin C for ten weeks) did not affect the phagocytosing or oxidative burst activities of neutrophils in any of the treatment groups of healthy volunteers. Nieman et al. [37] showed that breakfast cereal fortified with varying levels of micronutrients (low, medium and high groups containing 0.8, 20, and 100 mg/day of vitamin C respectively) given over two months to healthy children also did not affect the pattern of change in granulocyte phagocytosis or oxidative burst. Finally, Hunter et al. [36] supplemented healthy older adults with a vitamin C rich food (gold kiwifruit containing ~360 mg vitamin C daily for four weeks), however, this had no effect on neutrophil phagocytosing activity. Thus, micronutrient supplementation or fortification, or vitamin C-rich foods, do not appear to influence neutrophil function in healthy individuals.

3.3.3. Neutrophil Enzyme Activities

The enzymes catalase, superoxide dismutase and glutathione peroxidase scavenge reactive oxygen species and are therefore markers of neutrophil antioxidant defence [47]. Two studies investigated the effect of vitamin C, either alone or in an antioxidant cocktail, on neutrophil enzyme activities [32,39]. A study of a group of divers showed that oxidative stress induced by hypoxia can affect neutrophil function, specifically neutrophil antioxidant defences [32]. They showed that a group of divers supplemented with vitamin C (1 g/day for seven days) had significantly lower catalase and glutathione peroxidase enzyme activities compared to the placebo group at post-dive as well as during recovery. One interpretation was that vitamin C supplementation may have resulted in a higher rate of non-enzymatic scavenging of reactive oxygen species and hence a decrease in the activity of the antioxidant enzymes. In contrast, in a group of athletes, Tauler et al. [39] showed that three months of antioxidant supplementation (which included 500 mg/day vitamin C for the last fifteen days) significantly increased neutrophil enzyme activities, particularly of catalase, superoxide dismutase, glutathione peroxidase and glutathione reductase, relative to the placebo group. Once again, an antioxidant cocktail appeared to be more effective than monotherapy in athletes.

3.3.4. Neutrophil Apoptosis

One study investigated the effects of vitamin C supplementation on apoptosis in neutrophils isolated from the peripheral blood of septic abdominal surgery patients [33]. Although these investigators did not assess the vitamin C status of their patients, it is well known that low vitamin C status is a common feature of patients with sepsis [9]. Ferron-Celma et al. [33] found that administration of intravenous vitamin C (450 mg/day for six days) resulted in significantly lower levels of the pro-apoptotic factors caspase-3 and poly-ADP-ribose polymerase (PARP) in the vitamin C group compared to the placebo group. In addition, significantly higher levels of the anti-apoptotic factor (Bcl-2) were observed in the vitamin C group compared to the placebo group. Therefore, this study indicated that vitamin C supplementation may exert anti-apoptotic effects on the peripheral blood neutrophils of septic patients.

4. Discussion

Overall, nine of the 16 RCTs included in this review reported no effect of supplementation with vitamin C alone, or in combination with other micronutrients or antioxidants, on various neutrophil functions [19,26,28–31,36–38]. The seven studies which did show effects of supplementation on the neutrophil functions assessed (i.e., chemotaxis, oxidative burst activity, antioxidant enzyme activity and apoptosis) were in hospitalized patients or outpatients [25,27,33,34] or athletes [32,35,39]. None of the other studies carried out with healthy volunteers showed any effects of additional supplementation.

Eight of 10 RCTs showed no effect of supplementation on neutrophil phagocytosis and/or oxidative burst activity [19,28–31,36–38]. The two studies that showed an effect on oxidative burst activity used combination supplements and they showed opposite effects [34,35]. Herbaczynska-Cedro et al. [34] showed decreased oxidant burst activity in acute myocardial infarction patients treated with a combination of vitamins C and E. It is well known that vitamin C can recycle vitamin E and vitamin C has been proposed to interact with vitamin E in vivo, thus they appear to work synergistically [48]. Although another study also tested a combination of vitamins C and E, they saw no effect on oxidative burst activity [30]. However, this study was carried out in smokers and it is known that smoking causes enhanced oxidative stress and smokers require significantly higher intakes of vitamin C to reach the same circulating concentrations as non-smokers [49]. In contrast, Robson et al. [35] showed an increase in oxidative burst activity in trained runners supplemented with an antioxidant combination following prolonged exercise. Since the baseline vitamin C status of the participants was already at saturating levels (i.e., 70 μmol/L), this suggests that the observed effects may have been due to other components of the antioxidant mixture, although it does not rule out vitamin C acting synergistically with these components.

Eight of the 10 RCTs investigating oxidative burst activity and/or phagocytosis were carried out in healthy participants or athletes [19,28,29,31,35–38]. However, only one of these studies assessed baseline vitamin C status, which was already saturating [35]. It should also be noted that neutrophils saturate at lower vitamin C levels than plasma [50]. Therefore, it is unlikely that supplementing healthy volunteers or athletes with additional vitamin C over and above their normal baseline levels would have an effect on neutrophil function [51]. Exercise trials can also be complicated in that, depending on the exercise intensity, the effects on the immune system can vary such that moderate exercises may have immunopotentiating effects while intense exercise is potentially immunosuppressive [52]. Although two combination trials showed positive effects of supplementation on neutrophil function in athletes [35,39], with combination studies, it is not always possible to determine which of the component(s) is having the effects, or if there are synergistic interactions occurring between the components.

Four of the RCTs administered intravenous vitamin C in hospital or outpatient settings, three of which saw an effect of the intervention on neutrophil chemotaxis and apoptosis [25–27,33]. Intravenous vitamin C is known to provide significantly higher plasma concentrations of vitamin C than oral administration [53]. Anderson et al. showed that administration of intravenous vitamin C (1000 mg once daily) was associated with improved neutrophil chemotaxis in asthmatic patients. Maderazo et al. [27] reported an increase in plasma vitamin C status and enhanced neutrophil chemotaxis in trauma patients administrated the combination of vitamins C and E. Ferron-Celma et al. [33] observed a decrease in pro-apoptotic enzymes and an increase in anti-apoptotic proteins in septic patients administered vitamin C alone. The forth study was carried out in healthy children undergoing elective surgery and although their baseline vitamin C levels were not assessed, these may have already been adequate [26]. Furthermore, the vitamin C was administered as a single dose only (10 mg/kg bodyweight), which is less likely to have an effect than repeated dosing [54].

There are a number of limitations of using the RCT paradigm to assess the effectiveness of nutrients such as vitamin C [55]. RCTs were specifically developed and designed to test the safety and efficacy of pharmaceutical drugs, not nutrients. For example, it is not possible to have a true placebo group in RCTs of nutrients as all of the participants will be consuming variable amounts of the nutrient of interest. Of note, a number of the assessed studies did not control for dietary intake or the participants were asked to maintain their normal diet. More than half of the RCTs included in this review did not assess baseline plasma vitamin C status, and a majority of the studies were carried out in healthy individuals, who likely already had adequate plasma vitamin C status prior to beginning the supplementation, thus negating any effect of supplementation. Only one study measured the vitamin C content of the neutrophils pre- and post-supplementation [32]. There was also variability in the analysis of the neutrophil functions, with the chemotaxis, enzyme activity, and apoptosis assays being carried out with isolated cells in buffer or culture media, and the phagocytosis and/or oxidative burst assays being carried out with either whole blood or isolated cells. Furthermore, two of the studies used only a single dose of the vitamin [26,28]. Because vitamin C is water soluble, it is cleared rapidly from circulation by the kidneys, with a half-life of approximately two hours, therefore a regular intake is required to maintain adequate levels [53]. Finally, smoking status is well known to impact on vitamin C status and requirements, due to enhanced oxidative stress [43,49], however, this was not taken into account in a majority of the studies.

5. Conclusions

Overall, 44% of the RCTs assessed in this review showed effects of vitamin C supplementation on various neutrophil functions. The studies were very heterogeneous, comprising different participant cohorts (athletes, hospitalized patents or healthy volunteers) and different dosing regimens (oral or intravenous, monotherapy or multi-supplements, synthetic or food-derived, and from one-off to many months in duration). There were also a number of limitations inherent in the design of many of these RCTs. Unlike drug trials, evidence indicates that RCTs of vitamin C supplementation will be more likely to have a positive effect in participants who are suboptimal or deficient in the vitamin at baseline [55]. Therefore, future RCTs should incorporate prescreening of potential participants for low vitamin C status or utilize cohorts known to have low vitamin status, such as hospitalized patients. The effects of vitamin C administration on more recently discovered functions of neutrophils, such as the formation of neutrophil extracellular traps, should also be explored in future studies based on promising in vitro and preclinical data [16]. Meta-analyses have indicated that vitamin C intakes of at least 200 mg/day can decrease the risk of acquiring respiratory infections [56,57], however, gram doses of vitamin C are required once an infection has taken hold, due to increased requirements for the vitamin [10,58]. Therefore, future RCTs should also comprise appropriate vitamin C dosing for the specific cohort under investigation.

Author Contributions: Conceptualization, A.C.C. and M.L.; methodology, M.L. and A.C.C.; formal analysis and data curation, M.L.; writing—original draft preparation, M.L. and A.C.C.; supervision, A.C.C.

Funding: This research received no external funding.

Acknowledgments: A.C.C. is supported by a Health Research Council of New Zealand Sir Charles Hercus Health Research Fellowship. Thank you to Cate McCall for editing the initial report.

Conflicts of Interest: The authors declare no conflict of interest.

References

1. Ley, K.; Hoffman, H.M.; Kubes, P.; Cassatella, M.A.; Zychlinsky, A.; Hedrick, C.C.; Catz, S.D. Neutrophils: New insights and open questions. *Sci. Immunol.* **2018**, *3*, eaat4579. [CrossRef] [PubMed]
2. Borregaard, N. Neutrophils, from marrow to microbes. *Immunity* **2010**, *33*, 657–670. [CrossRef] [PubMed]
3. McCracken, J.M.; Allen, L.A. Regulation of human neutrophil apoptosis and lifespan in health and disease. *J. Cell Death* **2014**, *7*, 15–23. [CrossRef] [PubMed]
4. Weiss, S.J. Tissue destruction by neutrophils. *N. Engl. J. Med.* **1989**, *320*, 365–376. [PubMed]

5. Papayannopoulos, V. Neutrophil extracellular traps in immunity and disease. *Nat. Rev. Immunol.* **2017**, *18*, 134–147. [CrossRef] [PubMed]
6. Roos, D. Chronic granulomatous disease. *Br. Med. Bull.* **2016**, *118*, 50–63. [CrossRef] [PubMed]
7. Introne, W.; Boissy, R.E.; Gahl, W.A. Clinical, molecular, and cell biological aspects of Chediak-Higashi syndrome. *Mol. Genet. Metab.* **1999**, *68*, 283–303. [CrossRef] [PubMed]
8. Alves-Filho, J.C.; Spiller, F.; Cunha, F.Q. Neutrophil paralysis in sepsis. *Shock* **2010**, *34* (Suppl. 1), 15–21. [CrossRef] [PubMed]
9. Carr, A.C.; Rosengrave, P.C.; Bayer, S.; Chambers, S.; Mehrtens, J.; Shaw, G.M. Hypovitaminosis C and vitamin C deficiency in critically ill patients despite recommended enteral and parenteral intakes. *Crit. Care* **2017**, *21*, 300. [CrossRef] [PubMed]
10. Carr, A.C. Vitamin C in pneumonia and sepsis. In *Vissers*; Chen, M.Q., Ed.; Oxidative Stress and Disease; Boca Raton Taylor and Francis Group: Boca Raton, FL, USA, 2019; in press.
11. Carr, A.C.; Maggini, S. Vitamin C and immune function. *Nutrients* **2017**, *9*, 1211. [CrossRef]
12. Goldschmidt, M.C. Reduced bactericidal activity in neutrophils from scorbutic animals and the effect of ascorbic acid on these target bacteria in vivo and in vitro. *Am. J. Clin. Nutr.* **1991**, *54* (Suppl. 6), 1214S–1220S. [CrossRef] [PubMed]
13. Shilotri, P.G. Glycolytic, hexose monophosphate shunt and bactericidal activities of leukocytes in ascorbic acid deficient guinea pigs. *J. Nutr.* **1977**, *107*, 1507–1512. [CrossRef] [PubMed]
14. Shilotri, P.G. Phagocytosis and leukocyte enzymes in ascorbic acid deficient guinea pigs. *J. Nutr.* **1977**, *107*, 1513–1516. [CrossRef] [PubMed]
15. Vissers, M.C.; Wilkie, R.P. Ascorbate deficiency results in impaired neutrophil apoptosis and clearance and is associated with up-regulation of hypoxia-inducible factor 1alpha. *J. Leukoc. Biol.* **2007**, *81*, 1236–1244. [CrossRef] [PubMed]
16. Mohammed, B.M.; Fisher, B.J.; Kraskauskas, D.; Farkas, D.; Brophy, D.; Natarajan, R. Vitamin C: A novel regulator of neutrophil extracellular trap formation. *Nutrients* **2013**, *5*, 3131–3151. [CrossRef]
17. Washko, P.W.; Wang, Y.; Levine, M. Ascorbic acid recycling in human neutrophils. *J. Biol. Chem.* **1993**, *268*, 15531–15535.
18. Hume, R.; Weyers, E. Changes in leucocyte ascorbic acid during the common cold. *Scott. Med. J.* **1973**, *18*, 3–7. [CrossRef]
19. Nieman, D.C.; Henson, D.A.; Butterworth, D.E.; Warren, B.J.; Davis, J.M.; Fagoaga, O.R.; Nehlsen-Cannarella, S.L. Vitamin C supplementation does not alter the immune response to 2.5 hours of running. *Int. J. Sport Nutr.* **1997**, *7*, 173–184. [CrossRef]
20. Nieman, D.C.; Johanssen, L.M.; Lee, J.W.; Arabatzis, K. Infectious episodes in runners before and after the Los Angeles Marathon. *J. Sports Med. Phys. Fit.* **1990**, *30*, 316–328.
21. Peters, E.M.; Bateman, E.D. Ultramarathon running and upper respiratory tract infections. An epidemiological survey. *S. Afr. Med. J.* **1983**, *64*, 582–584.
22. Carr, A.C.; Vissers, M.C. Synthetic or food-derived vitamin C—Are they equally bioavailable? *Nutrients* **2013**, *5*, 4284–4304. [CrossRef]
23. Higgins, J.P.; Altman, D.G.; Gotzsche, P.C.; Juni, P.; Moher, D.; Oxman, A.D.; Savović, J.; Schulz, K.F.; Weeks, L.; Sterne, J.A. The Cochrane Collaboration's tool for assessing risk of bias in randomised trials. *BMJ* **2011**, *343*, d5928. [CrossRef]
24. Moher, D.; Liberati, A.; Tetzlaff, J.; Altman, D.G. Preferred reporting items for systematic reviews and meta-analyses: The PRISMA statement. *J. Clin. Epidemiol.* **2009**, *62*, 1006–1012. [CrossRef]
25. Anderson, R.; Hay, I.; van Wyk, H.A.; Theron, A. Ascorbic acid in bronchial asthma. *S. Afr. Med. J.* **1983**, *63*, 649–652. [PubMed]
26. Charlton, A.J.; Harvey, B.A.; Hatch, D.J.; Soothill, J.F. Neutrophil mobility during anaesthesia in children. A trial of ascorbate premedication. *Acta Anaesthesiol. Scand.* **1987**, *31*, 343–346. [CrossRef] [PubMed]
27. Maderazo, E.G.; Woronick, C.L.; Hickingbotham, N.; Jacobs, L.; Bhagavan, H.N. A randomized trial of replacement antioxidant vitamin therapy for neutrophil locomotory dysfunction in blunt trauma. *J. Trauma* **1991**, *31*, 1142–1150. [CrossRef]
28. Davison, G.; Gleeson, M. Influence of acute vitamin C and/or carbohydrate ingestion on hormonal, cytokine, and immune responses to prolonged exercise. *Int. J. Sport Nutr. Exerc. Metab.* **2005**, *15*, 465–479. [CrossRef]

29. Davison, G.; Gleeson, M. The effect of 2 weeks vitamin C supplementation on immunoendocrine responses to 2.5 h cycling exercise in man. *Eur. J. Appl. Physiol.* **2006**, *97*, 454–461. [CrossRef] [PubMed]
30. Fuller, C.J.; May, M.A.; Martin, K.J. The effect of vitamin E and vitamin C supplementation on LDL oxidizability and neutrophil respiratory burst in young smokers. *J. Am. Coll. Nutr.* **2000**, *19*, 361–369. [CrossRef]
31. Krause, R.; Patruta, S.; Daxbock, F.; Fladerer, P.; Biegelmayer, C.; Wenisch, C. Effect of vitamin C on neutrophil function after high-intensity exercise. *Eur. J. Clin. Investig.* **2001**, *31*, 258–263. [CrossRef] [PubMed]
32. Sureda, A.; Batle, J.M.; Tauler, P.; Aguilo, A.; Cases, N.; Tur, J.A.; Pons, A. Hypoxia/reoxygenation and vitamin C intake influence NO synthesis and antioxidant defenses of neutrophils. *Free Radic. Biol. Med.* **2004**, *37*, 1744–1755. [CrossRef] [PubMed]
33. Ferron-Celma, I.; Mansilla, A.; Hassan, L.; Garcia-Navarro, A.; Comino, A.M.; Bueno, P.; Ferrón, J.A. Effect of vitamin C administration on neutrophil apoptosis in septic patients after abdominal surgery. *J. Surg. Res.* **2009**, *153*, 224–230. [CrossRef] [PubMed]
34. Herbaczynska-Cedro, K.; Ko-W, B.; Cedro, K.; Wasek, W.; Panczenko-Kresowska, B.; Wartanowicz, M. Supplementation with vitamins C and E suppresses leukocyte oxygen free radical production in patients with myocardial infarction. *Eur. Heart J.* **1995**, *16*, 1044–1049. [CrossRef] [PubMed]
35. Robson, P.J.; Bouic, P.J.; Myburgh, K.H. Antioxidant supplementation enhances neutrophil oxidative burst in trained runners following prolonged exercise. *Int. J. Sport Nutr. Exerc. Metab.* **2003**, *13*, 369–381. [CrossRef] [PubMed]
36. Hunter, D.C.; Skinner, M.A.; Wolber, F.M.; Booth, C.L.; Loh, J.M.; Wohlers, M.; Stevenson, L.M.; Kruger, M.C. Consumption of gold kiwifruit reduces severity and duration of selected upper respiratory tract infection symptoms and increases plasma vitamin C concentration in healthy older adults. *Br. J. Nutr.* **2012**, *108*, 1235–1245. [CrossRef] [PubMed]
37. Nieman, D.C.; Henson, D.A.; Sha, W. Ingestion of micronutrient fortified breakfast cereal has no influence on immune function in healthy children: A randomized controlled trial. *Nutr. J.* **2011**, *10*, 36. [CrossRef] [PubMed]
38. Wolvers, D.A.; van Herpen-Broekmans, W.M.; Logman, M.H.; van der Wielen, R.P.; Albers, R. Effect of a mixture of micronutrients, but not of bovine colostrum concentrate, on immune function parameters in healthy volunteers: A randomized placebo-controlled study. *Nutr. J.* **2006**, *5*, 28. [CrossRef] [PubMed]
39. Tauler, P.; Aguilo, A.; Fuentespina, E.; Tur, J.A.; Pons, A. Diet supplementation with vitamin, E.; vitamin C and beta-carotene cocktail enhances basal neutrophil antioxidant enzymes in athletes. *Pflügers Arch.* **2002**, *443*, 791–797. [CrossRef] [PubMed]
40. Bagaitkar, J.; Demuth, D.R.; Scott, D.A. Tobacco use increases susceptibility to bacterial infection. *Tob. Induc. Dis.* **2008**, *4*, 12. [CrossRef]
41. Arcavi, L.; Benowitz, N.L. Cigarette smoking and infection. *Arch. Intern. Med.* **2004**, *164*, 2206–2216. [CrossRef]
42. Dietrich, M.; Block, G.; Norkus, E.P.; Hudes, M.; Traber, M.G.; Cross, C.E.; Packer, L. Smoking and exposure to environmental tobacco smoke decrease some plasma antioxidants and increase gamma-tocopherol in vivo after adjustment for dietary antioxidant intakes. *Am. J. Clin. Nutr.* **2003**, *77*, 160–166. [CrossRef] [PubMed]
43. Lykkesfeldt, J.; Loft, S.; Nielsen, J.B.; Poulsen, H.E. Ascorbic acid and dehydroascorbic acid as biomarkers of oxidative stress caused by smoking. *Am. J. Clin. Nutr.* **1997**, *65*, 959–963. [CrossRef] [PubMed]
44. Lykkesfeldt, J.; Christen, S.; Wallock, L.M.; Chang, H.H.; Jacob, R.A.; Ames, B.N. Ascorbate is depleted by smoking and repleted by moderate supplementation: A study in male smokers and nonsmokers with matched dietary antioxidant intakes. *Am. J. Clin. Nutr.* **2000**, *71*, 530–536. [CrossRef] [PubMed]
45. Wilson, R.; Willis, J.; Gearry, R.; Skidmore, P.; Fleming, E.; Frampton, C.; Carr, A. Inadequate vitamin C status in prediabetes and type 2 diabetes mellitus: Associations with glycaemic control, obesity, and smoking. *Nutrients* **2017**, *9*, 997. [CrossRef] [PubMed]
46. McCord, J.M. Oxygen-derived free radicals in postischemic tissue injury. *N. Engl. J. Med.* **1985**, *312*, 159–163.
47. Kinnula, V.L.; Soini, Y.; Kvist-Makela, K.; Savolainen, E.R.; Koistinen, P. Antioxidant defense mechanisms in human neutrophils. *Antioxid. Redox Signal.* **2002**, *4*, 27–34. [CrossRef]
48. Bruno, R.S.; Leonard, S.W.; Atkinson, J.; Montine, T.J.; Ramakrishnan, R.; Bray, T.M.; Traber, M.G. Faster plasma vitamin E disappearance in smokers is normalized by vitamin C supplementation. *Free Radic. Biol. Med.* **2006**, *40*, 689–697. [CrossRef]

49. Schectman, G.; Byrd, J.C.; Hoffmann, R. Ascorbic acid requirements for smokers: Analysis of a population survey. *Am. J. Clin. Nutr.* **1991**, *53*, 1466–1470. [CrossRef]
50. Levine, M.; Conry-Cantilena, C.; Wang, Y.; Welch, R.W.; Washko, P.W.; Dhariwal, K.R.; Park, J.B.; Lazarev, A.; Graumlich, J.F.; King, J.; et al. Vitamin C pharmacokinetics in healthy volunteers: Evidence for a recommended dietary allowance. *Proc. Natl. Acad. Sci. USA* **1996**, *93*, 3704–3709. [CrossRef]
51. Bozonet, S.M.; Carr, A.C. The role of physiological vitamin C concentrations on key functions of neutrophils isolated from healthy individuals. *Nutrients* **2019**, *11*, 1363. [CrossRef]
52. Hoffman-Goetz, L.; Pedersen, B.K. Exercise and the immune system: A model of the stress response? *Immunol. Today* **1994**, *15*, 382–387. [CrossRef]
53. Padayatty, S.J.; Sun, H.; Wang, Y.; Riordan, H.D.; Hewitt, S.M.; Katz, A.; Wesley, R.A.; Levine, M. Vitamin C pharmacokinetics: Implications for oral and intravenous use. *Ann. Intern. Med.* **2004**, *140*, 533–537. [CrossRef] [PubMed]
54. Carr, A.C. Duration of intravenous vitamin C therapy is a critical consideration. *Crit. Care Resusc.* **2019**, *21*, 220–221. [PubMed]
55. Lykkesfeldt, J.; Poulsen, H.E. Is vitamin C supplementation beneficial? Lessons learned from randomised controlled trials. *Br. J. Nutr.* **2010**, *103*, 1251–1259. [CrossRef] [PubMed]
56. Hemilä, H.; Chalker, E. Vitamin C for preventing and treating the common cold. *Cochrane Database Syst. Rev.* **2013**, *1*, CD000980. [CrossRef] [PubMed]
57. Hemilä, H.; Louhiala, P. Vitamin C for preventing and treating pneumonia. *Cochrane Database Syst. Rev.* **2013**, Cd005532. [CrossRef] [PubMed]
58. Ran, L.; Zhao, W.; Wang, J.; Wang, H.; Zhao, Y.; Tseng, Y.; Bu, H. Extra dose of vitamin C based on a daily supplementation shortens the common cold: A meta-analysis of 9 randomized controlled trials. *BioMed Res. Int.* **2018**, *2018*, 1837634. [CrossRef] [PubMed]

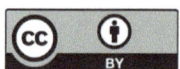

© 2019 by the authors. Licensee MDPI, Basel, Switzerland. This article is an open access article distributed under the terms and conditions of the Creative Commons Attribution (CC BY) license (http://creativecommons.org/licenses/by/4.0/).

Article

The Role of Physiological Vitamin C Concentrations on Key Functions of Neutrophils Isolated from Healthy Individuals

Stephanie M. Bozonet and Anitra C. Carr *

Department of Pathology and Biomedical Science, University of Otago, Christchurch, P.O. Box 4345, Christchurch 8140, New Zealand; stephanie.bozonet@otago.ac.nz
* Correspondence: anitra.carr@otago.ac.nz; Tel.: +643-364-0649

Received: 9 May 2019; Accepted: 6 June 2019; Published: 17 June 2019

Abstract: Vitamin C (ascorbate) is important for neutrophil function and immune health. Studies showing improved immune function have primarily used cells from scorbutic animals or from individuals with infectious conditions or immune cell disorders. Few studies have focused on the requirements of neutrophils from healthy adults. Therefore, we have investigated the role of vitamin C, at concentrations equivalent to those obtained in plasma from oral intakes (i.e., 50–200 µmol/L), on key functions of neutrophils isolated from healthy individuals. Cells were either pre-loaded with dehydroascorbic acid, which is rapidly reduced intracellularly to ascorbate, or the cells were activated in the presence of extracellular ascorbate. We measured the effects of enhanced ascorbate uptake on the essential functions of chemotaxis, oxidant production, programmed cell death and neutrophil extracellular trap (NET) formation. We found that neutrophils isolated from healthy individuals already had replete ascorbate status (0.35 nmol/10^6 cells), therefore they did not uptake additional ascorbate. However, they readily took up dehydroascorbic acid, thus significantly increasing their intracellular ascorbate concentrations, although this was found to have no additional effect on superoxide production or chemotaxis. Interestingly, extracellular ascorbate appeared to enhance directional mobility in the presence of the chemoattractant formyl-methionyl-leucyl-phenylalanine (fMLP). Stimulation of the cells in the presence of ascorbate significantly increased intracellular ascorbate concentrations and, although this exhibited a non-significant increase in phosphatidylserine exposure, NET formation was significantly attenuated. Our findings demonstrate the ability of neutrophils to regulate their uptake of ascorbate from the plasma of healthy humans to maintain an optimal level within the cell for proper functioning. Higher oral intakes, however, may help reduce tissue damage and inflammatory pathologies associated with NET formation.

Keywords: vitamin C; ascorbate; immunity; neutrophils; chemotaxis; neutrophil extracellular traps

1. Introduction

Vitamin C (ascorbate) is an essential nutrient which humans must acquire daily through the diet. It is a potent antioxidant, able to protect important biomolecules from the damaging effects of oxidants produced endogenously, during metabolism and inflammation, and from the environment [1]. It is also an essential cofactor for many enzymes involved in important biosynthetic and regulatory processes, including collagen and carnitine biosynthesis [2], hormone production [3], gene transcription [4] and epigenetic regulation [5]. Severe, prolonged vitamin C deficiency results in scurvy, a potentially fatal disease characterized by the breakdown of collagenous tissue. This leads to impaired wound healing and compromised immunity, leaving the individual vulnerable to life-threatening infections [6]. Severe respiratory infections, such as pneumonia, are a common complication of severe vitamin C deficiency and are one of the most common causes of mortality in vitamin C-deficient individuals [7]. Additionally, the enhanced oxidative stress and inflammation observed during infections can result in significant depletion of vitamin C due to increased requirements for the vitamin, and this depletion is also apparent in vital immune cells such as neutrophils [8].

In contrast to plasma ascorbate levels, which reflect what has been absorbed from the diet, neutrophils concentrate the vitamin through active uptake via the sodium-dependent vitamin C transporter-2 (SVCT2). Intracellular concentrations of ascorbate can therefore be in the millimolar range and are thought to be indicative of enhanced requirement by that particular cell type [9]. Once activated, neutrophils can further increase their intracellular concentration by the uptake of oxidized ascorbate, dehydroascorbate (DHA), via glucose transporters (GLUTs). Once inside the cell, DHA is immediately reduced to ascorbate, maintaining the concentration gradient and allowing further influx of DHA, thus resulting in increases of intracellular ascorbate by up to 20-fold [9]. This dramatic accumulation of ascorbate by activated neutrophils is thought to indicate an important requirement for their function.

Neutrophils are important mediators of the innate immune response whose primary function is to destroy invading pathogens. Upon detection of microbial products and inflammatory cytokines these cells migrate to sites of infection, a process known as chemotaxis, whereupon they engulf the pathogenic organisms, sequestering them in vesicles where they can be safely destroyed [10]. Microbial killing occurs by enzymatic as well as oxidative mechanisms, and it is thought that the antioxidant function of ascorbate is important in protecting the neutrophil during this process [11]. Attenuated chemotaxis, phagocytosis, oxidant production and microbial killing have been observed in neutrophils isolated from scorbutic animals, compared with controls, and dysfunctional activities were reversed by supplementation with ascorbate [12–14].

Following activation, neutrophils undergo a form of programmed cell death, known as phagocytosis-induced cell death, whereby oxidants generated in the phagosome result in phosphatidylserine exposure which facilitates clearance of the spent cells by macrophages [15]. This process occurs within hours of neutrophil stimulation and is critical for effective resolution of the immune response. Impaired resolution of the inflammatory response can result in tissue damage due to the release of proteases and pro-inflammatory mediators from necrotic cells, and is associated with autoimmune conditions and multiple organ failure [16,17]. Neutrophils can also generate extracellular traps (NETs), whereby DNA strands dotted with histones, proteases and oxidases are ejected from the cell [18]. Although NETs can trap invading pathogens, they are nonspecific and potentially inflammatory, damaging host tissues and resulting in various pathologies [19,20]. Dysfunctional neutrophil cell death and diminished uptake by macrophages has been reported in cells isolated from ascorbate-deficient gulonolactone oxidase (Gulo) knockout mice [21]. Furthermore, it has been demonstrated that vitamin C can decrease NET formation in septic Gulo knockout mice and in stimulated human neutrophils [22].

Although a number of studies have been carried out to explore the effects of vitamin C supplementation on neutrophil function, these have often used individuals with infectious or allergic conditions, or abnormal neutrophil function e.g., those with chronic granulomatous disease or Chédiak–Higashi syndrome [6]. However, very little information exists with respect to the potential for vitamin C supplementation, which provides physiological plasma concentrations, to enhance the function of neutrophils in healthy individuals [23]. Evidence suggests that plasma levels of ascorbate should be maintained above 50 µmol/L, a threshold viewed as adequate to maintain health [24]. In healthy individuals, a daily intake of 100–200 mg provides adequate to saturating steady-state levels of ascorbate in the plasma (i.e., 50–80 µmol/L) [25,26]. An intake of 200 mg/day is a suggested dietary target to reduce the risk of chronic disease [27], and meta-analyses have indicated that a vitamin C intake of at least 200 mg/day can decrease the risk of acquiring respiratory infections [28,29]. However, gram doses of vitamin C are required once an infection has taken hold, due to increased requirements for the vitamin [28–30]. Gram doses of oral vitamin C have been shown to provide peak plasma ascorbate concentrations of greater than 150 µmol/L [31].

The aim of this study was, therefore, to investigate whether increasing the intracellular ascorbate concentration, using physiologically relevant concentrations of ascorbate (i.e., 50–200 µmol/L), could improve essential functions of neutrophils isolated from healthy volunteers. The participants in this study were not asked to modify their eating habits in any way, nor were they fasting when blood was drawn, to more closely resemble normal day-to-day conditions. Neutrophils were isolated from whole blood and the intracellular ascorbate concentrations were measured before and after incubation with ascorbate or DHA. Analyses were carried out to determine the effects of pre-loading neutrophils with ascorbate, as well as co-incubation in the presence of extracellular ascorbate during activation, on the primary functions of chemotaxis, oxidant generation, programmed cell death and NET formation.

2. Materials and Methods

2.1. Materials

Vacutainer tubes were from Becton Dickinson (Auckland, NZ) and heparin was acquired through the Christchurch Hospital Pharmacy (Christchurch, NZ). Cell culture reagents (RPMI 1640 medium without phenol red, foetal bovine serum (FBS), penicillin and streptomycin), Sytox Green™ and the Annexin V-FITC antibody were from Life Technologies (Auckland, NZ). Ficoll-Hypaque was from Global Sciences (Auckland, NZ) and Calcein AM was from In Vitro Technologies (Auckland, NZ). Fluoroblok™ microtitre plates (96-well, 0.3 µm pore size) were from Becton Dickinson (Auckland, NZ). All other reagents (dextran, glucose, perchloric acid (PCA), dithiothreitol (DTT), diethylenetriaminepentaacetic acid (DTPA) cytochrome c, phorbol 12-myristate 13-acetate (PMA), catalase and formyl-methionyl-leucyl-phenylalanine (fMPL) were from Merck (formerly Sigma, Auckland, NZ).

2.2. Neutrophil Isolation

The collection of blood samples was approved by the Southern Health and Disability Ethics Committee, New Zealand (URA/06/12/083/AM05) and informed consent was obtained from all blood donors. Blood from healthy donors was collected into heparin tubes and neutrophils were isolated as described previously [32]. Briefly, neutrophils were obtained using Ficoll–Hypaque and dextran sedimentation, followed by hypotonic erythrocyte lysis. Neutrophils were resuspended in buffer (Hanks Buffered Saline Solution, HBSS, or phosphate buffered saline, PBS, with 5 mM glucose) or medium (RPMI with 2% or 10% fetal bovine serum) as indicated.

2.3. Ascorbate and DHA Loading of Neutrophils

Reagent ascorbate and DHA were prepared in HBSS for cell uptake experiments. The concentration of ascorbate was calculated from spectrophotometric measurement at 265 nm ($\varepsilon = 14{,}500$ M^{-1} cm^{-1}). The DHA was first reduced to ascorbate by incubation for 5 min at room temperature with DTT (2.5 mM). Due to the instability of DHA [33], this was made freshly before each use, was kept on ice at all stages, and was added immediately to the cells following standardization.

Cells were dispensed into sterile 1.7 mL tubes at 5×10^6/mL with either ascorbate or DHA (at indicated concentrations of 50–200 µmol/L, in 1 mL total volume) for indicated times (i.e., 7–90 min). Tubes were rotated gently end-over-end (6 rmp) at 37 °C. After incubation, the cells were centrifuged at 2300 rpm for 5 min and washed twice in PBS to remove any extracellular ascorbate or DHA before HPLC analysis.

2.4. Ascorbate Uptake by Stimulated Neutrophils

Neutrophils were resuspended at 1×10^6/mL in RPMI 1640 medium containing 10% FBS (2 mL final volume) and incubated in 12-well culture dishes, at 37 °C in a 5% CO_2 atmosphere. The cells were incubated in the presence of extracellular ascorbate (200 µmol/L), with and without PMA (100 ng/mL) for the indicated times (i.e., 10–60 min), and intracellular ascorbate was measured. Cells were similarly stimulated for 45 min in the presence of increasing concentrations of extracellular ascorbate (i.e., 50–200 µmol/L), in the presence of PMA (100 ng/mL), and intracellular ascorbate was measured.

2.5. Intracellular Ascorbate Analysis by HPLC

For intracellular ascorbate measurement, neutrophils ($2-5 \times 10^6$) were pelleted by centrifugation at 10,000 rpm for 1 min at room temperature. Cells were resuspended in PBS (100 µL) and an equal volume of ice cold PCA (0.54 M, containing the metal ion chelator DTPA, 100 µmol/L) was added. This was vortexed and samples kept on ice for 10 min before centrifugation (12,000 rpm for 2 min at 4 °C) to remove protein. Supernatants were stored at −80 °C and analyzed by HPLC with electrochemical detection as described previously [34].

2.6. Chemotaxis

Neutrophil chemotaxis was measured using a method modified from Kuijpers et al. [35]. Cells were resuspended at 5×10^6/mL in PBS with glucose (5 mM, PBS + G) and labelled by incubation with Calcein AM (1 µM) for 30 min at 37 °C. After washing twice with PBS + G, cells were resuspended in PBS + G at 1×10^6/mL, and 50 µL (50,000 cells) was delivered to the top compartment of a 96-well Fluoroblok™ microtitre plate. PBS + G with or without chemoattractant fMLP (100 nM), and with or without ascorbate, was added to the bottom compartment (225 µL/well). Directed cell migration into the lower chamber was monitored by measuring fluorescence (excitation 485 nm, emission 535 nm) over a 30 min period at 37 °C. The level of chemotaxis was determined as the amount of fluorescence measured in the lower compartment of the chamber after 30 min incubation.

2.7. Superoxide Generation

As described previously [36], the rate of superoxide generation by activated neutrophils was measured indirectly as a function of cytochrome c reduction. Neutrophils (0.5×10^6) were stimulated with PMA (100 ng/mL) in the presence of catalase (20 µg/mL) and cytochrome c (40 µM). Activity (µmol superoxide/min/10^6 cells) was calculated from the change in absorbance at 550 nm (over 5 min at 37 °C) using the extinction coefficient, 21.1×10^3 M^{-1} cm^{-1}.

2.8. Phosphatidylserine Exposure

The effect of ascorbate uptake on cell surface phosphatidylserine exposure of stimulated neutrophils was assessed using Annexin V-FITC binding and flow cytometry (Cytomics FC 500 Flow Cytometry system, Beckman Coulter Inc., North Shore City, New Zealand). After incubation in RPMI containing 10% FBS, with extracellular ascorbate (0, 100 or 200 µmol/L), in the presence or absence of PMA (100 ng/mL), cells (1×10^6 cells/mL) were resuspended in buffer containing Annexin V-FITC according to the manufacturer's instructions and the fluorescence of 10,000 cells was analyzed.

2.9. NET Production

NET production by PMA-stimulated neutrophils was measured using a fluorescent plate assay method [37]. Neutrophils (1×10^6/mL) were resuspended in RPMI 1640 medium, containing 2% FBS, and 100 µL/well was added, in triplicate, to a black 96-well tissue culture plate. Cells were incubated with extracellular ascorbate (0, 100 or 200 µmol/L) in the presence or absence of PMA (20 nM) for 4 h at 37 °C with 5% CO_2. Extracellular DNA (indicative of NET production) was then stained with Sytox Green™ (5 µmol/L) and the fluorescence measured (excitation 485 nm, emission 520 nm) using a PolarStar™ plate reader (BMG LABTECH, Alphatech Systems Ltd. Auckland, NZ). NET production was calculated as the difference in fluorescence between stimulated and unstimulated cells at 4 h.

2.10. Statistical Analysis

Data are presented as mean ± standard error of the mean (SEM), and analysis of paired data was carried out using two-tailed Student's t-test with significance determined as (*) $p < 0.05$ (SigmaPlot, Systat Software Inc., San Jose, CA, USA).

3. Results

3.1. Ascorbate and DHA Loading of Neutrophils

To ascertain whether neutrophils from healthy individuals would uptake additional ascorbate, we incubated cells with either ascorbate or DHA (200 µmol/L), for up to 90 min, and measured the intracellular ascorbate concentration. Mean plasma ascorbate concentrations were 82 ± 5 µmol/L ($n = 7$), indicating saturation, and the mean baseline concentration of the neutrophils was 0.35 ± 0.01 nmol/10^6 cells ($n = 13$). The isolated neutrophils did not uptake ascorbate, but did uptake DHA which increased their mean intracellular ascorbate concentration by 0.82 ± 0.13 nmol/10^6 cells compared to cells not incubated with DHA (Figure 1A). Incubation of cells for 15 min in the presence of increasing concentrations of DHA (25–200 µmol/L) showed a dose-dependent uptake (Figure 1B).

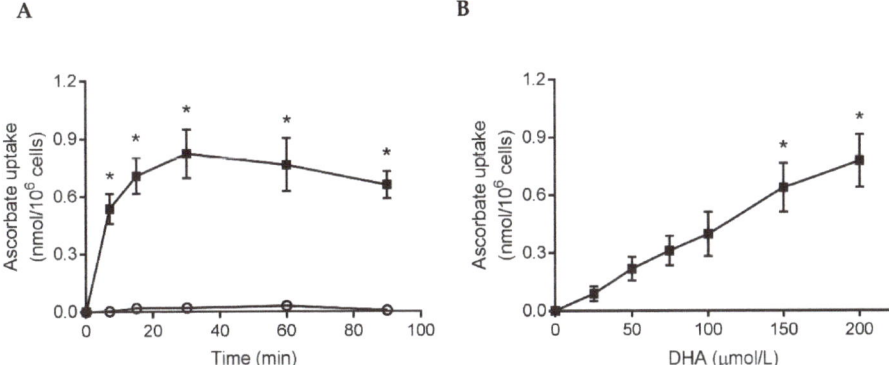

Figure 1. Uptake of ascorbate by neutrophils isolated from healthy individuals. (**A**) Cells were incubated with ascorbate (○) or DHA (■), 200 µmol/L, in HBSS for up to 90 min. Intracellular ascorbate was measured by HPLC and expressed as the increase above that of cells processed at 0 min (0.38 ± 0.05 nmol/10^6 cells), $n = 3$. (**B**) Cells were incubated with increasing concentrations of DHA for 15 min and the intracellular ascorbate concentration expressed as the increase above that of cells in HBSS (0.32 ± 0.01 nmol/10^6 cells), $n = 3$. Data represent mean ± SEM, * $p < 0.05$.

3.2. Chemotaxis

We measured the chemotactic response of neutrophils to a microbial signal (fMLP) after pre-loading the cells with DHA to increase their intracellular ascorbate concentration. There was no effect on chemotaxis (Figure 2A), despite increasing the intracellular ascorbate concentration (Figure 2B).

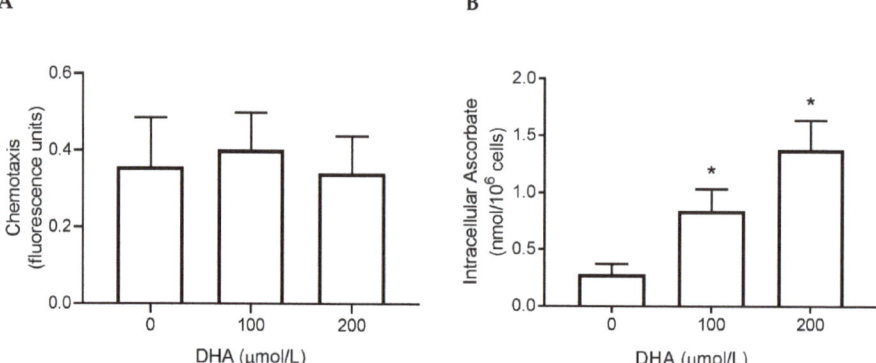

Figure 2. The effect of ascorbate uptake on neutrophil chemotaxis. (**A**) The directional motility of preloaded cells towards a microbial chemoattractant (fMLP). Graphical representation of the fluorescence detected in the lower assay compartment after 30 min. (**B**) The intracellular ascorbate concentration of the preloaded cells was measured using HPLC. Data represent mean ± SEM, $n = 3$, * $p < 0.05$.

We also measured the effect of extracellular ascorbate on the directional motility of neutrophils. We found that adding ascorbate (100 μmol/L) to the lower compartment further enhanced fMLP-stimulated directional motility of the cells, although this did not quite reach statistical significance (Figure 3).

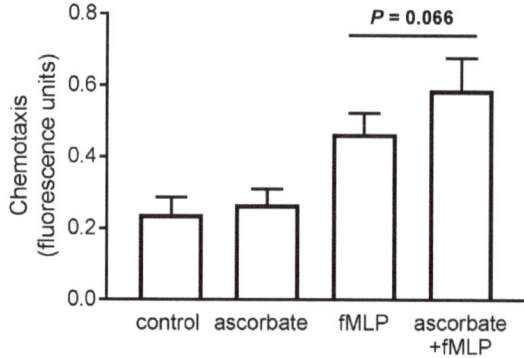

Figure 3. The effect of extracellular ascorbate on neutrophil chemotaxis. The directional motility of cells towards fMLP alone, or with extracellular ascorbate (100 μmol/L), was measured. Graphical representation of the fluorescence detected in the lower assay compartment after 30 min. Data represent mean ± SEM, $n = 3$.

3.3. Superoxide Generation

After pre-loading cells with DHA, superoxide generation was assessed as a measure of the oxidative burst, and potential microbicidal activity, of the isolated neutrophils. The cells were stimulated with the phorbol ester PMA, an agonist of the protein kinase C signal transduction pathway that results in superoxide generation by the NADPH oxidase complex. We observed a small, non-significant increase in oxidant production (Figure 4A) with increasing intracellular ascorbate concentration (Figure 4B).

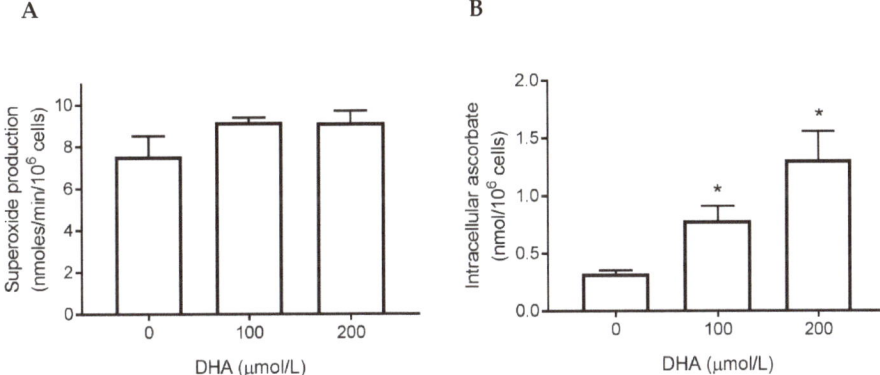

Figure 4. The effect of ascorbate uptake on superoxide generation by stimulated neutrophils. (**A**) Cells pre-loaded with DHA were stimulated with PMA (100 ng/mL) and the rate of superoxide generation measured over 5 min. (**B**) The intracellular ascorbate concentration of preloaded cells was measured by HPLC. Data represent mean ± SEM, $n = 3$. * $p < 0.05$.

3.4. Ascorbate Uptake by Stimulated Neutrophils

We assessed the ability of isolated neutrophils to uptake ascorbate, provided in the medium at a physiologically relevant concentration (100 μmol/L), over time. As expected, there was no increase in intracellular ascorbate without stimulation, but a mean increase of 0.55 ± 0.08 nmol/10^6 cells at 45 min was observed in the presence of PMA (Figure 5A). In support of this, ascorbate uptake by stimulated cells increased in a dose-dependent manner as the extracellular ascorbate concentration increased (Figure 5B). The mean intracellular ascorbate concentration, at 200 μmol/L, increased by 1.74 ± 0.51 nmol/10^6 cells after 45 min.

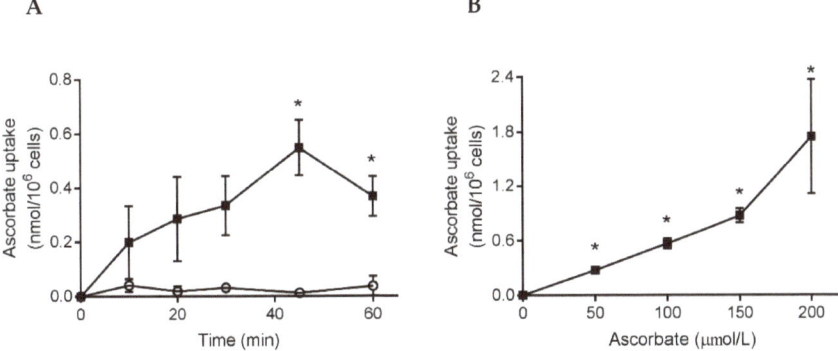

Figure 5. Ascorbate uptake by stimulated neutrophils. (**A**) Cells were incubated with extracellular ascorbate (100 μmol/L) for the indicated times, in the absence (○) or presence (■) of PMA (100 ng/mL). The time zero ascorbate concentration was 0.34 ± 0.134 nmol/10^6 cells, $n = 4$. (**B**) Cells were incubated with increasing concentrations of ascorbate for 45 min in the presence of PMA (100 ng/mL). The starting ascorbate concentration was 0.29 ± 0.11 nmol/10^6 cells, $n = 3$. The intracellular ascorbate concentration was measured by HPLC. Data represent mean ± SEM, * $p < 0.05$.

3.5. Effect of Ascorbate on Phosphatidylserine Exposure

Having established that the isolated neutrophils significantly increased their ascorbate content when stimulated in the presence of extracellular ascorbate (Figure 5), we investigated the effect of this on phosphatidylserine exposure as a measure of cell death and clearance. Cells were stimulated with PMA (100 ng/mL) for 2 or 4 h, in the presence of ascorbate, and the amount of Annexin-V FITC binding to externalized phosphatidylserine was measured by flow cytometry. There was no statistically significant effect of increased intracellular ascorbate on phosphatidylserine exposure after 2 or 4 h (Figure 6).

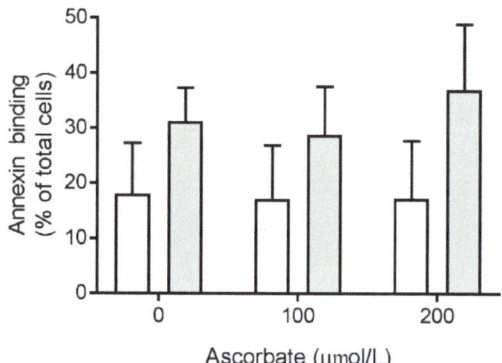

Figure 6. Effect of ascorbate on phosphatidylserine exposure of activated neutrophils. Cells were incubated with extracellular ascorbate (0, 100 or 200 μmol/L) and stimulated with PMA (100 ng/mL) for 2 h (white bars) or 4 h (grey bars). Phosphatidylserine exposure was measured by flow cytometry with Annexin-V FITC. Data represent mean ± SEM, $n = 5$.

3.6. Effect of Ascorbate on NET Production

We assessed the amount of DNA released by stimulated neutrophils, incubated in the presence of ascorbate, as an indicator of NET production. There was an attenuating effect of ascorbate on extracellular DNA released by neutrophils at the highest dose (200 μmol/L), which was statistically significant (Figure 7).

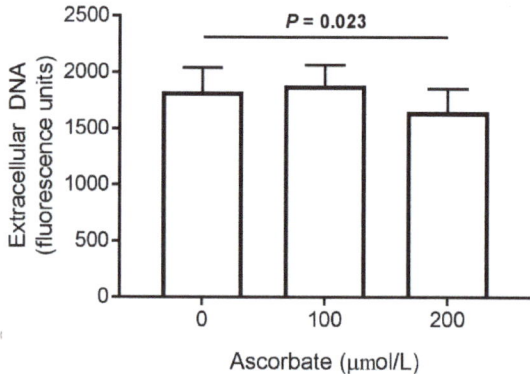

Figure 7. Effect of ascorbate on NET production by activated neutrophils. Cells were incubated with extracellular ascorbate (0, 100 or 200 μmol/L) and stimulated with PMA (2 μg/mL) for 4 h. Extracellular DNA was stained with SytoxGreen™ and fluorescence measured as a marker of NET production. Data represent mean ± SEM, $n = 5$.

4. Discussion

A number of studies have investigated the effects of vitamin C supplementation on neutrophils in conditions of vitamin C depletion, such as infectious disease, but little information exists with regard to neutrophils isolated from healthy adults with adequate plasma ascorbate levels [6]. In earlier trials we showed that supplementing participants who had a low dietary vitamin C intake could increase their neutrophil ascorbate concentrations [23,38,39], and a positive effect on neutrophil chemotaxis and oxidant production was observed [23]. In the current study we found that the baseline neutrophil ascorbate concentrations were comparable to those measured after supplementing participants with saturating levels of vitamin C [23]. Thus, the cells were fully replete, as confirmed by the saturating plasma concentrations, and would only take up additional ascorbate in the form of DHA when unstimulated. This is not unexpected given that ascorbate import by SVCT2 is regulated according to the intracellular concentration, whereas DHA enters the cells via GLUTs and is subsequently converted to ascorbate, thus maintaining a concentration gradient which facilitates further DHA uptake [9]. It is therefore possible to artificially raise intracellular ascorbate levels in already replete neutrophils. Although this is unlikely to occur under normal physiological conditions, as DHA is present at negligible levels in plasma [33,40], the oxidizing microenvironment of inflammatory loci could potentially result in extracellular ascorbate being oxidized to DHA in close proximity to sequestered neutrophils.

In our previous intervention study [23] we observed an increase in chemotaxis and superoxide production following supplementation of participants with low vitamin C status, yet there were no effects of ascorbate pre-loading on these functions in the current in vitro study. This may be due to baseline ascorbate levels in the isolated cells being already adequate for effective chemotaxis and oxidant production and suggests that maintaining neutrophil ascorbate levels around 0.35 nmol/10^6 cells may be an important factor in maintaining a healthy immune response. Another in vitro study reported ascorbate and DHA-dependent enhancement of superoxide generation by cells isolated from healthy non-fasting volunteers, however, they did not measure baseline cell ascorbate concentrations [41]. Anderson and Lukey [42] showed that ascorbate exhibited a dual role in isolated phagocytes, by enhancing intracellular oxidant generation, whilst scavenging oxidants released extracellularly, thus potentially protecting host tissues against oxidative damage.

Interestingly, although we saw no effect of ascorbate pre-loading on chemotaxis, we did observe a trend towards enhanced directional motility of the cells in response to extracellular ascorbate in the presence of the chemoattractant fMLP. This finding is comparable to an earlier study, which indicated that ascorbate, in combination with interleukin-8, enhanced the directional motility of neutrophils [43]. The mechanisms involved in ascorbate-stimulated chemotaxis are not yet understood, although enhanced microtubule formation has been suggested [44]. Recently, it was proposed that neutrophil motility could be used as an indication of vitamin C intake requirements [45], however, more research would need to be carried out in neutrophils that are ascorbate deficient in order to determine the minimum amounts of vitamin C required for optimal chemotactic activity.

In contrast to resting neutrophils, we showed that cells stimulated with PMA took up ascorbate from the medium in a time- and concentration-dependent manner. However, this provided only a non-significant increase in phosphatidylserine exposure in PMA-stimulated cells. In our earlier intervention study, there was no effect of vitamin C supplementation on spontaneous (unstimulated) neutrophil apoptosis, and it was concluded that the baseline concentrations of ascorbate may have already been sufficient to support programmed cell death [23]. It should be noted that neutrophils saturate at much lower vitamin C doses (~100 mg/day) than plasma saturation (~200 mg/day) [25]. In the current study, phosphatidylserine exposure after stimulation of cells in the presence of physiological concentrations of ascorbate was minimal, which suggests that the level of intracellular ascorbate upon isolation of the cells was adequate to allow efficient phosphatidylserine exposure and clearance of stimulated cells. Sharma et al. [41] observed a significant increase in neutrophil phosphatidylserine exposure following incubation with DHA and a bacterial stimulant, however, baseline ascorbate concentrations were not determined in that study. Efficient clearance of spent neutrophils is critical for maintaining physiological homeostasis and preventing tissue damage associated with cell necrosis and poor uptake by macrophages [16,46].

One function where we did see a significant effect of increased ascorbate uptake by stimulated cells was in NET production; when cells were co-incubated with ascorbate and PMA, NET formation was significantly decreased. NET components such as histones can act as damage-associated molecular pattern proteins (DAMP) which stimulate inflammation and have been linked with autoimmune conditions and organ damage in sepsis [19,20]. Indeed, sepsis patients have elevated levels of circulating cell-free DNA [47,48] and a preclinical study has shown ascorbate to be a negative regulator of NET formation in a murine sepsis model and in human neutrophils in vitro [22]. Interestingly, the transcription factor hypoxia-inducible factor (HIF)-1 has been associated with NET production [49] and ascorbate is a key cofactor for the enzymes that downregulate HIF-1 [50]. HIF-1 has also been shown to prolong the survival of neutrophils in regions of localized hypoxia [51], thus, the regulation of HIF-1 may be one mechanism by which ascorbate affects neutrophil function and death [21].

For our earlier intervention study, the participants were screened and selected for having low plasma ascorbate and also underwent a 3-week lead-in period, during which time they limited their vitamin C intake still further [23]. Despite this, neutrophil ascorbate levels remained at around 0.21 nmol/10^6 cells, even when plasma levels fell well below the adequate threshold to 26 µmol/L. This supports the premise that neutrophils retain their ascorbate levels, even when plasma levels drop, because it serves critical roles within the cell. During infectious episodes, however, neutrophils are known to become depleted of ascorbate, and this appears to impact negatively on their functions [6,8]. Supplementation of individuals with respiratory infections with saturating doses of vitamin C results in enhanced neutrophil ascorbate status and improved neutrophil functions in many cases [6,8,52].

Overall, our study has shown that although a low dose vitamin C intake, which provides <100 µmol/L plasma concentration, may not impact on neutrophil functions in healthy individuals, higher (gram) doses may provide sufficiently high peak concentrations to impact on some functions, such as NET formation, which was decreased in the presence of 200 µmol/L ascorbate. Two intervention studies have demonstrated beneficial effects of gram dose vitamin C supplementation on the function of neutrophils from healthy donors. In a double-blind cross-over trial, enhanced chemotaxis was observed following supplementation with 2 g/day for one week [53]. In a similar study, chemotaxis was enhanced in neutrophils isolated from healthy adults after ingestion of 2 or 3 g/day of vitamin C for one week [54]. Interestingly, 1 g/day had no effect when administered orally, however the same group observed increased neutrophil motility 1 h after a single 1 g intravenous dose of ascorbate, which is known to provide significantly higher peak ascorbate concentrations [31,55].

5. Conclusions

In this study we have shown that whilst it is possible to artificially increase the intracellular ascorbate content of neutrophils isolated from healthy volunteers by incubation with DHA, this does not significantly enhance their functions of chemotaxis and superoxide generation. This suggests that neutrophils isolated from individuals with saturating plasma ascorbate concentrations already contained sufficient intracellular ascorbate to carry out these functions. We did, however, show that co-incubation of neutrophils with ascorbate in the high physiological range (i.e., 200 µmol/L) did attenuate PMA-stimulated NET generation, consistent with another study [22], and may support a role for ascorbate in protecting against inflammatory and autoimmune conditions [19]. Therefore, it is critical to ensure an adequate daily intake of vitamin C to maintain plasma ascorbate concentrations sufficient to support optimal neutrophil function. Although saturation of neutrophils can be achieved by consumption of around 100 mg/day in healthy adults [25,26], we observed decreased NET formation in the presence of 200 µmol/l ascorbate, which is only achieved during peak dietary uptake of gram doses of ascorbate [31].

Author Contributions: S.M.B.; methodology, investigation, writing—original draft preparation A.C.C.; conceptualization, funding acquisition, project administration, supervision, writing—review & editing.

Funding: This research was funded by Bayer Consumer Care. A.C.C. is supported by a Health Research Council of New Zealand Sir Charles Hercus Health Research Fellowship.

Acknowledgments: We thank the volunteers for providing blood samples for neutrophil isolations and we thank Margreet Vissers for methodological advice.

Conflicts of Interest: The authors declare no conflict of interest. The funders had no role in the design of the study; in the collection, analyses, or interpretation of data; in the writing of the manuscript, or in the decision to publish the results.

References

1. Carr, A.C.; Frei, B. Toward a new recommended dietary allowance for vitamin C based on antioxidant and health effects in humans. *Am. J. Clin. Nutr.* **1999**, *69*, 1086–1107. [CrossRef] [PubMed]
2. Englard, S.; Seifter, S. The biochemical functions of ascorbic acid. *Annu. Rev. Nutr.* **1986**, *6*, 365–406. [CrossRef] [PubMed]
3. Carr, A.C.; Shaw, G.M.; Fowler, A.A.; Natarajan, R. Ascorbate-dependent vasopressor synthesis: A rationale for vitamin C administration in severe sepsis and septic shock? *Crit. Care.* **2015**, *19*, e418. [CrossRef] [PubMed]
4. Kuiper, C.; Vissers, M.C. Ascorbate as a co-factor for Fe- and 2-oxoglutarate dependent dioxygenases: Physiological activity in tumor growth and progression. *Front. Oncol.* **2014**, *4*, 359. [CrossRef] [PubMed]
5. Young, J.I.; Zuchner, S.; Wang, G. Regulation of the epigenome by vitamin C. *Annu. Rev. Nutr.* **2015**, *35*, 545–564. [CrossRef] [PubMed]
6. Carr, A.C.; Maggini, S. Vitamin C and immune function. *Nutrients* **2017**, *9*, 1211. [CrossRef] [PubMed]
7. Hemilä, H. Vitamin C and infections. *Nutrients* **2017**, *9*, 339. [CrossRef]
8. Hume, R.; Weyers, E. Changes in leucocyte ascorbic acid during the common cold. *Scott. Med. J.* **1973**, *18*, 3–7. [CrossRef] [PubMed]
9. Washko, P.W.; Wang, Y.; Levine, M. Ascorbic acid recycling in human neutrophils. *J. Biol. Chem.* **1993**, *268*, 15531–15535.
10. Ley, K.; Hoffman, H.M.; Kubes, P.; Cassatella, M.A.; Zychlinsky, A.; Hedrick, C.C.; Catz, S.D. Neutrophils: New insights and open questions. *Sci. Immunol.* **2018**, *3*, eaat4579. [CrossRef]
11. Parker, A.; Cuddihy, S.L.; Son, T.G.; Vissers, M.C.; Winterbourn, C.C. Roles of superoxide and myeloperoxidase in ascorbate oxidation in stimulated neutrophils and H_2O_2-treated HL60 cells. *Free Radic. Biol. Med.* **2011**, *51*, 1399–1405. [CrossRef] [PubMed]
12. Shilotri, P.G. Glycolytic, hexose monophosphate shunt and bactericidal activities of leukocytes in ascorbic acid deficient guinea pigs. *J. Nutr.* **1977**, *107*, 1507–1512. [CrossRef] [PubMed]
13. Shilotri, P.G. Phagocytosis and leukocyte enzymes in ascorbic acid deficient guinea pigs. *J. Nutr.* **1977**, *107*, 1513–1516. [CrossRef] [PubMed]
14. Goldschmidt, M.C. Reduced bactericidal activity in neutrophils from scorbutic animals and the effect of ascorbic acid on these target bacteria in vivo and in vitro. *Am. J. Clin. Nutr.* **1991**, *54* (Suppl. 6), 1214S–1220S. [CrossRef]
15. McCracken, J.M.; Allen, L.A. Regulation of human neutrophil apoptosis and lifespan in health and disease. *J. Cell Death* **2014**, *7*, 15–23. [CrossRef] [PubMed]
16. Fox, S.; Leitch, A.E.; Duffin, R.; Haslett, C.; Rossi, A.G. Neutrophil apoptosis: Relevance to the innate immune response and inflammatory disease. *J. Innate Immun.* **2010**, *2*, 216–227. [CrossRef] [PubMed]
17. Brown, K.A.; Brain, S.D.; Pearson, J.D.; Edgeworth, J.D.; Lewis, S.M.; Treacher, D.F. Neutrophils in development of multiple organ failure in sepsis. *Lancet* **2006**, *368*, 157–169. [CrossRef]
18. Papayannopoulos, V. Neutrophil extracellular traps in immunity and disease. *Nat. Rev. Immunol.* **2017**, *18*, 134–147. [CrossRef] [PubMed]
19. Lee, K.H.; Kronbichler, A.; Park, D.D.; Park, Y.; Moon, H.; Kim, H.; Choi, J.H.; Choi, Y.; Shim, S.; Lyu, I.S.; et al. Neutrophil extracellular traps (NETs) in autoimmune diseases: A comprehensive review. *Autoimmun. Rev.* **2017**, *16*, 1160–1173. [CrossRef] [PubMed]
20. Czaikoski, P.G.; Mota, J.M.; Nascimento, D.C.; Sonego, F.; Castanheira, F.V.; Melo, P.H.; Scortegagna, G.T.; Silva, R.L.; Barroso-Sousa, R.; Souto, F.O.; et al. Neutrophil extracellular traps induce organ damage during experimental and clinical sepsis. *PLoS ONE* **2016**, *11*, e0148142. [CrossRef] [PubMed]

21. Vissers, M.C.; Wilkie, R.P. Ascorbate deficiency results in impaired neutrophil apoptosis and clearance and is associated with up-regulation of hypoxia-inducible factor 1alpha. *J. Leukoc. Biol.* **2007**, *81*, 1236–1244. [CrossRef] [PubMed]
22. Mohammed, B.M.; Fisher, B.J.; Kraskauskas, D.; Farkas, D.; Brophy, D.F.; Fowler, A.A.; Natarajan, R. Vitamin C: A novel regulator of neutrophil extracellular trap formation. *Nutrients* **2013**, *5*, 3131–3151. [CrossRef] [PubMed]
23. Bozonet, S.M.; Carr, A.C.; Pullar, J.M.; Vissers, M.C.M. Enhanced human neutrophil vitamin C status, chemotaxis and oxidant generation following dietary supplementation with vitamin C-rich SunGold kiwifruit. *Nutrients* **2015**, *7*, 2574–2588. [CrossRef]
24. German Nutrition Society (DGE). New reference values for vitamin C intake. *Ann. Nutr. Metab.* **2015**, *67*, 13–20. [CrossRef] [PubMed]
25. Levine, M.; Conry-Cantilena, C.; Wang, Y.; Welch, R.W.; Washko, P.W.; Dhariwal, K.R.; Park, J.B.; Lazarev, A.; Graumlich, J.F.; King, J.; et al. Vitamin C pharmacokinetics in healthy volunteers: Evidence for a recommended dietary allowance. *Proc. Natl. Acad. Sci. USA* **1996**, *93*, 3704–3709. [CrossRef] [PubMed]
26. Levine, M.; Wang, Y.; Padayatty, S.J.; Morrow, J. A new recommended dietary allowance of vitamin C for healthy young women. *Proc. Natl. Acad. Sci. USA* **2001**, *98*, 9842–9846. [CrossRef] [PubMed]
27. National Health and Medical Research Council. *Nutrient Reference Values for Australia and New Zealand Including Recommended Dietary Intakes*; NHMRC Publications: Canberra, Australia, 2006.
28. Hemilä, H.; Chalker, E. Vitamin C for preventing and treating the common cold. *Cochrane Database Syst. Rev.* **2013**, *1*, CD000980.
29. Hemilä, H.; Louhiala, P. Vitamin C for preventing and treating pneumonia. *Cochrane Database Syst. Rev.* **2013**, *1*, Cd005532.
30. Ran, L.; Zhao, W.; Wang, J.; Wang, H.; Zhao, Y.; Tseng, Y.; Bu, H. Extra dose of vitamin C based on a daily supplementation shortens the common cold: A meta-analysis of 9 randomized controlled trials. *BioMed Res. Int.* **2018**, *2018*, 1837634. [CrossRef]
31. Padayatty, S.J.; Sun, H.; Wang, Y.; Riordan, H.D.; Hewitt, S.M.; Katz, A.; Wesley, R.A.; Levine, M. Vitamin C pharmacokinetics: Implications for oral and intravenous use. *Ann. Intern. Med.* **2004**, *140*, 533–537. [CrossRef]
32. Boyum, A. Isolation of mononuclear cells and granulocytes from human blood. Isolation of monuclear cells by one centrifugation, and of granulocytes by combining centrifugation and sedimentation at 1 g. *Scand. J. Clin. Lab. Investig. Suppl.* **1968**, *97*, 77–89.
33. Pullar, J.M.; Bayer, S.; Carr, A.C. Appropriate handling, processing and analysis of blood samples is essential to avoid oxidation of vitamin C to dehydroascorbic acid. *Antioxidants* **2018**, *7*, 29. [CrossRef] [PubMed]
34. Lee, W.; Hamernyik, P.; Hutchinson, M.; Raisys, V.A.; Labbe, R.F. Ascorbic acid in lymphocytes: Cell preparation and liquid-chromatographic assay. *Clin. Chem.* **1982**, *28*, 2165–2169.
35. Kuijpers, T.W.; Maianski, N.A.; Tool, A.T.; Smit, G.P.; Rake, J.P.; Roos, D.; Visser, G. Apoptotic neutrophils in the circulation of patients with glycogen storage disease type 1b (GSD1b). *Blood* **2003**, *101*, 5021–5024. [CrossRef] [PubMed]
36. Vissers, M.C.; Day, W.A.; Winterbourn, C.C. Neutrophils adherent to a nonphagocytosable surface (glomerular basement membrane) produce oxidants only at the site of attachment. *Blood* **1985**, *66*, 161–166. [PubMed]
37. Parker, H.; Albrett, A.M.; Kettle, A.J.; Winterbourn, C.C. Myeloperoxidase associated with neutrophil extracellular traps is active and mediates bacterial killing in the presence of hydrogen peroxide. *J. Leukoc. Biol.* **2012**, *91*, 369–376. [CrossRef] [PubMed]
38. Carr, A.C.; Pullar, J.M.; Moran, S.; Vissers, M.C. Bioavailability of vitamin C from kiwifruit in non-smoking males: Determination of 'healthy' and 'optimal' intakes. *J. Nutr. Sci.* **2012**, *1*, e14. [CrossRef]
39. Carr, A.C.; Bozonet, S.M.; Pullar, J.M.; Simcock, J.W.; Vissers, M.C. Human skeletal muscle ascorbate is highly responsive to changes in vitamin C intake and plasma concentrations. *Am. J. Clin. Nutr.* **2013**, *97*, 800–807. [CrossRef]
40. Dhariwal, K.R.; Hartzell, W.O.; Levine, M. Ascorbic acid and dehydroascorbic acid measurements in human plasma and serum. *Am. J. Clin. Nutr.* **1991**, *54*, 712–716. [CrossRef]
41. Sharma, P.; Raghavan, S.A.; Saini, R.; Dikshit, M. Ascorbate-mediated enhancement of reactive oxygen species generation from polymorphonuclear leukocytes: Modulatory effect of nitric oxide. *J. Leukoc. Biol.* **2004**, *75*, 1070–1078. [CrossRef]

42. Anderson, R.; Lukey, P.T. A biological role for ascorbate in the selective neutralization of extracellular phagocyte-derived oxidants. *Ann. N. Y. Acad. Sci.* **1987**, *498*, 229–247. [CrossRef] [PubMed]
43. Schwager, J.; Bompard, A.; Weber, P.; Raederstorff, D. Ascorbic acid modulates cell migration in differentiated HL-60 cells and peripheral blood leukocytes. *Mol. Nutr. Food Res.* **2015**, *59*, 1513–1523. [CrossRef] [PubMed]
44. Boxer, L.A.; Vanderbilt, B.; Bonsib, S.; Jersild, R.; Yang, H.H.; Baehner, R.L. Enhancement of chemotactic response and microtubule assembly in human leukocytes by ascorbic acid. *J. Cell Physiol.* **1979**, *100*, 119–126. [CrossRef]
45. Elste, V.; Troesch, B.; Eggersdorfer, M.; Weber, P. Emerging evidence on neutrophil motility supporting its usefulness to define vitamin C intake requirements. *Nutrients* **2017**, *9*, 503. [CrossRef]
46. Weiss, S.J. Tissue destruction by neutrophils. *N. Engl. J. Med.* **1989**, *320*, 365–376. [PubMed]
47. Margraf, S.; Logters, T.; Reipen, J.; Altrichter, J.; Scholz, M.; Windolf, J. Neutrophil-derived circulating free DNA (cf-DNA/NETs): A potential prognostic marker for posttraumatic development of inflammatory second hit and sepsis. *Shock* **2008**, *30*, 352–358. [CrossRef] [PubMed]
48. Hashiba, M.; Huq, A.; Tomino, A.; Hirakawa, A.; Hattori, T.; Miyabe, H.; Tsuda, M.; Takeyama, N. Neutrophil extracellular traps in patients with sepsis. *J. Surg. Res.* **2015**, *194*, 248–254. [CrossRef] [PubMed]
49. McInturff, A.M.; Cody, M.J.; Elliott, E.A.; Glenn, J.W.; Rowley, J.W.; Rondina, M.T.; Yost, C.C. Mammalian target of rapamycin regulates neutrophil extracellular trap formation via induction of hypoxia-inducible factor 1 alpha. *Blood* **2012**, *120*, 3118–3125. [CrossRef] [PubMed]
50. Du, J.; Cullen, J.J.; Buettner, G.R. Ascorbic acid: Chemistry, biology and the treatment of cancer. *Biochim. Biophys. Acta* **2012**, *1826*, 443–457. [CrossRef] [PubMed]
51. Elks, P.M.; van Eeden, F.J.; Dixon, G.; Wang, X.; Reyes-Aldasoro, C.C.; Ingham, P.W.; Whyte, M.K.; Walmsley, S.R.; Renshaw, S.A. Activation of hypoxia-inducible factor-1alpha (Hif-1alpha) delays inflammation resolution by reducing neutrophil apoptosis and reverse migration in a zebrafish inflammation model. *Blood* **2011**, *118*, 712–722. [CrossRef] [PubMed]
52. Hunt, C.; Chakravorty, N.K.; Annan, G.; Habibzadeh, N.; Schorah, C.J. The clinical effects of vitamin C supplementation in elderly hospitalised patients with acute respiratory infections. *Int. J. Vitam. Nutr. Res.* **1994**, *64*, 212–219. [PubMed]
53. Johnston, C.S.; Martin, L.J.; Cai, X. Antihistamine effect of supplemental ascorbic acid and neutrophil chemotaxis. *J. Am. Coll. Nutr.* **1992**, *11*, 172–176. [PubMed]
54. Anderson, R.; Oosthuizen, R.; Maritz, R.; Theron, A.; Van Rensburg, A.J. The effects of increasing weekly doses of ascorbate on certain cellular and humoral immune functions in normal volunteers. *Am. J. Clin. Nutr.* **1980**, *33*, 71–76. [CrossRef] [PubMed]
55. Anderson, R. Ascorbate-mediated stimulation of neutrophil motility and lymphocyte transformation by inhibition of the peroxidase/H$_2$O$_2$/halide system in vitro and in vivo. *Am. J. Clin. Nutr.* **1981**, *34*, 1906–1911. [CrossRef] [PubMed]

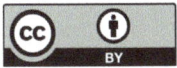

© 2019 by the authors. Licensee MDPI, Basel, Switzerland. This article is an open access article distributed under the terms and conditions of the Creative Commons Attribution (CC BY) license (http://creativecommons.org/licenses/by/4.0/).

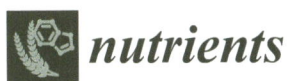

Article

Plasma Vitamin C Levels: Risk Factors for Deficiency and Association with Self-Reported Functional Health in the European Prospective Investigation into Cancer-Norfolk

Stephen J. McCall [1,2], Allan B. Clark [3], Robert N. Luben [4], Nicholas J. Wareham [5], Kay-Tee Khaw [4] and Phyo Kyaw Myint [2,*]

1. National Perinatal Epidemiology Unit, Nuffield Department of Population Health, University of Oxford, Richard Doll Building, Old Road Campus, Oxford OX3 7LF, UK
2. Ageing Clinical & Experimental Research Group, Institute of Applied Health Sciences, University of Aberdeen, Foresterhill, Aberdeen AB25 2ZD, UK
3. Norwich Medical School, University of East Anglia, Norwich NR4 7TJ, UK
4. Department of Public Health and Primary Care, University of Cambridge, Cambridge CB2 0SR UK
5. MRC Epidemiology Unit, University of Cambridge School of Clinical Medicine, Cambridge CB2 0QQ, UK
* Correspondence: phyo.myint@abdn.ac.uk; Tel.: +44-(0)-1224-437841; Fax: +44-(0)-1224-437911

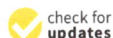

Received: 6 May 2019; Accepted: 2 July 2019; Published: 9 July 2019

Abstract: Background: To investigate the demographic and lifestyles factors associated with vitamin C deficiency and to examine the association between plasma vitamin C level and self-reported physical functional health. Methods: A population-based cross-sectional study using the European Prospective Investigation into Cancer-Norfolk study. Plasma vitamin C level < 11 µmol/L indicated vitamin C deficiency. Unconditional logistic regression models assessed the association between vitamin C deficiency and potential risk factors. Associations between quartiles of vitamin C and self-reported functional health measured by the 36-item short-form questionnaire (SF-36) were assessed. Results: After adjustment, vitamin C deficiency was associated with older age, being male, lower physical activity, smoking, more socially deprived area (Townsend index) and a lower educational attainment. Compared to the highest, those in the lowest quartile of vitamin C were more likely to score in the lowest decile of physical function (adjusted odds ratio (aOR): 1.43 (95%CI: 1.21–1.70)), bodily pain (aOR: 1.29 (95% CI: 1.07–1.56)), general health (aOR: 1.4 (95%CI: 1.18–1.66)), and vitality (aOR: 1.23 (95%CI: 1.04–1.45)) SF-36 scores. Conclusions: Simple public health interventions should be aimed at populations with risk factors for vitamin C deficiency. Poor self-reported functional health was associated with lower plasma vitamin C levels, which may reflect symptoms of latent scurvy.

Keywords: vitamin C; self-reported health; risk factors; EPIC-Norfolk

1. Introduction

Vitamin C (ascorbic acid) is a co-substrate for many enzymatic reactions. It is essential for the synthesis of collagen proteins and has a vital role in the prevention of bleeding and wound repair [1,2]. Unlike plants and other species, humans cannot synthesise ascorbic acid due to a lack of the functional gulonolactone oxidase enzyme. As a result, it has to be supplemented through the dietary intake of fruit and vegetables [1].

It is important to maintain a sufficient intake of vitamin C to avoid illness. For instance, prolonged deficiency of vitamin C over a 2–3 month period can result in scurvy, a recognised clinical disease [3,4]. The symptoms of scurvy include poor wound repair, haemorrhage, oedema of lower limbs, and fatigue [2]. If the vitamin C deficiency is less severe, latent scurvy can occur without many of the extreme clinical symptoms of scurvy. Latent scurvy presents with more common and non-specific symptoms, such as fatigue, irritability, and muscle pain [5,6]. The non-specificity of the symptoms may cause latent scurvy in the general population to be underreported and underdiagnosed [4,7]. While adult reports of scurvy are very rare in developed nations, 7.1% of a representative sample of the US population were described as having a vitamin C deficiency (<11.4 µmol/L) [7] and other studies define a deficiency as <11 µmol/L [8,9]. Further still, other studies have examined marginal vitamin C deficiency defined as either 11–40 µmol/L [10] or ≥11–28 µmol/L [9,11], where one-fifth of a deprived population, from the United Kingdom, had a suboptimal level of vitamin C [8].

Previous research, in a Western background, has shown that smokers and populations with low socioeconomic status were at increased risk of vitamin C deficiency [8,12]. However, these studies were limited in the number of possible covariates that could be examined for their association with vitamin C deficiency; for example, potential risk factors such as physical activity, educational status, alcohol intake, and prevalent disease were not explored together. The European Prospective Investigation into Cancer (EPIC)-Norfolk cohort study has a wide range of factors that can be explored, which thus offers a more comprehensive exploration of the risk factors of vitamin C.

Symptoms of latent scurvy, such as fatigue, irritability, and muscle pain, are likely to impact self-reported functional health, and if they are caused by vitamin C deficiency, they are easily preventable through supplementation of vitamin C [4,13]. Vitamin C has been shown to be an objective biomarker of fruit and vegetable intake [14]. Low vegetable and fruit intake has been shown to be associated with low self-reported health with regard to summary component scores in the EPIC-Norfolk study [14,15]. However, the association between the level of plasma vitamin C as an objective marker of fruit and vegetable consumption and self-reported health focusing on physical health domains of functional health has yet to be examined.

Therefore, this study has two objectives; firstly, to examine the risk factors for vitamin C deficiency and, secondly, using the 36-item short-form questionnaire (SF-36), to examine the association between plasma vitamin C level and physical functional health in the general population.

2. Material and Methods

The study population was drawn from the EPIC-Norfolk cohort study. The study methodology has been previously described [16]. In brief, men and women aged 40–79 were identified from general practices from Norfolk, UK, and were asked to participate in the study by mail. The baseline survey was conducted during 1993–1997 and 30,445 out of 77,630 invited individuals consented to participation. Norwich Local Research Ethics Committee approved the study.

2.1. Assay for Vitamin C Measurements

The methods of laboratory analyses and specifically for plasma vitamin C have been previously described [17–19]. Non-fasting blood samples were taken from participants at baseline. Venous blood was drawn into plain and citrate bottles and stored overnight in a dark box stored at 4–7 °C. Sample bottles were then centrifuged at 2100g at 4 °C for 15 minutes. About 1 year after the initiation of the study, extra blood samples from participants were taken for ascorbic acid assays. Plasma vitamin C was measured from blood taken into citrate bottles, and plasma was stabilized in a standardized volume of metaphosphoric acid and later stored at −70 °C. Plasma vitamin C concentration was estimated ≤1 week after blood sampling using a fluorometric assay [20]. The coefficient of variation was 5.6% at the lower end of the range (mean: 33.2 mol/L) and 4.6% at the upper end (102.3 mol/L). Blood samples for ascorbic acid assays were taken approximately a year into the study.

2.2. Baseline Measurements

At the baseline assessment, height and weight were measured using a standardised protocol [21] and these were used to derive baseline BMI. The participants answered a detailed health and lifestyle questionnaire at baseline, including questions on smoking, socioeconomic measures, physical activity, self-reported comorbidities, and a food frequency questionnaire.

Socioeconomic measurements included the Registrar General's occupation-based classification scheme, educational attainment, and the Townsend index [22]. The Registrar General's occupation-based classification was reclassified into manual (social classes III manual, IV, and V) and non-manual (or professional) occupations (social classes I, II, III non-manual) [23,24]. Highest educational attainment was included as no attainment, O-level (educational attainment at 16 years), A-level (educational attainment at 18 years), and degree-level or beyond.

The Townsend index is an area level-based deprivation measure. Using the 1991 UK census at enumeration district level, Z-scores were obtained for the following: the percentage of economically active residents aged over 16 years old; percentage of households without a car; percentage of household, not owner-occupied; and percentage of households with more than one person per room were used to calculate the score for enumeration districts. The sum of the Z-scores was used to calculate the Townsend score for each postcode area. The postcodes of participants were used to assign a Townsend score for each participant.

Participants were asked about previous medical conditions using the following question: 'Has the doctor ever told you that you have any of the following?'. The following prevalent illnesses included in this study were as follows: cancer, stroke, myocardial infarction, diabetes mellitus, and asthma. A food frequency questionnaire was used to derive the alcohol intake [25]. Physical activity was measured using the EPIC short physical activity questionnaire. From this questionnaire, a validated 4-level physical index was created, which was used as a measure of physical activity [26].

2.3. Functional Health

The study population was asked to complete the Health and Life Experiences Questionnaire (HLEQ), which included the SF-36 [27]. The questionnaire was sent 18 months after the baseline questionnaire via mail, and the response rate was 73.2% (20,921 participants) of the EPIC-Norfolk sample. Not all participants who attended the baseline health check responded to the SF-36 and vice versa.

The SF-36 contains 36 items, which measures self-reported physical and mental health across a number of domains. These are physical functioning; pain; role limitation due to physical problems; social functioning; role limitation due to emotional problems; mental health; energy/vitality; and general health perception. For the purpose of this study, we chose to examine only those domains related to physical health and vitality. The scoring for each domain is based on the participants' perceived wellbeing. Each participant is given a score between 0 and 100 for each domain, where a score of 100 represents good health and 0 represents poor health.

2.4. Statistical Analysis

Participants with missing data on vitamin C were excluded from the sample. Complete case analysis was used in the analysis. All analyses were completed using STATA 13 SE (College Station, Texas).

2.4.1. Risk Factors for Vitamin C Deficiency

The primary analysis identified risk factors for vitamin C deficiency in the UK setting. This study defined vitamin C deficiency as <11 µmol/L, suboptimal plasma vitamin C levels as ≥11–28 µmol/L, and adequate levels of plasma vitamin C as >28 µmol/L. Unconditional logistic regression models were used, and the dependent variable was vitamin C deficiency (<11 vs. >28 µmol/L) [9]. Log likelihood ratio tests were used to assess linearity in continuous variables. Stepwise methods were used to assess which variables best-predicted vitamin C deficiency. Covariates were chosen for the multivariable model if they had a *p-value* < 0.1 at the univariable level. Covariates were included if they statistically improved the model fit, which was assessed by likelihood ratio tests (<0.05) and if they were associated with the outcome (*p-value* for Wald test < 0.05). Vitamin C supplementation was not assessed as a risk factor for vitamin C deficiency and occupation social class was excluded due to collinearity with educational status (Pearson correlation coefficient > 0.3).

2.4.2. Plasma Vitamin C and Physical Domains of Self-Reported Functional Health

From the 25,639 participants in the baseline question, 18,249 participants also completed HLEQ and, of these, 16,056 had plasma vitamin C samples collected. Histograms were used to assess normality in continuous variables. Descriptive analyses such as chi-square tests (global and test for trend), rank sum tests and Student's *t*-test were used to assess the difference between participants characteristics, outcomes, and quartiles of vitamin C.

Vitamin C quartiles were the exposure and physical domain scores of SF-36 were the outcomes in this analysis. The physical domains of SF-36 included in this analysis were 'physical functioning', 'role limitation due to a physical problem', 'bodily pain', 'vitality' (fatigue), and 'general health'. These continuous measures of self-reported health were categorised because the distribution was biased to the nearest ten or five. All SF-36 domains were categorised into deciles apart from 'role limitation due to physical problem' and this was categorised into quintiles, which was due to the distribution of values.

Multiple logistic regression models were created for each SF-36 physical domain assessed. The physical domains were categorised into a binary variable that compared the bottom decile/quintile to all the other deciles/quintiles. A sensitivity analysis was completed stratifying the fully adjusted model by vitamin C supplementation.

2.4.3. Sensitivity Analyses

In the primary analysis, linear regression models estimated the association between a standard deviation change in vitamin C and each SF-36 domain (continuous). This analysis was further stratified by vitamin C supplementation. A post hoc analysis was completed in participants who did not take vitamin C supplementation; this was completed using spline models. Across the range of vitamin C values, it appeared that the linear association between vitamin C was made up of a number of slopes. As a result, four linear terms were fitted to each SF-36 domain.

3. Results

Out of 30,445 participants who agreed to be part of the study, 22,474 attended the second health check and had a plasma vitamin C sample available in the EPIC-Norfolk study.

3.1. Risk Factors for Vitamin C Deficiency Analysis

Table 1 shows the sample characteristics according to vitamin C deficiency, and suboptimal and adequate levels of vitamin C. There were 315 (1.4%) participants with a plasma vitamin C < 11 µmol/L and 2410 (10.7%) participants with a plasma vitamin C ≥ 11–28 µmol/L in the EPIC-Norfolk study. At the univariable level, participants with a vitamin C deficiency as compared to those with a normal vitamin C level were older, male, more likely to smoke, be physically inactive, live in a deprived area, have a manual occupation, not take vitamin C supplementation, and have a lower educational status. Other than myocardial infarction, there appeared to be no statistically significant association between vitamin C deficiency and prevalent illness at baseline.

Table 1. Sociodemographic, lifestyle, and self-reported comorbidities by vitamin C deficiency status.

		Deficiency in Vitamin C Concentration < 11 mol/L; n = 315		Suboptimal Vitamin C Concentration ≥ 11–28 mol/L; n = 2410		Adequate Vitamin C Concentration > 28 mol/L; n = 19,749		Odds Ratio (Deficient vs. Adequate Vitamin C)	95% CI	p-Value
Age (mean SD)		62.5	(9.5)	60.7	(9.6)	59.0	(9.2)	1.04	(1.03–1.06)	<0.01
BMI (median IQR)		25.9	(23.4–28.5)	26.4	(24.2–29.1)	25.8	(23.7–28.2)	0.99	(0.96–1.02)	0.57
Number (%)										
Sex	Male	222	(70.5)	1554	(64.5)	8491	(43)	3.16	(2.48–4.04)	<0.01
	Female	93	(29.5)	856	(35.5)	11,258	(57)	1		
Smoking status	Current smoker	120	(38.7)	638	(26.7)	1797	(9.2)	8.82	(6.56–11.86)	<0.01
	Former smoker	118	(38.1)	1045	(43.8)	8298	(42.3)	1.88	(1.40–2.52)	<0.01
	Non-smoker	72	(23.2)	703	(29.5)	9510	(48.5)	1		
Physical activity	Inactive	156	(49.5)	982	(40.7)	5643	(28.6)	3.22	(2.20–4.72)	<0.01
	Moderately inactive	75	(23.8)	581	(24.1)	5764	(29.2)	1.52	(1.00–2.30)	0.05
	Moderately active	52	(16.5)	464	(19.3)	4612	(23.4)	1.31	(0.84–2.05)	0.23
	Active	32	(10.2)	383	(15.9)	3729	(18.9)	1		
Alcohol intake	None	101	(33.3)	568	(24.7)	3594	(18.8)	2.17	(1.66–2.84)	<0.01
	1 to ≤7 units a week	115	(38)	1024	(44.5)	8882	(46.4)	1		
	>7 to ≤14 units a week	41	(13.5)	361	(15.7)	3812	(19.9)	0.83	(0.58–1.19)	0.31
	>14 units a week	46	(15.2)	349	(15.2)	2862	(14.9)	1.24	(0.88–1.75)	0.22
Sociodemographic										
Townsend score	Least deprived (<−3.82)	53	(16.9)	401	(16.7)	3994	(20.3)	1		
	2 (−3.82 to −2.96)	38	(12.1)	421	(17.5)	4034	(20.5)	0.71	(0.47–1.08)	0.11
	3 (−2.96 to −2.16)	52	(16.6)	472	(19.6)	3922	(19.9)	1.00	(0.68–1.47)	0.99
	4 (−2.16 to −0.74)	62	(19.7)	507	(21.1)	3917	(19.9)	1.19	(0.82–1.73)	0.35
	Most deprived (>−0.74)	109	(34.7)	605	(25.1)	3797	(19.3)	2.16	(1.55–3.01)	<0.01
Education below	Lower than O-level	160	(50.8)	1121	(46.5)	6959	(35.3)	4.48	(2.59–7.75)	<0.01
	O-level	23	(7.3)	224	(9.3)	2050	(10.4)	2.19	(1.12–4.26)	0.02
	A-level or equivalent	118	(37.5)	890	(36.9)	8003	(40.5)	2.87	(1.65–5.01)	<0.01
	Degree or equivalent	14	(4.4)	174	(7.2)	2727	(13.8)	1		
Vitamin C supplementation	No supplementation	242	(77.3)	1824	(76.2)	10,883	(55.4)	2.75	(2.11–3.58)	<0.01
	Taking supplementation	71	(22.7)	570	(23.8)	8772	(44.6)	1		
Social class	Non-manual occupations	112	(37.1)	1116	(47.9)	12,030	(62.1)	1		
	Manual	190	(62.9)	1213	(52.1)	7337	(37.9)	2.78	(2.20–3.52)	<0.01
Self-reported prevalent illness	Cerebrovascular incident	7	(2.2)	61	(2.5)	242	(1.2)	1.83	(0.86–3.91)	0.12
	Myocardial infarction	18	(5.7)	127	(5.3)	551	(2.8)	2.12	(1.31–3.43)	0.002
	Cancer	17	(5.4)	131	(5.4)	1053	(5.3)	1.01	(0.62–1.66)	0.96
	Diabetes mellitus	5	(1.6)	88	(3.7)	411	(2.1)	0.76	(0.31–1.84)	0.54
	Asthma	25	(8)	204	(8.5)	1664	(8.4)	0.94	(0.62–1.42)	0.76

Linear trend between categories. Physical activity shows that there is statistical evidence for a linear trend and no evidence for education level.

The final regression model included seven risk factors that were statistically associated with vitamin C deficiency; these were older age, being male, physically inactive or current smoking, and having higher Townsend index (higher level of area deprivation), no alcohol intake, or lower educational attainment (see Table 2). Current smokers had a considerably higher risk of vitamin C deficiency than non-smokers (adjusted odds ratio (aOR): 7.38 (95%CI: 5.39–10.12)). Those who were physically inactive had over twice the odds of vitamin C deficiency compared to being physically active (aOR: 2.85 (95%CI: 1.87–4.33)). Similarly, there were twice the odds of vitamin C deficiency in those who did not drink compared to those who had a moderate consumption of alcohol. In addition, after adjusting for confounders, the positive association between excessive drinking and vitamin C deficiency was not statistically significant. Males had over four times the odds of vitamin C deficiency compared to females (aOR: 4.09 (95%CI: 3.11–5.37)). Participants living in the most deprived area had an increased likelihood of vitamin C deficiency compared to those living in the least deprived areas. Furthermore, participants with a lower than O-level educational attainment had over three times the odds of vitamin C deficiency compared to those who had attained a degree (aOR: 3.12 (95%CI: 1.76–5.51)). The adjusted odds for vitamin C deficiency increased by 2% per year increase in age (aOR: 1.02 (95%CI: 1.01–1.04)).

Table 2. Risk factors for vitamin C deficiency in EPIC-Norfolk cohort study.

		Adjusted Odds Ratio	95% CI	p-Value
Lifestyle				
Smoking status	Current smoker	7.38	(5.39–10.12)	<0.01
	Former smoker	1.26	(0.92–1.73)	0.15
	Non-smoker	1		
Physical activity	Inactive	2.85	(1.87–4.33)	<0.01
	Moderately inactive	1.88	(1.20–2.93)	0.01
	Moderately active	1.58	(0.99–2.52)	0.05
	Active	1		
Alcohol intake	None	2.06	(1.55–2.73)	<0.01
	1 to ≤7 units a week	1		
	>7 to ≤14 units a week	0.74	(0.51–1.07)	0.1
	>14 units a week	0.9	(0.62–1.30)	0.57
Sociodemographic				
Townsend score	Least deprived (<−3.82)	1		
	2 (−3.82 to −2.96)	0.67	(0.43–1.03)	0.07
	3 (−2.96 to − 2.16)	0.9	(0.60–1.35)	0.62
	4 (−2.16 to −0.74)	1.07	(0.73–1.57)	0.74
	Most deprived (> −0.74)	1.68	(1.18–2.38)	<0.01
Age		1.02	(1.01–1.04)	<0.01
Sex	Male	4.09	(3.11–5.37)	<0.01
	Female	1		
Education	Lower than O level	3.12	(1.76–5.51)	<0.01
	O-level	1.81	(0.90–3.63)	0.1
	A-level or equivalent	2.33	(1.32–4.11)	<0.01
	Degree or equivalent	1		

These are the factors remaining in the model after forward stepwise regression method. All factors are mutually adjusted for each other.

These are the factors remaining in the model after forward stepwise regression method. All factors are mutually adjusted for each other.

3.2. Association between Plasma Vitamin C and Self-Reported Physical Health Domains

The characteristics of participants by quartiles of vitamin C are presented in Table S1. The range of vitamin C in each quartile are as follows: quartile one, <41.0 µmol/L; quartile two, 41.0–53.9 µmol/L; quartile three, 54.0–65.9 µmol/L; and quartile four, ≥66.0 µmol/L. In brief, those in the lowest quartile of vitamin C had very similar characteristics to those with vitamin C deficiency. Table 3 shows the association between quartiles of vitamin C and SF-36 physical functional health domains. In all four models, those in the bottom quartile of vitamin C, compared to the highest, had statistically significant increased odds of having a poor physical functional health SF-36 score. After adjustment for potential confounders, those in the lowest quartile of vitamin C compared the highest quartile had increased odds of having a poor physical functional health score (aOR: 1.43 (95%CI: 1.21–1.70)), a poor bodily pain score (aOR: 1.29 (95%CI: 1.07–1.56)), having poor self-reported general health (aOR:1.4 (95%CI: 1.18–1.66)) and a poor vitality score (aOR:1.23 (95%CI: 1.04–1.45)) (defined as the bottom decile). In addition, after adjustment, those in the lowest quartile of vitamin C had a 1.26 (95%CI: 1.10–1.45) times increased odds of scoring in the lowest quintile of role of physical health score. This trend was more varied when the populations were stratified by those who used vitamin C supplementation (see Table 4). In particular, in those who had a vitamin C supplementation, the results were not statistically significant for two SF-36 physical functional health domains, while the results were more consistent for participants with no vitamin C supplementation.

Table S2 presents the coefficients and 95% confidence intervals of the linear regression models, which treated both vitamin C and SF-36 domains as continuous variables. An increase in one standard deviation (SD) of vitamin C levels was statistically associated with an improved score in all-physical functional health domains assessed (0.65–1.68 unit increase in SF-36 per SD increase in vitamin C) with a larger effect size observed in those who were not taking vitamin C supplementation (1.4–3.5 unit increase in SF-36 per SD increase in vitamin C). Spline models in those without supplementation showed that low vitamin C levels were associated with low SF-36 levels; in particular, the linear association was only present in those below 40 µmol/L.

Table 3. Association between plasma vitamin C quartile and SF-36 domain (physical functions and vitality).

	Vitamin Quartile	Unadjusted			Model A			Model B			Model C			Model D		
		Odds ratio	95% CI	p-value	Odds ratio	95% CI	p-value	Odds ratio	95% CI	p-value	Odds ratio	95% CI	p-value	Odds ratio	95% CI	p-value
Physical function*	1 (Lowest)	2.03	(1.75–2.35)	<0.01	2.17	(1.85–2.54)	<0.01	1.75	(1.48–2.06)	<0.01	1.56	(1.32–1.84)	<0.01	1.43	(1.21–1.70)	<0.01
	2	1.28	(1.10–1.51)	<0.01	1.42	(1.21–1.68)	<0.01	1.3	(1.09–1.54)	<0.01	1.16	(0.97–1.38)	0.1	1.11	(0.93–1.32)	0.24
	3	0.91	(0.77–1.07)	0.24	0.99	(0.84–1.17)	0.92	0.96	(0.80–1.14)	0.61	0.89	(0.75–1.06)	0.2	0.88	(0.73–1.05)	0.15
	4 (Highest)	1			1			1			1			1		
Role physical health**	1 (Lowest)	1.6	(1.41–1.81)	<0.01	1.63	(1.43–1.87)	<0.01	1.41	(1.23–1.62)	<0.01	1.33	(1.16–1.53)	<0.01	1.26	(1.10–1.45)	0.001
	2	1.16	(1.02–1.32)	0.02	1.23	(1.07–1.41)	<0.01	1.15	(1.00–1.32)	0.05	1.09	(0.95–1.25)	0.23	1.06	(0.92–1.22)	0.42
	3	0.98	(0.86–1.12)	0.74	1.04	(0.91–1.18)	0.60	1	(0.88–1.15)	0.95	0.98	(0.85–1.12)	0.72	0.97	(0.84–1.11)	0.62
	4 (Highest)	1			1			1			1			1		
Bodily Pain*	1 (Lowest)	1.68	(1.42–2.00)	<0.01	1.83	(1.53–2.18)	<0.01	1.49	(1.24–1.79)	0.001	1.37	(1.13–1.65)	<0.01	1.29	(1.07–1.56)	0.01
	2	1.19	(0.99–1.42)	0.06	1.29	(1.08–1.55)	0.01	1.19	(0.99–1.44)	0.07	1.1	(0.91–1.33)	0.34	1.07	(0.89–1.30)	0.47
	3	1	(0.84–1.20)	0.98	1.06	(0.88–1.27)	0.54	0.99	(0.82–1.20)	0.94	0.95	(0.79–1.15)	0.59	0.95	(0.78–1.14)	0.57
	4 (Highest)	1			1			1			1			1		
Vitality*	1 (Lowest)	1.35	(1.17–1.57)	<0.01	1.6	(1.38–1.87)	<0.01	1.34	(1.14–1.58)	<0.01	1.29	(1.10–1.52)	<0.01	1.23	(1.04–1.45)	0.01
	2	1.12	(0.96–1.30)	0.15	1.26	(1.08–1.47)	<0.01	1.16	(0.99–1.36)	0.07	1.12	(0.95–1.32)	0.17	1.1	(0.94–1.30)	0.23
	3	0.98	(0.85–1.15)	0.84	1.04	(0.90–1.22)	0.59	1.03	(0.88–1.20)	0.75	1.01	(0.86–1.18)	0.92	1	(0.85–1.17)	0.96
	4 (Highest)	1			1			1			1			1		
General health*	1 (Lowest)	2.01	(1.72–2.35)	<0.01	1.92	(1.64–2.26)	<0.01	1.56	(1.32–1.84)	<0.01	1.48	(1.25–1.75)	<0.01	1.4	(1.18–1.66)	<0.01
	2	1.38	(1.17–1.62)	<0.01	1.36	(1.15–1.60)	<0.01	1.23	(1.04–1.46)	0.02	1.17	(0.99–1.39)	0.07	1.14	(0.96–1.36)	0.13
	3	1	(0.84–1.19)	0.99	1	(0.84–1.19)	0.99	0.95	(0.79–1.13)	0.54	0.92	(0.77–1.10)	0.37	0.91	(0.76–1.09)	0.31
	4 (Highest)	1			1			1			1			1		

* Outcome defined as bottom decile vs. all other deciles; ** Outcome defined as the bottom quintile vs. rest; Model A: Basic model + age and sex. Model B: model A + smoking, physical activity and alcohol intake. Model C: model B + BMI. Model D: model C + education status, Townsend index and previous medical history (cancer, diabetes, cerebrovascular incident, myocardial infarction, asthma).

Table 4. Association between plasma vitamin C quartile and SF-36 domain (physical function and vitality) stratified by supplementation of vitamin C.

	Vitamin Quartile	With Vitamin C Supplementation			No Vitamin C Supplementation		
		Odds Ratio	95% CI	p-Value	Odds Ratio	95% CI	p-Value
Physical function	1 (Lowest)	1.62	(1.26–2.08)	<0.01	1.45	(1.12–1.86)	<0.01
	2	1.05	(0.82–1.35)	0.68	1.26	(0.97–1.64)	0.08
	3	0.93	(0.74–1.19)	0.58	0.88	(0.66–1.16)	0.36
	4 (Highest)	1			1		
Role physical health	1 (Lowest)	1.19	(0.96–1.48)	0.11	1.47	(1.20–1.81)	<0.01
	2	0.97	(0.80–1.19)	0.8	1.24	(1.01–1.54)	0.04
	3	0.98	(0.82–1.18)	0.85	1.01	(0.81–1.25)	0.94
	4 (Highest)	1			1		
Bodily Pain	1 (Lowest)	1.36	(1.02–1.81)	0.03	1.32	(1.00–1.73)	0.05
	2	1.15	(0.88–1.51)	0.3	1.08	(0.81–1.43)	0.6
	3	1.07	(0.83–1.38)	0.59	0.84	(0.63–1.14)	0.27
	4 (Highest)	1			1		
Vitality	1 (Lowest)	1.2	(0.92–1.56)	0.17	1.34	(1.06–1.69)	0.01
	2	0.98	(0.77–1.25)	0.9	1.28	(1.01–1.61)	0.04
	3	0.99	(0.80–1.22)	0.9	1.04	(0.82–1.33)	0.72
	4 (Highest)	1			1		
General health	1 (Lowest)	1.52	(1.16–2.00)	<0.01	1.34	(1.05–1.71)	0.02
	2	1.05	(0.81–1.37)	0.71	1.21	(0.94–1.55)	0.14
	3	1.03	(0.81–1.31)	0.8	0.81	(0.62–1.05)	0.12
	4 (Highest)	1			1		

Adjusted for age, sex, smoking, physical activity, alcohol intake, BMI, education status, Townsend index, and previous medical history (cancer, diabetes, cerebrovascular incident, myocardial infarction, asthma)). All outcomes compared the bottom decile vs. all other deciles except role physical health, which was defined the comparison as the bottom quintile vs. rest.

4. Discussion

4.1. Main Findings

In this British population-based study, seven factors were associated with vitamin C deficiency. These were older age, being male, lower socioeconomic status measured by higher Townsend index, lower educational attainment, no alcohol intake, smoking, and physical inactivity. This study also showed that lower vitamin C levels were associated with significantly poorer self-reported physical functional health, such as self-reported fatigue, increased bodily pain, and poorer general health. In addition, poorer self-reported health appeared to be worse in those who were not taking vitamin C supplementation and in those who had lower levels plasma of vitamin C at baseline.

4.2. Findings in Context—Factors Associated with Vitamin C Deficiency

Consistent with previous research, this study showed that manual occupation as an indicator of low socioeconomic status, smoking, and being male was associated with vitamin C deficiency [8]. In contrast to previous studies [7,8], this study found older age was linearly associated with vitamin C deficiency, where a quadratic trend was shown in the US study [7] and was not examined as a risk factor [8]. In addition to these known risk factors, we also found that physical inactivity increased the risk of vitamin C deficiency. Although no previous research examined this association, this finding is consistent with a wider body of work. Woolcott, et al. (2013) showed that those who were more physically active tended to have a higher fruit and vegetable intake [28].

Conversely, there was no association between excessive alcohol intake and vitamin C deficiency. This is contrast to a previous study which showed an association between excessive alcohol intake and scurvy [29]. A recent review [11] has called for future RCTs to examine vitamin C supplementation in excessive drinkers, which would robustly test this intervention.

Interestingly, in contrast to previous research, BMI was not associated with vitamin C deficiency [7]. This may relate to a relatively narrow range of BMI in this population with very few people in low BMI range (median 25.8 kg/m^2 (IQR: 23.7–28.3)). Furthermore, this may also be a reflection of inconsistent evidence surrounding the magnitude of the association between BMI and fruit and vegetable intake [15,30].

Our findings showed that no vitamin C supplementation was associated with increased likelihood of a vitamin C deficiency, although this was completed at the univariable level. It should be noted that vitamin C supplementation did not reduce mortality in large-scale RCTs [31,32]; thus, it is probable that vitamin C supplementation may only be beneficial in those with clinical disease as a consequence of a vitamin C deficiency.

4.3. Self-Reported Health and Vitamin C

Even after adjustment for sociodemographic factors, lifestyle factors, and comorbidities, an association with low vitamin C quartile and poor functional health remained. This finding was consistent with a wider body of previous work [15] which showed that fruit and vegetable intake was positively associated with improved self-reported functional health using the component summary scores of SF-36. We have further explored this existing knowledge by examining the objective marker of fruit and vegetable intake, vitamin C levels, and individual domains of physical health. The relationship between physical self-reported functional health and vitamin C was most pronounced in low values of plasma vitamin C and in those without supplementation. This is biologically plausible as symptoms of latent scurvy include fatigue, irritability, and muscle pain [4,6,7]. From the outset, those with latent scurvy presenting with bodily pain and fatigue would have low levels of vitamin C, while the association with bodily pain and fatigue would be attenuated at higher levels of vitamin C. Thus, it is likely that supplementation of vitamin C would only have an impact in those with the lowest levels of vitamin C.

4.4. Limitations and Strengths

There are a number of limitations to this study. Firstly, the study population had to volunteer to participate, which is shown by a 40% response rate to the baseline questionnaire. As a result, this study may be healthier than the UK population as a whole. However, compared to the general population, the EPIC-Norfolk study was similar to other representative samples other than having a slightly lower proportion of smokers [16]. Furthermore, the external validity of the results may be limited due to the low prevalence of vitamin C deficiency in the EPIC-Norfolk population. Only a single measurement of vitamin C was taken from participants; therefore, the measurements are prone to random error and regression dilution bias. However, random error will only attenuate the relationship between vitamin C and self-reported health. Furthermore, the relationship between vitamin C and self-reported functional health may be biased by residual confounding.

There are a number of limitations regarding the storage of the assays and processing of plasma vitamin C. In particular, recent evidence, which was not known at the time of the study, showed that overnight storage of the sample at 4 °C may result in loss of ascorbate from the sample [33]. As this occurred for all the samples, it will not have caused any differential bias but may likely to have biased estimates towards the null. It could be argued that the vitamin C level in a plasma blood test may fluctuate according to dietary intake and, thus, a fasting blood test may provide a better representation of an individual's vitamin C level. Furthermore, since this study was completed, there are now more specific methods of plasma vitamin C quantification, such as HPLC, which may improve the accuracy of future studies examining vitamin C [34].

This study has several strengths. We used self-reported physical functional health measures of SF-36, which is a widely validated tool, and we have previously demonstrated that SF-36 is linked to objective health outcomes of mortality, cardiovascular disease, and stroke [35–38]. In addition, mean age–sex-standardised SF-36 scores from the Health Survey for England and Oxford Healthy Life Survey showed similar values to the EPIC-HLEQ SF-36 scores [39]. Other strengths include a large sample size with the ability to control for a myriad of socioeconomic and lifestyle factors, the ability to examine relationships based on vitamin C supplement use, and use of plasma vitamin C as a measure of dietary vitamin C.

5. Conclusions

Low plasma vitamin C levels were associated with poor physical functioning, an established risk factor of objective health outcomes as well as a valid quality of life outcome in its own right. We have also identified risk factors for vitamin C deficiency. Vitamin C deficiency was associated with poor self-reported functional health, which may reflect that this population has symptoms of vitamin C deficiency. Whilst scurvy is rare, populations with poor general health are likely to be micronutrient-deficit and may benefit from increased fruit and vegetable intake.

Supplementary Materials: The following are available online at http://www.mdpi.com/2072-6643/11/7/1552/s1. Table S1: Characteristics of EPIC Norfolk in quartiles of plasma vitamin C level. Table S2: Linear regression models for the association between vitamin C and self-reported health.

Author Contributions: S.J.M. and P.K.M. conceived the study. K.-T.K. and N.J.W. are PIs of EPIC-Norfolk. R.N.L. performed data linkage. A.B.C. provided statistical advice. S.J.M. performed analysis and drafted the manuscript. All authors contributed to the interpretation of the results and writing of the paper. P.K.M. is the guarantor.

Funding: EPIC-Norfolk is supported by Cancer Research UK and MRC, UK. Funders had no role in design, analysis and interpretation of the study results.

Acknowledgments: We would like to thank the participants of the EPIC-Norfolk and collaborating General Practices and the staff of EPIC-Norfolk. We would also like to thank Robert House and Carrie Stewart for proofreading the article.

Conflicts of Interest: The authors declare no conflict of interest. The sponsors had no role in the design, execution, interpretation, or writing of the study.

References

1. Mandl, J.; Szarka, A.; Bánhegyi, G. Vitamin C: Update on physiology and pharmacology. *Br. J. Pharmacol.* **2009**, *157*, 1097–1110. [CrossRef] [PubMed]
2. Combs, J.P., Jr.; Gerald, F. Vitamin C. In *The Vitamins: Fundamental Aspects in Nutrition and Health*, 5th ed.; Combs, J.P., Jr., Gerald, F., Eds.; Academic Press: London, UK, 2017; pp. 267–295.
3. Wilson, L.G. The clinical definition of scurvy and the discovery of vitamin C. *J. Hist. Med. Allied Sci.* **1975**, *30*, 40–60. [CrossRef] [PubMed]
4. Prinzo, Z. *Scurvy and Its Prevention and Control in Major Emergencies*; World Health Organization: Geneva, Switzerland, 1999.
5. Price, K.; Price, C.; Reynolds, R. Hyperglycemia-induced latent scurvy and atherosclerosis: The scorbutic-metaplasia hypothesis. *Med. Hypotheses* **1996**, *46*, 119–129. [CrossRef]
6. Lux-Battistelli, C.; Battistelli, D. Latent scurvy with tiredness and leg pain in alcoholics: An underestimated disease three case reports. *Medicine* **2017**, *96*, e8861. [CrossRef] [PubMed]
7. Schleicher, R.L.; Carroll, M.D.; Ford, E.S.; Lacher, D.A. Serum vitamin C and the prevalence of vitamin C deficiency in the United States: 2003–2004 National Health and Nutrition Examination Survey (NHANES). *Am. J. Clin. Nutr.* **2009**, *90*, 1252–1263. [CrossRef] [PubMed]
8. Mosdøl, A.; Erens, B.; Brunner, E.J. Estimated prevalence and predictors of vitamin C deficiency within UK's low-income population. *J. Public Health* **2008**, *30*, 456–460. [CrossRef] [PubMed]
9. Ravindran, R.D.; Vashist, P.; Gupta, S.K.; Young, I.S.; Maraini, G.; Camparini, M.; Jayanthi, R.; John, N.; Fitzpatrick, K.E.; Chakravarthy, U. Prevalence and risk factors for vitamin C deficiency in north and south India: A two centre population based study in people aged 60 years and over. *PLoS ONE* **2011**, *6*, e28588. [CrossRef]
10. Richardson, T.; Ball, L.; Rosenfeld, T. Will an orange a day keep the doctor away? *Postgrad. Med. J.* **2002**, *78*, 292–294. [CrossRef]
11. Lim, D.J.; Sharma, Y.; Thompson, C.H. Vitamin C and alcohol: A call to action. *BMJ Nutr. Prev. Health.* 2018. Available online: http://dx.doi.org/10.1136/bmjnph-2018-000010 (accessed on 10 June 2019).
12. Hampl, J.S.; Taylor, C.A.; Johnston, C.S. Vitamin C deficiency and depletion in the United States: The third national health and nutrition examination survey, 1988 to 1994. *Am. J. Public Health* **2004**, *94*, 870–875. [CrossRef]
13. Weber, P.; Bendich, A.; Schalch, W. Vitamin C and human health—A review of recent data relevant to human requirements. *Int. J. Vitam. Nutr Res.* **1996**, *66*, 19–30.
14. Khaw, K.-T.; Bingham, S.; Welch, A.; Luben, R.; Wareham, N.; Oakes, S.; Day, N. Relation between plasma ascorbic acid and mortality in men and women in EPIC-Norfolk prospective study: A prospective population study. *Lancet* **2001**, *357*, 657–663. [CrossRef]
15. Myint, P.K.; Welch, A.A.; Bingham, S.A.; Surtees, P.G.; Wainwright, N.W.; Luben, R.N.; Wareham, N.J.; Smith, R.D.; Harvey, I.M.; Day, N.E. Fruit and vegetable consumption and self-reported functional health in men and women in the European Prospective Investigation into Cancer–Norfolk (EPIC–Norfolk): A population-based cross-sectional study. *Public Health Nutr.* **2007**, *10*, 34–41. [CrossRef] [PubMed]
16. Day, N.; Oakes, S.; Luben, R.; Khaw, K.-T.; Bingham, S.; Welch, A.; Wareham, N. EPIC-Norfolk: Study design and characteristics of the cohort. *Br. J. Cancer* **1999**, *80*, 95–103. [PubMed]
17. Myint, P.K.; Luben, R.N.; Welch, A.A.; Bingham, S.A.; Wareham, N.J.; Khaw, K.-T. Plasma vitamin C concentrations predict risk of incident stroke over 10 y in 20,649 participants of the European Prospective Investigation into Cancer–Norfolk prospective population study. *Am. J. Clin. Nutr.* **2008**, *87*, 64–69. [CrossRef] [PubMed]
18. Myint, P.K.; Luben, R.N.; Wareham, N.J.; Khaw, K.-T. Association between plasma vitamin C concentrations and blood pressure in the European prospective investigation into cancer-Norfolk population-based study. *Hypertension* **2011**, *58*, 372–379. [CrossRef] [PubMed]
19. Ros, M.M.; Bueno-de-Mesquita, H.B.; Kampman, E.; Aben, K.K.; Büchner, F.L.; Jansen, E.H.; van Gils, C.H.; Egevad, L.; Overvad, K.; Tjønneland, A. Plasma carotenoids and vitamin C concentrations and risk of urothelial cell carcinoma in the European Prospective Investigation into Cancer and Nutrition. *Am. J. Clin. Nutr.* **2012**, *96*, 902–910. [CrossRef] [PubMed]

20. Vuilleumier, J.; Keck, E. Fluorometric assay of vitamin C in biological materials using a centrifugal analyser with fluorescence attachment. *J. Micronutr. Anal.* **1989**, *5*, 25–34.
21. Dettwyler, K.A. *ANTHROPOMETRIC Standardization Reference Manual*, abridged ed.; Lohman, T.G., Roche, A.F., Martoll, R., Eds.; Human Kinetic Books; Wiley Online Library: Champaign, IL, USA, 1993; p. 90.
22. Townsend, P.; Phillimore, P.; Beattie, A. *Health and Deprivation: Inequality and the North*; Routledge: London, UK, 1988.
23. Szreter, S.R. The genesis of the Registrar-General's social classification of occupations. *Br. J. Sociol.* **1984**, *35*, 522–546. [CrossRef]
24. Brewer, R.I. A note on the changing status of the Registrar General's classification of occupations. *Br. J. Sociol.* **1986**, *37*, 131–140. [CrossRef]
25. Welch, A.A.; Luben, R.; Khaw, K.; Bingham, S. The CAFE computer program for nutritional analysis of the EPIC-Norfolk food frequency questionnaire and identification of extreme nutrient values. *J. Hum. Nutr. Diet.* **2005**, *18*, 99–116. [CrossRef] [PubMed]
26. Wareham, N.J.; Jakes, R.W.; Rennie, K.L.; Schuit, J.; Mitchell, J.; Hennings, S.; Day, N.E. Validity and repeatability of a simple index derived from the short physical activity questionnaire used in the European Prospective Investigation into Cancer and Nutrition (EPIC) study. *Public Health Nutr.* **2003**, *6*, 407–413. [CrossRef]
27. Brazier, J.E.; Harper, R.; Jones, N.; O'cathain, A.; Thomas, K.; Usherwood, T.; Westlake, L. Validating the SF-36 health survey questionnaire: New outcome measure for primary care. *BMJ* **1992**, *305*, 160–164. [CrossRef] [PubMed]
28. Woolcott, C.G.; Dishman, R.K.; Motl, R.W.; Matthai, C.H.; Nigg, C.R. Physical activity and fruit and vegetable intake: Correlations between and within adults in a longitudinal multiethnic cohort. *Am. J. Health Promot.* **2013**, *28*, 71–79. [CrossRef] [PubMed]
29. Fain, O.; Pariés, J.; Jacquart, B.t.; Le Moël, G.; Kettaneh, A.; Stirnemann, J.; Héron, C.; Sitbon, M.; Taleb, C.; Letellier, E. Hypovitaminosis C in hospitalized patients. *Eur. J. Int. Med.* **2003**, *14*, 419–425. [CrossRef]
30. Pérez, C.E. Fruit and vegetable consumption. *Health Rep.* **2002**, *13*, 23. [PubMed]
31. Group, H.P.S.C. MRC/BHF Heart Protection Study of antioxidant vitamin supplementation in 20 536 high-risk individuals: A randomised placebo-controlled trial. *Lancet* **2002**, *360*, 23–33.
32. Hercberg, S.; Galan, P.; Preziosi, P.; Bertrais, S.; Mennen, L.; Malvy, D.; Roussel, A.-M.; Favier, A.; Briançon, S. The SU. VI. MAX Study: A randomized, placebo-controlled trial of the health effects of antioxidant vitamins and minerals. *Arch. Int. Med.* **2004**, *164*, 2335–2342. [CrossRef]
33. Pullar, J.; Bayer, S.; Carr, A. Appropriate handling, processing and analysis of blood samples is essential to avoid oxidation of vitamin C to dehydroascorbic acid. *Antioxidants* **2018**, *7*, 29. [CrossRef] [PubMed]
34. Grotzkyj Giorgi, M.; Howland, K.; Martin, C.; Bonner, A.B. A novel HPLC method for the concurrent analysis and quantitation of seven water-soluble vitamins in biological fluids (plasma and urine): A validation study and application. *Sci. World J.* **2012**. [CrossRef]
35. Myint, P.K.; Luben, R.N.; Surtees, P.G.; Wainwright, N.W.; Welch, A.A.; Bingham, S.A.; Day, N.E.; Wareham, N.J.; Khaw, K.T. Relation between self-reported physical functional health and chronic disease mortality in men and women in the european prospective investigation into cancer (EPIC–Norfolk): A prospective population study. *Ann. Epidemiol.* **2006**, *16*, 492–500.
36. Myint, P.K.; Luben, R.N.; Surtees, P.G.; Wainwright, N.W.; Welch, A.A.; Bingham, S.A.; Wareham, N.J.; Smith, R.D.; Harvey, I.M.; Khaw, K.T. Self-reported mental health-related quality of life and mortality in men and women in the European Prospective Investigation into Cancer (EPIC-Norfolk): A prospective population study. *Psychosom. Med.* **2007**, *69*, 410–414. [PubMed]
37. Myint, P.K.; Surtees, P.G.; Wainwright, N.W.; Luben, R.N.; Welch, A.A.; Bingham, S.A.; Wareham, N.J.; Khaw, K.T. Physical health-related quality of life predicts stroke in the EPIC-Norfolk. *Neurology* **2007**, *69*, 2243–2248. [CrossRef] [PubMed]

38. Myint, P.K.; Luben, R.N.; Surtees, P.G.; Wainwright, N.W.; Wareham, N.J.; Khaw, K.T. Physical functional health predicts the incidence of coronary heart disease in the European Prospective Investigation into Cancer-Norfolk prospective population-based study. *Int. J. Epidemiol.* **2010**, *39*, 996–1003. [CrossRef] [PubMed]
39. Surtees, P.G.; Wainwright, N.W.; Khaw, K.-T. Obesity, confidant support and functional health: Cross-sectional evidence from the EPIC-Norfolk cohort. *Int. J. Obes.* **2004**, *28*, 748–758. [CrossRef] [PubMed]

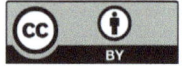

© 2019 by the authors. Licensee MDPI, Basel, Switzerland. This article is an open access article distributed under the terms and conditions of the Creative Commons Attribution (CC BY) license (http://creativecommons.org/licenses/by/4.0/).

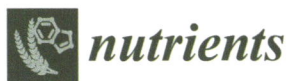

Article

Vitamin C Inhibits Triple-Negative Breast Cancer Metastasis by Affecting the Expression of YAP1 and Synaptopodin 2

Liping Gan [1,2,†], Vladimir Camarena [1,†], Sushmita Mustafi [1] and Gaofeng Wang [1,3,*]

1. John P. Hussman Institute for Human Genomics, Dr. John T. Macdonald Foundation Department of Human Genetics, University of Miami Miller School of Medicine, Miami, FL 33136, USA; ganliping@cau.edu.cn (L.G.); vcamarena@med.miami.edu (V.C.); sxm1241@med.miami.edu (S.M.)
2. State Key Laboratory of Animal Nutrition, College of Animal Science and Technology, China Agricultural University, Beijing 100193, China
3. Sylvester Comprehensive Cancer Center, University of Miami Miller School of Medicine, Miami, FL 33136, USA
* Correspondence: gwang@med.miami.edu; Tel.: +01-305-243-5381
† These authors contributed equally.

Received: 21 October 2019; Accepted: 3 December 2019; Published: 6 December 2019

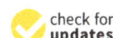

Abstract: Vitamin C supplementation has been shown to decrease triple-negative breast cancer (TNBC) metastasis. However, the molecular mechanism whereby vitamin C inhibits metastasis remains elusive. It has been postulated that vitamin C reduces the levels of HIF-1α, the master regulator of metastasis, by promoting its hydroxylation and degradation. Here, we show that vitamin C at 100 µM, a concentration achievable in the plasma in vivo by oral administration, blocks TNBC cell migration and invasion in vitro. The protein level of HIF-1α remains largely unchanged in cultured TNBC cells and xenografts, partially due to its upregulated transcription by vitamin C, suggesting that HIF-1α unlikely mediates the action of vitamin C on metastasis. Vitamin C treatment upregulates the expression of synaptopodin 2 and downregulates the expression of the transcription coactivator YAP1, both genes in the Hippo pathway. The changes in SYNPO2 and YAP1 expression were subsequently validated at mRNA and protein levels in cultured TNBC cells and xenografts. Further experiments showed that vitamin C treatment inhibits F-actin assembly and lamellipodia formation, which correlates with the changes in SYNPO2 and YAP1 expression. Overall, these results suggest that vitamin C inhibits TNBC metastasis by affecting the expression of SYNPO2 and YAP1. Vitamin C may thus have a potential role in the prevention and treatment of TNBC metastasis.

Keywords: vitamin C; triple-negative breast cancer; metastasis; HIF-1α; YAP1; synaptopodin 2; lamellipodia; F-actin; hippo pathway

---

1. Introduction

Metastatic invasion to organs such as bone marrow and lung is the major cause of death for breast cancer patients. Hypoxia-inducible factor 1α (HIF-1α) is the master regulator of cancer cell metastasis [1]. The hydroxylation of HIF-1α, which is a key step toward its degradation, requires vitamin C as a cofactor for HIF prolyl-hydroxylase [2]. Humans cannot synthesize vitamin C de novo due to a mutant and nonfunctional L-gulonolactone oxidase (*Gulo*), the enzyme catalyzing the final step of vitamin C biosynthesis [3]. Vitamin C is thus an essential micronutrient for humans and needs to be consumed by a vitamin C-rich diet or supplements. Vitamin C enters breast epithelial cells mainly through sodium-dependent vitamin C transporters (SVCT). However, the expression of sodium-dependent vitamin C transporter 2 (SVCT2) is decreased in breast cancer cells compared to normal breast epithelial cells from the same patients [4]. Lower SVCT2 expression is shown to cause intracellular vitamin C deficiency in cancer cells [5], suggesting that there is likely intracellular vitamin C deficiency in breast cancer. Taken together, there is a possibility that in breast cancer, lack of vitamin C hinders the degradation of HIF-1α, which in turn promotes metastasis. Thus, supplementation of vitamin C could help decrease HIF-1α levels in breast cancer, which may be beneficial for blocking metastasis.

Although studies on vitamin C and breast cancer metastasis in human patients are still lacking, in vivo animal models confirm the inhibition of metastasis by vitamin C supplementation. For example, oral vitamin C supplementation blocks murine breast cancer metastasis in *Gulo* knockout mice, which like humans, cannot synthesize vitamin C [6]. High doses of vitamin C via intraperitoneal injection inhibit metastasis of human breast cancer xenografts in nude mice [7], which, like the *Gulo* wild-type mice, maintain endogenous vitamin C at ~50 μM in the plasma [8]. Our earlier work also showed that oral vitamin C supplementation blocks human triple-negative breast cancer (TNBC) xenograft metastasis in mice [9]. Due to the lack of targeted therapy, TNBC is usually associated with a more aggressive clinical course and poor survival [10]. Vitamin C, a readily available micronutrient, has been shown to be beneficial in TNBC treatment by inhibiting metastasis in animal models. However, whether HIF-1α is involved in this action of vitamin C remains unclear.

The pharmacokinetics of vitamin C shows a unique, nonlinear relationship between doses and levels in the blood [11]. The average concentration of vitamin C in the plasma of healthy humans is ~50 μM, similar to the levels in *Gulo* wild-type mice. Intravenous infusion of high doses of vitamin C can increase the plasma concentration to mM levels, which quickly drops to ~200 μM. Oral delivery of vitamin C can maintain plasma vitamin C at ~100 μM, which cannot be further elevated by higher doses. Elevating vitamin C by oral delivery, intravenous infusion, or intraperitoneal injection could in principle help compensate for the downregulated SVCT2 expression and increase the uptake of vitamin C by breast cancer cells.

In addition to promoting the degradation of HIF-1α, vitamin C has a previously unrecognized function in epigenetic regulation, identified and verified by different groups, specifically enhancing the demethylation of DNA and histones [12]. Furthermore, our previous study showed that vitamin C suppresses histone acetylation (H3ac and H4ac) in TNBC cells mainly by upregulating the expression of histone deacetylase 1 (HDAC1) [9]. Vitamin C thus is poised to affect the transcriptome of TNBC cells via HIF-1α, DNA demethylation, histone deacetylation, and potentially histone demethylation and other secondary mechanisms. In an attempt to understand the molecular mechanism by which vitamin C inhibits TNBC metastasis, we examined the expression of HIF-1α and other potential candidate genes in cultured TNBC cells and xenografts. Contrary to our initial reasoning, the results showed that inhibition of TNBC metastasis by vitamin C is largely independent of HIF-1α.

2. Materials and Methods

2.1. Cell Culture and Treatment

MDA-MB-231 and BT-549 TNBC cell lines were purchased from ATCC and maintained under a 5% CO_2 atmosphere in RPMI medium (Lonza, Walkersville, MD, USA) with 10% heat-inactivated fetal bovine serum (FBS), 100 Units/mL of penicillin, and 100 μg/mL of streptomycin. The cells were incubated for 24 h after seeding and subsequently treated with vitamin C (sodium ascorbate, Sigma-Aldrich, St. Louis, MO, USA). The medium was changed daily to ensure the presence of fresh vitamin C.

2.2. Cell Invasion Assay and Migration Assay

A cell invasion assay was performed using the CytoSelect-24 well cell assay (Cell Biolabs, San Diego, CA, USA). Briefly, the cells were pretreated with 0, 50, or 100 μM vitamin C for 2 days. After pretreatment, 2.5×10^4 cells were transferred into an invasion chamber containing membrane inserts with 8 μM pores coated with extracellular matrix (protein matrix isolated from tumor cells, collagen, and laminin). The cells were allowed to invade across the membrane for 48 h and then stained with crystal violet. Five random fields of view (cells that penetrated the membrane) were counted per well. Data are presented as mean ± SEM. A scratch assay was conducted to evaluate cell migratory ability. Briefly, 1×10^5 cells were plated into 6-well plates and pretreated for 5 days with 50 µM or 100 µM vitamin C. Linear wounds were created in cell monolayers using a sterile pipette tip. Images were captured and documented at 0.5 or 20 hours (h) using an Olympus 1 × 50 inverted microscope with a 10× objective lens. Eight images per treatment were analyzed to determine the average position of the migrating cells at the edges of the scratch. Closure was determined by calculating the percentage of distance that cells had migrated.

2.3. Immunoblot

MDA-MB-231 cells were seeded into 6-well plates and treated for 5 days with either 0 or 100 µM vitamin C. Cell lysates were collected in radioimmunoprecipitation assay (RIPA) buffer (Thermo Scientific, Waltham, MA, USA) containing a protease inhibitor cocktail (Sigma-Aldrich, St. Louis, MO, USA), 1% SDS, and 0.5 mM dithiothreitol (DTT). The protein concentration was determined by the BCA protein assay (Thermo Scientific, Waltham, MA, USA). Cell lysates were resolved by SDS-PAGE, transferred to polyvinylidene fluoride (PVDF) membranes (Bio-Rad Laboratories, Hercules, CA, USA), and immunoblotted with anti-HIF-1α antibody, anti-YAP1 antibody, anti-cyclophilin B (PPIB) antibody and, anti-β-actin antibody (Cell Signaling Technology, Danvers, MA, USA). Proteins were visualized by using chemiluminescence ECL (Thermo Scientific, Waltham, MA, USA). Specific band densities were quantified by using ImageJ and analyzed by Student's t-test, at $\alpha = 0.05$.

2.4. Immunofluorescence

MDA-MB-231 cells were pretreated with either 0 or 100 µM vitamin C for 3 days in 10 cm dishes before splitting and seeding on coverslips in a 24-well plate. Vitamin C treatment was continued for two additional days. The cells were then washed with cold PBS and fixed for 30 min at room temperature with 4% paraformaldehyde, permeabilized with 0.4% Triton X-100 for 20 min, and blocked with 3% BSA at room temperature for 30 min. The cells were incubated with primary antibodies overnight at 4 °C. After washing with PBS, the cells were incubated with secondary antibodies (Alexa Fluor 488-conjugated donkey anti-rabbit) and 4′,6-diamidino-2-phenylindole (DAPI) for 1 h at room temperature. The cells where washed 3 times with PBS, and the coverslips were mounted with mowiol 4-88 mounting medium (Polysciences, Warrington, PA, USA). The primary antibodies used include anti-SYNPO2 (#HPA030665, Sigma-Aldrich, St. Louis, MO, USA), anti-HIF-1alpha, and anti-YAP1 (#3716S, and #14074; Cell Signaling, Danvers, MA, USA). CF640R phalloidin (Biotium, Fremont, CA, USA) was used to visualize F-actin. All fluorescence images were acquired using a Zeiss LSM 710 confocal microscope and captured into a 1024 × 1024 or 2048 × 2048 frame size by averaging 4 times at a bit depth of 16. The intensities of the images were quantified using ImageJ. The average intensity of each cell within the image field was measured from a minimum of five 20× images per condition. The intensity values of individual cells were plotted and statistically analyzed by Student's t-test, at $\alpha = 0.05$. The lamellipodia extent was quantified as described previously [13]. Briefly, F-actin was stained with phalloidin, and the flattened F-actin-rich leading edge of the cell was outlined and measured. The summed length of the lamellipodia was normalized to the total cell circumference. Quantification was done using the average of 50 cells per condition.

2.5. Xenograft Immunohistochemistry

Xenografts of MDA-MB-231 were collected from previous published experiments [9]. The tumors were fixed in 4% paraformaldehyde overnight at room temperature, and subsequently, 6 µM paraffin-embedded sections were used for staining. For histological examination, the sections were stained with hematoxylin and eosin (H&E). For immunohistochemistry, the above described primary antibodies for immunofluorescence were used. After incubation with biotinylated secondary antibodies and horse radish peroxidase (Vectastain® Elite ABC Reagent, Vector, Peterborough, UK), diaminobenzidine (Vector ImmPACT DAB substrate, Vector, Peterborough, UK) was applied for 5 min before mounting in Permount (Fisher Scientific, Hampton, NH, USA). The sections were subsequently imaged using a Nikon eclipse 50i microscope and a Qimaging micropublisher 5.0 rtv camera.

2.6. Gene Silencing

SiRNA against human TET1, TET2, and TET3 were purchased from Dharmacon (Lafayettte, CO, USA) and transfected following the manufacturer's instruction. Briefly, MDA-MB-231 cells were plated and grown until achieving ~50% confluence. Transfection of siRNA was performed using Lipofectamine 2000 (Thermo Fisher, Waltham, MA, USA). The medium was changed after 6 h of transfection to eliminate the possible toxicity of the transfecting reagents. The cells were then used for invasion assays or harvested after 3 days for RNA extraction.

2.7. Quantitative Real-Time PCR

Total RNA was extracted from TNBC cells using RNeasy kits (Qiagen). A nanodrop 8000 photospectrometer was used to quantify the RNA (Thermo Scientific, Waltham, MA, USA). The qScript Flex cDNA kit (Quanta Biosciences, Beverly, MA, USA) was used for reverse transcription, according to the manufacturer's instructions. Quantitative real-time RT-PCR (qRT-PCR) was performed in triplicate on a Quantstudio 12K flex system (Thermo Scientific, Waltham, MA, USA), using the PowerUp SYBR green master mix (Thermo Scientific, Waltham, MA, USA). Primers were designed to span introns (*SDHA* forward 5′-GCCAGGGAAGACTACAAGGTGCG-3′, reverse 5′-GAATGGCTGGCGGGACGGTG-3′; *HIF-1α* forward 5′-GGTTCACTTTTTCAAGCAGTAGG-3′, reverse 5′-GTGGTAATCCACTTTCATCCATT-3′; *SYNPO2* forward 5′-CTCGCCCCTGTCAAGACTG-3′, reverse 5′-CCAGGCTGTACCGCTTCTA-3′; *YAP1* forward 5′-GAACTCGGCTTCAGGTCCTC-3′, reverse 5′-GGTTCATGGCAAAACGAGGG-3′). The transcript amplification results were analyzed with the QuantStudio 12K Flex software, and all values were normalized to the levels of the SDHA gene using the $2^{-(\Delta\Delta Ct)}$ method. Statistical significance of differences in expression levels was assessed by Student's t-test, at $\alpha = 0.05$.

2.8. Actin Segmentation

The actin segmentation analysis was done using a method described previously [14]. Briefly, cells were lysed directly using actin stabilization buffer (50 mM PIPES (pH 6.9), 50 mM NaCl, 5 mM $MgCl_2$, 5 mM EGTA, 2 mM ATP, 5% glycerol, 0.1% Nonidet P-40, 0.1% Triton X-100, 0.1% Tween 20, 0.1% β-mercaptoethanol, 1:100 protease inhibitor mixture, and 1:100 phosphatase inhibitor mixture (Sigma-Aldrich, St. Louis, MO, USA). The cells were collected into tubes, homogenized with a 28G syringe, and incubated at 37 °C for 10 min, followed by centrifugation at 300 × g at room temperature to remove insoluble particles. The lysate was centrifuged at 100,000 × g at 37 °C for 1 h to precipitate F-actin and to separate the G-actin that remained soluble in the supernatant. The pellet containing F-actin was resuspended and dissociated with 10 μM cytochalasin D (Sigma-Aldrich, St. Louis, MO, USA). Both fractions were resolved by SDS-PAGE and probed with an anti-β-actin antibody. The ratio of F-actin over G-actin was determined and analyzed by Student's t-test.

2.9. Statistical Analysis

All data were normalized to those of inner controls, such as housekeeping peptidylpropyl isomerase B (PPIB) expression level. Data are presented as mean ± standard error of the mean (SEM.). Statistically significant changes amongst treatments were assessed by Student t tests at $\alpha = 0.05$.

3. Results

3.1. Vitamin C Inhibits the Invasion of TNBC Cells

Our earlier work showed that oral vitamin C supplementation alone did not affect the growth of MDA-MB-231 xenografts but significantly inhibited metastasis to the liver in NOD severe combined immune deficiency (scid) gamma (NSG) mice [9]. To verify the effect of vitamin C on TNBC metastasis, we conducted an in vitro invasion assay. MDA-MB-231 and BT-549 TNBC cells were pretreated with vitamin C (0, 50, 100 μM) for 3 days and then seeded into invasion chambers. In the presence of different doses of vitamin C, the cells were allowed to invade for two additional days. The number of invading cells were significantly decreased ($p < 0.001$) for both MDA-MB-231 and BT-549 cells treated with vitamin C, as shown by imaging (Figure 1A) and quantification (Figure 1B). Vitamin C at 100 μM further decreased the number of MDA-MB-231 invading cells compared to 50 μM. To test if TET-mediated DNA demethylation is involved in the effect of vitamin C on cell invasion, TETs were silenced in MDA-MB-231 cells by siRNA. Vitamin C only moderately inhibited the invasion of cells transfected with TETs siRNA, while it markedly blocked the invasion of cells transfected with scramble siRNA (Figure S1). These results suggest that TETs could partially mediate the effect of vitamin C on TNBC metastasis.

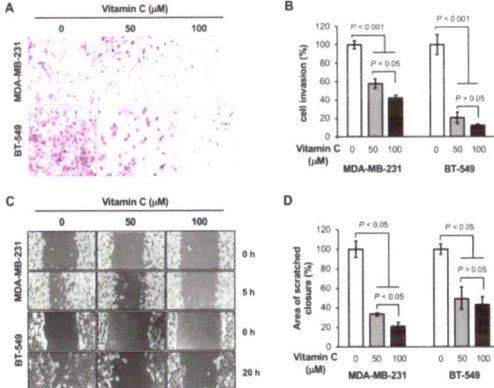

Figure 1. Vitamin C blocks the invasion and migration of triple-negative breast cancer (TNBC) cells. (**A,B**) Representative images and quantification show that vitamin C treatment inhibits the invasion of MDA-MB-231 and BT549 cells; (**C,D**) representative images and quantification show that vitamin C treatment delays the migration of MDA-MB-231 and BT-549 cells.

To further validate the effect of vitamin C on TNBC metastasis, a scratch assay was performed. As shown in Figure 1C,D, vitamin C treatment inhibited the migration of both MDA-MB-231 and BT-549 cells after scratching ($p < 0.05$). Vitamin C at 100 μM further blocked migration of MDA-MB-231 cells compared to the concentration of 50 μM. A cell survival assay was then performed to examine if the effect of vitamin C on invasion and migration was influenced by cell growth. Treatment with vitamin C (50 or 100 μM) did not significantly change the growth of the two TNBC cell lines (Figure S2). Overall, these results suggest that vitamin C at 100 μM, a concentration achievable in the plasma in vivo by oral supplementation, blocks the migration and invasion of TNBC cells in vitro, confirming the inhibitory effect of oral vitamin C on TNBC metastasis in vivo [6,9].

3.2. The Level of HIF-1α Protein is Not Altered in TNBC Cells by Vitamin C Treatment

HIF-1α is the master regulator of metastasis, and vitamin C promotes HIF-1α degradation [2], suggesting that vitamin C could inhibit metastasis by decreasing HIF-1α protein level. Even under normal cell culture condition (5% CO_2 atmosphere), the transcripts of HIF-1α were relatively highly expressed in MDA-MB-231 cells, and their expression increased by ~1.5-fold after vitamin C (100 µM) treatment for 3 days on the basis of our published RNA-seq data [4]. Subsequently qRT-PCR showed that HIF-1α RNA level was indeed increased in MDA-MB-231 cells by ~1.5-fold after treatment with 100 µM vitamin C for 5 days ($p < 0.05$, Figure 2A). However, no obvious changes were detected in HIF-1α protein level after this latter vitamin C treatment, as shown by immunoblotting (Figure 2B,C) and immunofluorescence (Figure 2D,E). The housekeeper protein PPIB was used as a loading control. We then examined MDA-MB-231 xenografts collected in our previous study, which showed that oral vitamin C supplementation alone inhibited metastasis to the liver of mice [9]. We found that HIF-1α immunostaining remained at a similar level in MDA-MB-231 xenografts collected from mice supplemented with or without vitamin C (3.3 g/L in the drinking water, Figure 2F,G). These results suggest that vitamin C supplementation does not alter the level of HIF-1α protein in TNBC cells, which may be explained by the counteractions of an increased transcription and enhanced degradation by vitamin C.

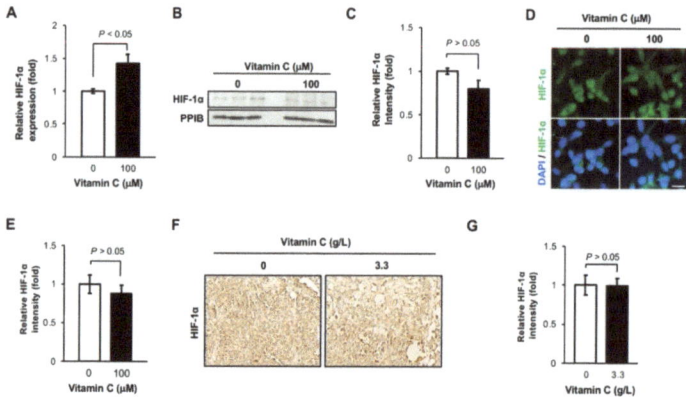

Figure 2. Hypoxia-inducible factor 1α (HIF-1α) protein level remains largely unchanged after vitamin C treatment. (**A**) qRT-PCR shows that HIF-1α RNA is increased in MDA-MB-231 cells after vitamin C treatment for 5 days; (**B,C**) HIF-1α protein level remains unchanged in MDA-MB-231 cells after vitamin C treatment, as shown by immunoblotting and semi-quantification; (**D,E**) no obvious changes are found in HIF-1α immunofluorescence in MDA-MB-231 cells after vitamin C treatment, as shown by imaging and semi-quantification. Bar = 20 µM; (**F,G**) immunostaining (40×) and semi-quantification show no differences in HIF-1α expression in MDA-MB-231 xenografts from NOD combined immune deficiency (scid) gamma (NSG) mice administered or not vitamin C (3.3 g/L) in the drinking water.

3.3. Vitamin C Increases Synaptopodin 2 Expression in TNBC Cells

No obvious changes in HIF-1α protein level after vitamin C treatment indicated that other genes, at least within the transcriptome, could underpin the observed reduced TNBC metastasis. By reviewing the known genes involved in breast cancer metastasis [15–17] and our available MDA-MB-231 cell RNA-seq data [4], we identified synaptopodin 2 (SYNPO2), with a known function in metastasis, which showed the highest fold change (2.05-fold increase) in MDA-MB-231 cells after vitamin C treatment. Studies have shown that breast cancer has a reduced amount of SYNPO2, which is associated with higher TNBC metastasis and lower patient survival [18]. Using qRT-PCR, we found that the RNA level of SYNPO2 was elevated in MDA-MB-231 cells after vitamin C (100 µM) treatment for 5 days ($p < 0.05$, Figure 3A). The upregulated expression of SYNPO2 after this vitamin C treatment was then verified at the protein level by immunofluorescence ($p < 0.05$, Figure 3B,C). Furthermore, SYNPO2 expression was also higher in MDA-MB-231 xenografts from mice administered vitamin C (3.3 g/L) compared to mice receiving water without vitamin C (Figure 3D,E). Collectively, these results suggest that vitamin C upregulates the expression of SYNPO2, which is known to inhibit TNBC metastasis.

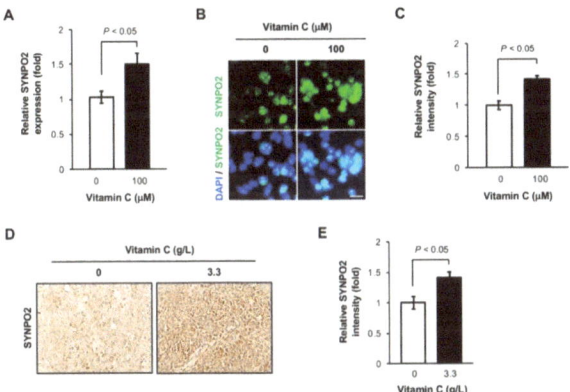

Figure 3. Vitamin C upregulates the expression of synaptopodin (SYNPO2). (**A**) SYNPO2 RNA is increased in MDA-MB-231 cells after treatment with vitamin C for 5 days, as shown by qRT-PCR; (**B**,**C**) immunofluorescence and semi-quantification show increased SYNPO2 protein level in MDA-MB-231 cells after vitamin C treatment. Bar = 20 µM; (**D**,**E**) the level of SYNPO2 protein is higher in MDA-MB-231 xenografts from NSG mice supplemented with vitamin C (3.3 g/L) compared to mice without supplementation, as shown by immunostaining (40×) and semi-quantification.

3.4. Vitamin C Decreases YAP1 Expression in TNBC Cells

SYNPO2 has been found to suppress metastasis by inhibiting the activity of the transcriptional coactivator YAP1, also known as yes-associated protein 1 [19]. As a key regulator in the Hippo pathway, YAP1 promotes focal adhesion formation and metastasis [20]. By inquiring our RNA-seq data, we found that YAP1 was downregulated in MDA-MB-231 cells by vitamin C (100 µM) treatment. qRT-PCR validated the downregulation of YAP1 in MDA-MB-231 cells after treatment with vitamin C (100 µM) for 5 days ($p < 0.05$, Figure 4A). Subsequently, immunoblotting and immunofluorescence analyses showed that the protein level of YAP1 was also reduced in MDA-MB-231 cells after the same treatment ($p < 0.05$, Figure 4B–E). It is known that YAP1 shuttles into the nucleus and promotes the transcription of genes responsible for metastasis [21]. We then evaluated the subcellular location of YAP1 by comparing its immunofluorescence signal in the nucleus with the its overall signal. The results showed that vitamin C treatment decreased the ratio of YAP1 in the nucleus, suggesting the inhibition of YAP1 nuclear translocation (Figure S3). Further experiments confirmed that there was a significant YAP1 expression decrease in MDA-MB-231 xenografts from mice supplemented with vitamin C (Figure 4F,G). Taken together, these results suggest that vitamin C treatment inhibits the expression of YAP1, which may underpin at least partially the observed reduced TNBC metastasis.

3.5. Vitamin C Reduces Lamellipodia in MDA-MB-231 Cells

YAP1 promotes metastasis by regulating actin dynamics [14], which involves the assembly of filamentous actin (F-actin) from monomeric actin (G-actin) to form lamellipodia to the advantage of cell motility [22,23]. To understand how vitamin C blocks metastasis, we first examined the impact of vitamin C on F-actin and lamellipodia, which were visualized by phalloidin labeling. After vitamin C treatment, we observed an obvious reduction in lamellipodia compared with non-treated cells (Figure 5A,B). We then evaluated the ratio of F-actin over G-actin to examine if vitamin C changed the assembly of actin. There was a significant reduction of the F-actin/G-actin ratio after vitamin C treatment (Figure 5C,D). These results indicate that vitamin C treatment inhibits the formation of

F-actin and lamellipodia, which is correlated with the upregulation of *SYNPO2* and the downregulation of *YAP1*. These events could underlie at least partially the action of vitamin C on TNBC cell invasion in vitro and xenograft metastasis in vivo.

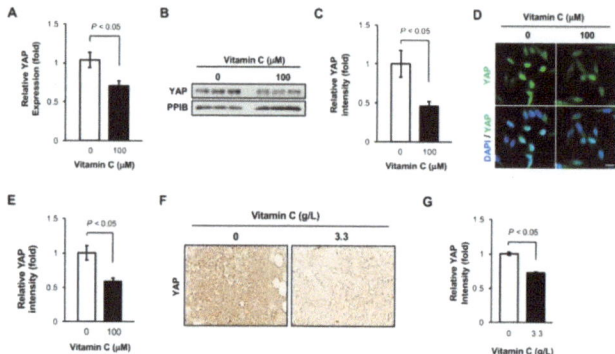

Figure 4. Vitamin C downregulates yes-associated protein 1 (*YAP1*) expression. (**A**) q-RT-PCR shows that *YAP1* RNA level is decreased in MDA-MB-231 cells after treatment with vitamin C; (**B,C**) immunoblot and semi-quantification show decreased *YAP1* protein in MDA-MB-231 cells after vitamin C treatment; (**D,E**) vitamin C treatment reduces *YAP1* immunofluorescence signal in MDA-MB-231 cells, as shown by imaging and semi-quantification. Bar = 20 µM; (**F,G**) The level of *YAP1* protein is lower in MDA-MB-231 xenografts from NSG mice supplemented with vitamin C (3.3 g/L) compared to mice without supplementation, as shown by immunostaining (40×) and semi-quantification.

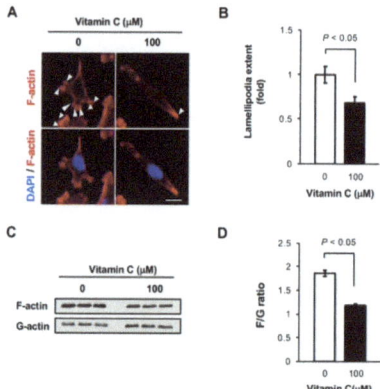

Figure 5. Vitamin C inhibits the formation of F-actin and lamellipodia. (**A,B**) Vitamin C treatment reduces F-actin assembly, labeled by phalloidin, and lamellipodia (arrow heads) in MDA-MB-231 cells, as shown by imaging and semi-quantification; (**C,D**) the F-actin/G-actin ratio is decreased after vitamin C treatment for 5 days, as shown by immunoblot of fractionated MDA-MB-231 cell samples and semi-quantification.

4. Discussion

Inadequate vitamin C intake has been associated with the risk of breast cancer and the mortality of breast cancer patients. For instance, a meta-analysis of 17,696 patients showed a statistically significant association between the use of vitamin C supplements and reduced mortality [24]. The downregulated expression of SVCT2 in breast cancer could underpin the requirement of additional vitamin C supplementation in breast cancer patients [4]. While vitamin C can be administered orally or by intravenous infusion or intraperitoneal injection, oral vitamin C is easily accessible and more convenient for patients. Possibly due to the difficulty to control vitamin C consumption quantitatively in human subjects, the benefit of oral vitamin C against breast cancer metastasis has remained unclear in patient care. TNBC is often associated with early metastasis and short overall survival [10]. In animal models, oral vitamin C supplementation has been shown to inhibit TNBC metastasis to other organs [6,9], indicating the benefit of oral vitamin C for TNBC metastasis inhibition and calling for further examination of the molecular mechanisms by which vitamin C blocks metastasis.

Intratumoral hypoxia, a common condition in cancer, triggers the expression of HIF-1α which in turn initiates the progression of breast cancer toward metastasis [25]. HIF-1α is thus a prime candidate to mediate the inhibition of TNBC metastasis by vitamin C, because of its known role in HIF-1α hydroxylation and further degradation [2]. However, our results showed that vitamin C does not change the overall HIF-1α protein level. This likely results from the combined effects of enhanced degradation of HIF-1α and upregulated transcription of HIF-1α by vitamin C treatment. It was shown that the transcription of HIF-1α is enhanced by KDM4C-mediated histone demethylation, such as of H3K9me3 and H3K9me2, as well as by TET-1-mediated DNA demethylation [26,27], both of which can be promoted by vitamin C, which thus serves as a cofactor for these iron- and 2-oxoglutarate-dependent demethylases [12]. Therefore, vitamin C increases HIF-1α transcription on one hand and augments HIF-1α protein degradation on the other hand, which results in a largely unaltered HIF-1α protein level, as we discovered in cultured TNBC cells and xenografts. Overall, HIF-1α unlikely mediates the role of vitamin C in blocking TNBC metastasis.

Oral vitamin C administration can easily maintain the plasma level of vitamin C at 100 μM, a concentration which markedly inhibited TNBC xenograft metastasis in vivo [6,9] and TNBC cell invasion in vitro, as shown above. Loss of 5-hydroxymethylcytosine (5hmC) is an epigenetic hallmark of breast cancer and other cancers [28]. Treatment with vitamin C at 100 μM restored 5hmC content in TNBC cells toward the level of non-cancerous breast epithelial cells and shifted the transcriptome [4]. We found that after silencing TETs, vitamin C less effectively inhibited TNBC invasion, suggesting that TETs-mediated DNA demethylation is likely involved in the action of vitamin C on TNBC metastasis. In addition to TET-mediated DNA demethylation, vitamin C can modulate transcription in TNBC cells by enhancing histone deacetylation, as shown in our earlier work [9], and potentially histone demethylation as well. Some of the genes whose expression was altered by vitamin C could in principle underpin the action of vitamin C on metastasis. In this study, we examined *SYNPO2*, which whose expression in MDA-MB-231 cells was most significantly changed by vitamin C treatment, and subsequently its related partner *YAP1*. Both proteins are key players in the Hippo pathway and have known functions in metastasis formation, consistently with the changes we observed in cultured TNBC cells and xenografts after vitamin C treatment. Activation of *YAP1* promotes F-actin assembly and lamellipodia formation, which are essential to cell mobility and invasion [19]. Our results show that vitamin C treatment downregulates the expression of *YAP1* and upregulates that of *SYNPO2*, which further inhibits the activity of *YAP1*. Subsequently, vitamin C treatment inhibits both F-actin assembly and lamellipodia formation, which correlates with the changes in *YAP1* and *SYNPO2* and likely underpin the effect of vitamin C, at least partially, on TNBC invasion and metastasis.

5. Conclusions

In summary, vitamin C inhibits TNBC metastasis independently of HIF-1α and, likely, by affecting the expression of *YAP1* and *SYNPO2*, two genes in the Hippo pathway which regulate cell mobility and cancer metastasis. These results suggest a potential role of oral vitamin C supplementation in the prevention and treatment of TNBC metastasis.

Supplementary Materials: The following are available online at http://www.mdpi.com/2072-6643/11/12/2997/s1, Figure S1: The inhibition of TNBC cell invasion by vitamin C is partially abolished by TETs siRNA; Figure S2: Vitamin C (100 μM) does not affect TNBC cell proliferation; Figure S3: Vitamin C increases YAP1 nuclear translocation.

Author Contributions: G.W. conceived, designed, and supervised the study. L.G. executed most of cell-based assays. V.C. examined xenografts and assisted in statistical analysis. S.M. conducted the invasion assays. G.W. and L.G. drafted the manuscript. All authors edited, commented and approved the final manuscript.

Funding: This research was funded by Florida Breast Cancer Foundation, Florida Academic Cancer Center Alliance (FACCA), and Sylvester Comprehensive Cancer Center at the University of Miami.

Acknowledgments: L.G. acknowledges gratefully the support by the China Scholarship Council.

Conflicts of Interest: The authors declare no conflict of interest

References

1. Rankin, E.B.; Giaccia, A.J. Hypoxic control of metastasis. *Science* **2016**, *352*, 175–180. [CrossRef] [PubMed]
2. Knowles, H.J.; Raval, R.R.; Harris, A.L.; Ratcliffe, P.J. Effect of ascorbate on the activity of hypoxia-inducible factor in cancer cells. *Cancer Res.* **2003**, *63*, 1764–1768. [PubMed]
3. Linster, C.L.; Van Schaftingen, E. Vitamin C Biosynthesis, recycling and degradation in mammals. *FEBS J.* **2007**, *274*, 1–22. [CrossRef] [PubMed]
4. Sant, D.W.; Mustafi, S.; Gustafson, C.B.; Chen, J.; Slingerland, J.M.; Wang, G. Vitamin C promotes apoptosis in breast cancer cells by increasing TRAIL expression. *Sci. Rep.* **2018**, *8*, 5306. [CrossRef]
5. Spielholz, C.; Golde, D.W.; Houghton, A.N.; Nualart, F.; Vera, J.C. Increased facilitated transport of dehydroascorbic acid without changes in sodium-dependent ascorbate transport in human melanoma cells. *Cancer Res.* **1997**, *57*, 2529–2537.
6. Cha, J.; Roomi, M.W.; Ivanov, V.; Kalinovsky, T.; Niedzwiecki, A.; Rath, M. Ascorbate supplementation inhibits growth and metastasis of B16FO melanoma and 4T1 breast cancer cells in vitamin C-deficient mice. *Int. J. Oncol.* **2013**, *42*, 55–64. [CrossRef]
7. Zeng, L.H.; Wang, Q.M.; Feng, L.Y.; Ke, Y.D.; Xu, Q.Z.; Wei, A.Y.; Zhang, C.; Ying, R.B. High-dose vitamin C suppresses the invasion and metastasis of breast cancer cells viainhibiting epithelial-mesenchymal transition. *OncoTargets Ther.* **2019**, *12*, 7405–7413.
8. Tsao, C.S.; Leung, P.Y.; Young, M. Effect of dietary ascorbic acid intake on tissue vitamin C in mice. *J. Nutr.* **1987**, *117*, 291–297.
9. Mustafi, S.; Camarena, V.; Qureshi, R.; Yoon, H.; Volmar, C.H.; Huff, T.C.; Sant, D.W.; Zheng, L.; Brothers, S.P.; Wahlestedt, C.; et al. Vitamin C supplementation expands the therapeutic window of BETi for triple negative breast cancer. *EBioMedicine* **2019**, *43*, 201–210. [CrossRef]
10. Pal, S.K.; Childs, B.H.; Pegram, M. Triple negative breast cancer: Unmet medical needs. *Breast Cancer Res. Treat.* **2011**, *125*, 627–636. [CrossRef]
11. Levine, M.; Padayatty, S.J.; Espey, M.G. Vitamin C: A concentration-function approach yields pharmacology and therapeuticdiscoveries. *Adv. Nutr.* **2011**, *2*, 78–88. [CrossRef] [PubMed]
12. Young, J.I.; Züchner, S.; Wang, G. Regulation of the Epigenome by Vitamin C. *Annu. Rev. Nutr.* **2015**, *35*, 545–564. [CrossRef] [PubMed]
13. Xie, Y.; Wolff, D.W.; Wei, T.; Wang, B.; Deng, C.; Kirui, J.K.; Jiang, H.; Qin, J.; Abel, P.W.; Tu, Y. Breast cancer migration and invasion depend on proteasome degradation of regulator of G-protein signaling 4. *Cancer Res.* **2009**, *69*, 5743–5751. [CrossRef] [PubMed]
14. Qiao, Y.; Chen, J.; Lim, Y.B.; Finch-Edmondson, M.L.; Seshachalam, V.P.; Qin, L.; Jiang, T.; Low, B.C.; Singh, H.; Lim, C.T.; et al. YAP Regulates Actin Dynamics through ARHGAP29 and Promotes Metastasis. *Cell Rep.* **2017**, *19*, 1495–1502. [CrossRef]
15. Minn, A.J.; Gupta, G.P.; Siegel, P.M.; Bos, P.D.; Shu, W.; Giri, D.D.; Viale, A.; Olshen, A.B.; Gerald, W.L.; Massagué, J. Genes that mediate breast cancer metastasis to lung. *Nature* **2005**, *436*, 518–524. [CrossRef]
16. Daves, M.H.; Hilsenbeck, S.G.; Lau, C.C.; Man, T.K. Meta-analysis of multiple microarray datasets reveals a common gene signature of metastasis in solid tumors. *BMC Med. Genom.* **2011**, *4*, 56. [CrossRef]
17. Hartung, F.; Wang, Y.; Aronow, B.; Weber, G.F. A core program of gene expression characterizes cancer metastases. *Oncotarget* **2017**, *8*, 60.
18. Jing, L.; Liu, L.; Yu, Y.P. Expression of myopodin induces suppression of tumor growth and metastasis. *Am. J. Pathol.* **2004**, *164*, 1799–1806. [CrossRef]

19. Liu, J.; Ye, L.; Li, Q.; Wu, X.; Wang, B.; Ouyang, Y.; Yuan, Z.; Li, J.; Lin, C. Synaptopodin-2 suppresses metastasis of triple-negative breast cancer via inhibition of YAP/TAZ activity. *J. Pathol.* **2018**, *244*, 71–83. [CrossRef]
20. Abylkassov, R.; Xie, Y. Role of Yes-associated protein in cancer: An update. *Oncol. Lett.* **2016**, *12*, 2277–2282. [CrossRef]
21. Nair, P.R.; Wirtz, D. Enabling migration by moderation: YAP/TAZ are essential for persistent migration. *J. Cell Biol.* **2019**, *218*, 1092–1093. [CrossRef]
22. Raz-Ben Aroush, D.; Ofer, N.; Abu-Shah, E.; Allard, J.; Krichevsky, O.; Mogilner, A.; Keren, K. Actin Turnover in Lamellipodial Fragments. *Curr. Biol.* **2017**, *27*, 2963–2973. [CrossRef]
23. Gardel, M.L.; Schneider, I.C.; Aratyn-Schaus, Y.; Waterman, C.M. Mechanical integration of actin and adhesion dynamics in cell migration. *Annu. Rev. Cell Dev. Biol.* **2010**, *26*, 315–333. [CrossRef]
24. Harris, H.R.; Bergkvist, L.; Wolk, A. Vitamin C intake and breast cancer mortality in a cohort of Swedish women. *Br. J. Cancer* **2013**, *109*, 257–264. [CrossRef]
25. Semenza, G.L. The hypoxic tumor microenvironment: A driving force for breast cancer progression. *Biochim. Biophys. Acta.* **2016**, *1863*, 382–391. [CrossRef]
26. Luo, W.; Chang, R.; Zhong, J.; Pandey, A.; Semenza, G.L. Histone demethylase JMJD2C is a coactivator for hypoxia-inducible factor 1 that is required for breast cancer progression. *Proc. Natl. Acad. Sci. USA* **2012**, *109*, E3367–E3376. [CrossRef]
27. Tsai, Y.P.; Chen, H.F.; Chen, S.Y.; Cheng, W.C.; Wang, H.W.; Shen, Z.J.; Song, C.; Teng, S.C.; He, C.; Wu, K.J. TET1 regulates hypoxia-induced epithelial-mesenchymal transition by acting as a co-activator. *Genome Biol.* **2014**, *15*, 513. [CrossRef]
28. Hsu, C.H.; Peng, K.L.; Kang, M.L.; Chen, Y.R.; Yang, Y.C.; Tsai, C.H.; Chu, C.S.; Jeng, Y.M.; Chen, Y.T.; Lin, F.M.; et al. TET1 suppresses cancer invasion by activating the tissue inhibitors of metalloproteinases. *Cell Rep.* **2012**, *2*, 568–579. [CrossRef]

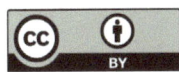

© 2019 by the authors. Licensee MDPI, Basel, Switzerland. This article is an open access article distributed under the terms and conditions of the Creative Commons Attribution (CC BY) license (http://creativecommons.org/licenses/by/4.0/).

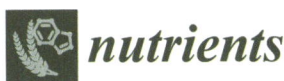

Article

Patients Undergoing Myeloablative Chemotherapy and Hematopoietic Stem Cell Transplantation Exhibit Depleted Vitamin C Status in Association with Febrile Neutropenia

Anitra C. Carr [1,*], Emma Spencer [1], Andrew Das [2], Natalie Meijer [3], Carolyn Lauren [3], Sean MacPherson [3] and Stephen T. Chambers [4]

1. Nutrition in Medicine Research Group, Department of Pathology and Biomedical Science, University of Otago, Christchurch 8011, New Zealand; emma.spencer@otago.ac.nz
2. Centre for Free Radical Research, Department of Pathology and Biomedical Science, University of Otago, Christchurch 8011, New Zealand; andrew.das@otago.ac.nz
3. Department of Haematology, Christchurch Hospital, Christchurch 8011, New Zealand; natalie.meijer@cdhb.health.nz (N.M.); carolyn.lauren@cdhb.health.nz (C.L.); sean.macpherson@cdhb.health.nz (S.M.)
4. The Infection Group, Department of Pathology and Biomedical Science, University of Otago, Christchurch 8011, New Zealand; steve.chambers@otago.ac.nz
* Correspondence: anitra.carr@otago.ac.nz; Tel.: +643-364-0649

Received: 26 May 2020; Accepted: 20 June 2020; Published: 24 June 2020

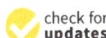

Abstract: Patients undergoing myeloablative chemotherapy and hematopoietic stem cell transplantation (HSCT) experience profound neutropenia and vulnerability to infection. Previous research has indicated that patients with infections have depleted vitamin C status. In this study, we recruited 38 patients with hematopoietic cancer who were undergoing conditioning chemotherapy and HSCT. Blood samples were collected prior to transplantation, at one week, two weeks and four weeks following transplantation. Vitamin C status and biomarkers of inflammation (C-reactive protein) and oxidative stress (protein carbonyls and thiobarbituric acid reactive substances) were assessed in association with febrile neutropenia. The vitamin C status of the study participants decreased from 44 ± 7 µmol/L to 29 ± 5 µmol/L by week one ($p = 0.001$) and 19 ± 6 µmol/L by week two ($p < 0.001$), by which time all of the participants had undergone a febrile episode. By week four, vitamin C status had increased to 37 ± 10 µmol/L ($p = 0.1$). Pre-transplantation, the cohort comprised 19% with hypovitaminosis C (i.e., <23 µmol/L) and 8% with deficiency (i.e., <11 µmol/L). At week one, those with hypovitaminosis C had increased to 38%, and at week two, 72% had hypovitaminosis C, and 34% had outright deficiency. C-reactive protein concentrations increased from 3.5 ± 1.8 mg/L to 20 ± 11 mg/L at week one ($p = 0.002$), and 119 ± 25 mg/L at week two ($p < 0.001$), corresponding to the development of febrile neutropenia in the patients. By week four, these values had dropped to 17 ± 8 mg/L ($p < 0.001$). There was a significant inverse correlation between C-reactive protein concentrations and vitamin C status ($r = -0.424$, $p < 0.001$). Lipid oxidation (thiobarbituric acid reactive substances (TBARS)) increased significantly from 2.0 ± 0.3 µmol/L at baseline to 3.3 ± 0.6 µmol/L by week one ($p < 0.001$), and remained elevated at week two ($p = 0.003$), returning to baseline concentrations by week four ($p = 0.3$). Overall, the lowest mean vitamin C values (recorded at week two) corresponded with the highest mean C-reactive protein values and lowest mean neutrophil counts. Thus, depleted vitamin C status in the HSCT patients coincides with febrile neutropenia and elevated inflammation and oxidative stress.

Keywords: vitamin C; ascorbate; ascorbic acid; immune compromised; conditioning chemotherapy; hematopoietic stem cell transplantation; inflammation; C-reactive protein; febrile neutropenia; oxidative stress

1. Introduction

Hematopoietic stem cell transplantation (HSCT), using stem cells derived from bone marrow or peripheral blood, is reserved for patients with life-threatening diseases such as hematopoietic malignancies (e.g., leukemia, lymphoma, and myeloma). Disease free survival is low, with recurrence of underlying disease the main cause of death post-transplant [1]. HSCT has major treatment-related complications. Patients are typically treated with high-dose chemotherapy, with or without radiotherapy, to destroy the bone marrow's ability to produce new blood cells, called myeloablative conditioning. Allogeneic transplant recipients also require immunosuppressive agents to prevent rejection of the donor stem cells. Infection is a common complication of both myeloablative conditioning and immunosuppressive agents.

Vitamin C is an essential nutrient with antioxidant and anti-inflammatory properties [2]. Since the middle of the last century, it has been known that patients with hematological cancers have significantly lower vitamin C status than healthy controls [3,4]; findings which have been confirmed in more recent case-control studies [5–7]. The reasons for these differences are uncertain, although elevated biomarkers of oxidative stress have been detected in patients with hematological cancer compared with healthy controls [6,7]. Myeloablative chemotherapy causes oxidative stress, inflammation, and tissue damage, which contribute to common side effects such as gastrointestinal mucositis [8–10]. Vitamin C concentrations have been shown to drop dramatically following conditioning chemotherapy [11–13]. These values continued to decline by week two and took at least one month to recover to pre-chemotherapy concentrations [12,13].

An explanation for the continued decrease in vitamin C status two weeks following myeloablative conditioning is acute infection developing in the presence of neutropenia (febrile neutropenia). Our previous research has indicated that depleted vitamin C status and enhanced biomarkers of oxidative stress (protein carbonyls) are frequently found in patients with severe infections [14,15]. Elevated oxidative stress may be both a cause and a consequence of the low vitamin C status of these patients. We also observed an association between depleted vitamin C status and elevated C-reactive protein, a marker of infection severity [16]. Similarly, Nannya and colleagues observed an inverse correlation between vitamin C and C-reactive protein in 15 patients undergoing allogeneic stem cell transplantation [12]. Thus, development of infection in the immune-compromised patients may contribute to further inflammation and oxidative stress and result in additional loss of vitamin C. Therefore, we tested this hypothesis in a cohort of HSCT recipients undergoing myeloablative conditioning by measuring vitamin C status in association with febrile neutropenia and markers of inflammation and oxidative stress.

2. Materials and Methods

2.1. Study Participants

Patients undergoing myeloablative conditioning and HSCT were recruited for this observational study (July 2017 to June 2018). All patients were cared for by the Hematology Department of Christchurch Hospital, a tertiary referral hospital servicing more than 600,000 people. Ethical approval was obtained from the New Zealand Southern Health and Disability Ethics Committee (#16STH235). All patients aged ≥18 years who were undergoing autologous or allogeneic transplants and able to provide signed informed consent were eligible. Patient data collected included the following: demographics (age, sex, ethnicity); hematological cancer diagnosis (multiple myeloma, Hodgkin and non-Hodgkin lymphoma, acute myeloid leukemia); transplant type (autologous or allogeneic); and conditioning chemotherapy regimen. Other data collected included the following: comorbidities; febrile episodes using Systemic Inflammatory Response Syndrome (SIRS) criteria (tachycardia (heart rate > 90 beats/min), tachypnea (respiratory rate > 20 breaths/min), and fever (temperature > 38 °C)); neutropenia (neutrophil counts < 1.5×10^9/L); type and dose of antimicrobial agents used; blood culture information; and whether the patient was taking vitamin C-containing supplements or receiving enteral or parenteral nutrition, including type and dose.

2.2. Blood Sampling and Processing

Blood samples were collected the day prior to transplant (baseline, week 0), seven days later (week 1), at day 10–14 (week 2), when the patients were exhibiting febrile neutropenia, and at approximately day 28 (week 4). The non-fasting blood samples (with heparin anticoagulant) were placed on ice and immediately transferred to the laboratory for centrifugation to separate plasma for vitamin C and oxidative stress biomarker analysis. An aliquot of the plasma was treated with an equal volume of 0.54 M perchloric acid and 100 µmol/L of the metal chelator diethylenetriamine-pentaacetic acid (DTPA) to precipitate protein and stabilize the vitamin C. The supernatant and spare plasma samples were stored at −80 °C until analysis.

2.3. Analysis of Blood Analytes

Routine hematological, kidney function, and liver function tests were carried out at Canterbury Health Laboratories, an International Accreditation New Zealand (IANZ) laboratory. C-reactive protein concentrations were assessed using endpoint nephelometry. The vitamin C content of the processed plasma samples was determined using HPLC with electrochemical detection, as described previously [17]. Systemic protein oxidation was determined by measuring plasma protein carbonyl content using a sensitive ELISA method, as described previously [18]. Plasma lipid oxidation was measured using the thiobarbituric acid reactive substances (TBARS) assay [19]. Fluorometric detection at 540 nm excitation and 590 nm emission provided greater sensitivity and specificity than spectrophotometric detection at 532 nm. Icteric samples were excluded from TBARS analyses due to interference [20].

2.4. Statistical Analysis

Data are presented as mean and *SD* or mean and 95% CI, as indicated. Statistical analyses were carried out using Microsoft Excel data analysis add-in (Microsoft, Auckland, NZ) and GraphPad Prism 8.0 software (Graphpad, San Diego, CA, USA). Differences between groups were determined using Student's *t*-test or Mann–Whitney U test for non-parametric variables. Linear regression analyses were carried out using Pearson correlations. Statistical significance was set at $p < 0.05$.

3. Results

3.1. Participant Characteristics

We recruited 38 patients undergoing conditioning chemotherapy and HSCT. The participant characteristics are indicated in Table 1 below. Of the total cohort, 88% identified as European and 12% as Māori. The predominant diagnoses were multiple myeloma and lymphoma, with a majority of the patients undergoing autologous transplant. Melphalan monotherapy was used for patients with multiple myeloma and carmustine combination therapy for patients with lymphoma.

Table 1. Participant characteristics.

Characteristic	Total Cohort ($n = 38$)
Age, years [1]	57 (8)
Male sex, n (%)	22 (58)
Diagnosis, n (%)	
Multiple myeloma	23 (61)
Lymphoma	12 (32)
Acute myeloid leukemia	3 (8)
Transplant, n (%)	
Autologous	32 (86)
Allogeneic	5 (14)
Conditioning regimen, n (%)	
Melphalan	23 (61)
Carmustine, Cytarabine, Etoposide, Melphalan	8 (22)
Carmustine, Thiotepa	1 (3)
Alemtuzumab, Fludarabine, Melphalan	1 (3)
Fludarabine, Cytarabine, Amsacrine, Busulfan, Anti-thymocyte globulin	1 (3)

[1] Data is presented as mean (SD) unless specified otherwise.

3.2. Vitamin C Status of Study Participants

The vitamin C status of the non-fasting participants pre-transplantation was 44 ± 7 µmol/L (Figure 1). This dropped to 29 ± 5 µmol/L one week following transplantation ($p = 0.001$); three of the participants had developed febrile neutropenia. Vitamin C concentrations dropped further to 19 ± 6 µmol/L another week later ($p < 0.001$), by which time all but one of the participants had developed febrile neutropenia. By week four, the vitamin C status of the participants had started to recover (38 ± 10 µmol/L) and was no longer significantly different to the pre-transplantation values ($p = 0.1$).

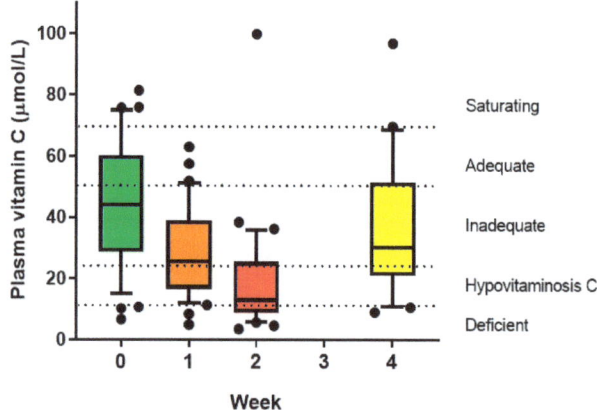

Figure 1. Vitamin C status of individuals undergoing myeloablative conditioning and hematopoietic stem cell transplantation (HSCT). Box plots show median with 25th and 75th percentiles as boundaries, and whiskers are the 10th and 90th percentiles, with symbols indicating outlying data points. Vitamin C category cut-offs are indicated by dotted lines. The mean values for weeks 1 and 2 were significantly lower than baseline ($p \leq 0.001$).

One of the participants (with multiple myeloma, treated with melphalan and autologous transplant) had unusually high vitamin C status (~100 µmol/L) at weeks two and four follow-up; the reason for this is unknown, as the patient did not report any vitamin C supplementation during this period.

Of note, this was the only patient who did not experience an episode of febrile neutropenia (neutrophil counts at week two were 2.2×10^9/L, and temperature and heart rate did not meet SIRS criteria).

Pre-transplantation, 53% of the patients had an inadequate vitamin C status (i.e., <50 µmol/L), 19% had hypovitaminosis C (i.e., <23 µmol/L), and 8% had vitamin C deficiency (i.e., <11 µmol/L) (Figure 2). One week post-transplantation, the number of patients with inadequate status had increased to 88% and those with hypovitaminosis C to 38%. Another week later, when all but one of the patients had developed febrile neutropenia, 72% had hypovitaminosis C and 34% had outright vitamin C deficiency. Although there was a decrease in these values by week four, to 75% with inadequate vitamin C status, 30% with hypovitaminosis C, and 10% with vitamin C deficiency, these were still higher than baseline values.

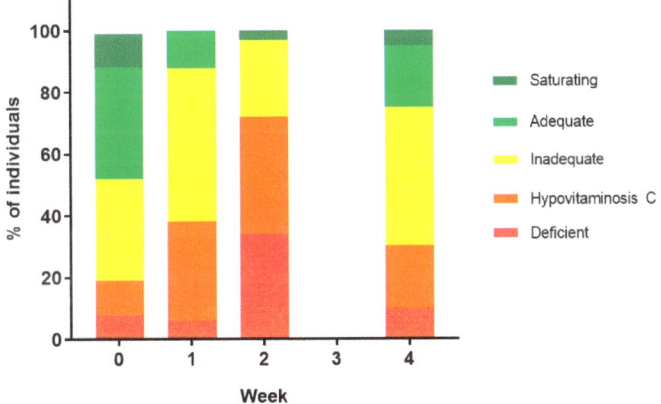

Figure 2. Percentage of individuals in different vitamin C categories. Vitamin C categories are presented as follows: saturating (>70 µmol/L), adequate (>50 µmol/L), inadequate (<50 µmol/L), hypovitaminosis C (<23 µmol/L), and deficient (<11 µmol/L).

3.3. C-Reactive Protein Concentrations Relative to Vitamin C Status

C-reactive protein mean plasma concentrations increased from 4 ± 2 mg/L (normal < 3 mg/L) at baseline to 20 ± 11 mg/L one week following transplantation ($p = 0.002$; Figure 3a). By week two, there was a large increase in mean C-reactive protein concentrations (119 ± 25 mg/L, $p < 0.001$), corresponding to development of febrile neutropenia in the patients (Table 2). By week four, these values had dropped to 17 ± 8 mg/L, although these were still significantly higher than baseline values ($p < 0.001$). There was an inverse correlation between C-reactive protein concentrations and vitamin C status, with higher vitamin C corresponding to lower C-reactive protein ($r = -0.424$, $p < 0.001$). At concentrations of vitamin C < 23 µmol/L (hypovitaminosis C), all but one patient had elevated C-reactive protein values (i.e., ≥3 mg/L); mean C-reactive protein was 71 ± 20 mg/L at <23 µmol/L vitamin C versus 21 ± 12 mg/L at >23 µmol/L vitamin C ($p < 0.001$). At concentrations of vitamin C < 50 µmol/L, mean C-reactive protein concentrations were 52 ± 14 mg/L versus 4 ± 4 mg/L at vitamin C concentrations > 50 µmol/L ($p < 0.001$; Figure 3b).

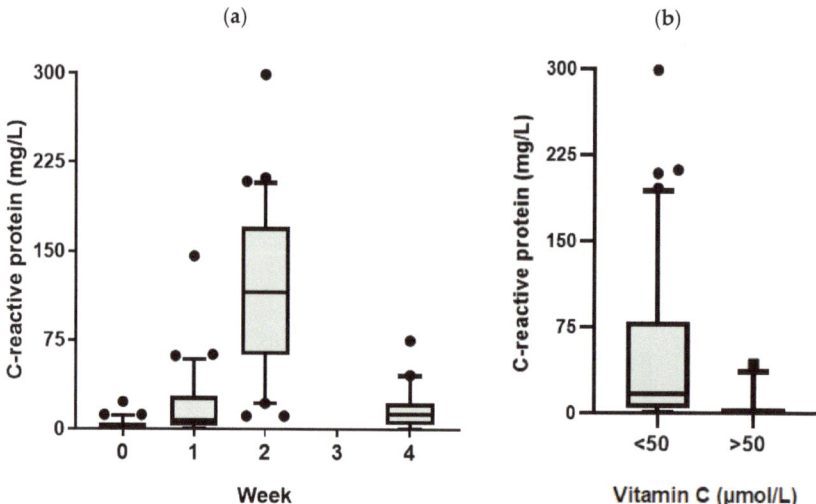

Figure 3. C-reactive protein concentrations in the patients. The C-reactive protein concentrations were assessed relative to (**a**) time of sampling, and (**b**) vitamin C concentration (< or >50 µmol/L, i.e., adequate). Box plots show median with 25th and 75th percentiles as boundaries, and whiskers are the 10th and 90th percentiles, with symbols indicating outlying data points. The mean values of weeks 1, 2, and 4 were significantly higher than baseline ($p < 0.01$); <50 µmol/L values were significantly higher than >50 µmol/L values ($p < 0.001$).

Table 2. Vitamin C status relative to febrile neutropenia and oxidative stress.

Analyte	Week 0	Week 1	Week 2	Week 4
Vitamin C (µmol/L)	44 (7) [1]	29 (5) *	19 (6) *	38 (10)
C-reactive protein (mg/L)	3.5 (1.8)	20 (11) *	119 (25) *	17 (8) *
Neutrophils (×10^9/L)	3.2 (0.5)	1.8 (1.0) *	0.1 (0.1) *	2.1 (0.6) *
TBARS (µmol/L) [2]	2.0 (0.3)	3.3 (0.6) *	2.9 (0.5) *	2.5 (0.6)

[1] Data is presented as mean (95% CI); [2] TBARS, thiobarbituric acid reactive substances: one participant had icteric samples, so their data was excluded from TBARS analyses; * Significantly different to week 0 values ($p < 0.01$).

3.4. Oxidative Stress Biomarkers

Protein carbonyls were 172 ± 19 pmol/mg protein at baseline (week 0). These did not differ significantly over the time course ($p > 0.05$), and were not significantly different to a healthy cohort of comparable age (57 ± 17 years, $n = 50$) that we have previously measured (i.e., 159 ± 11 pmol/mg protein) [14]. In contrast, TBARS increased significantly from 2.0 ± 0.3 µmol/L at baseline to 3.3 ± 0.6 µmol/L by week one ($p < 0.001$), and remained elevated at week two ($p = 0.003$), returning to baseline concentrations by week four ($p = 0.3$). The elevated TBARS were comparable to values we have previously observed in critically ill patients [15]. There was a significant inverse correlation between vitamin C status and TBARS ($r = -0.306$, $p < 0.001$).

4. Discussion

Our study showed profound depletion of plasma vitamin C concentrations in patients undergoing conditioning chemotherapy and HSCT. This reached a nadir at week two (19 µmol/L), with 72% developing hypovitaminosis C and 34% with outright deficiency. These values are directly comparable to those observed in critically ill patients in intensive care [16]. The vitamin C concentrations had not quite recovered to baseline values by week four. This confirms earlier reports that showed similar vitamin C profiles in smaller patient cohorts [11–13]. Despite recovery to near baseline concentrations by week four, these values are still considered inadequate (i.e., <50 µmol/L). Although the blood samples were non-fasting, low vitamin C status moderates potential fluctuations in plasma concentrations, as a result of recent dietary intake, due to uptake of the vitamin by depleted tissues. C-reactive protein concentrations increased dramatically by week two, in association with neutropenia and infection. We showed an inverse correlation between vitamin C status and C-reactive protein, with lower vitamin C status associated with higher C-reactive protein concentrations, an association also reported by Nannya and coworkers [12].

We have previously observed elevated protein carbonyls in patients with severe infections [14,15]. However, no increase in protein carbonyls was observed in the current study, despite patients exhibiting evidence of infection at week two. We have previously hypothesized that reactive oxygen species generated by activated neutrophils could contribute to the elevated protein carbonyls observed in patients with severe infections [15]. As such, the lack of an increase in protein carbonyls at week two in our current study may be a reflection of neutropenia in the patients. We did, however, observe elevated TBARS, a marker of lipid peroxidation, at weeks one and two. Others have reported similar findings, with elevated TBARS observed in patients versus healthy controls [6,7], and in patients following conditioning chemotherapy [8]. Administration of high-dose vitamin C to the patients was found to enhance the vitamin C status of the patients and decrease the elevated TBARS [8]. Whether this was through the vitamin's antioxidant or enzyme cofactor functions is unknown.

Due to the important and varied functions of vitamin C in the body, and the significant depletion of vitamin C in the hematopoietic cancer patients, it is anticipated that supplementation of these patients with vitamin C to restore adequate concentrations would be of benefit to the patients [21]. Up to 80% of HSCT recipients experience gastrointestinal mucositis, which is an ablation-related injury of the mucosal lining of the gastrointestinal tract, including the mouth and throat [22]. Oral mucositis is a painful and debilitating inflammatory condition that can prevent eating and drinking. Oral mucositis is thought to be initiated by free radical damage that activates an inflammatory response [23], and preliminary findings indicate an inverse association between vitamin C status and the severity of mucositis [13]. Supplementation of allogeneic HSCT recipients with vitamin C at doses of 2000 mg/d resulted in saturating vitamin C status (i.e., >70 µmol/L) and was associated with an improvement in graft versus host symptoms of the mucous membranes [24]. High-dose vitamin C administration to oncology patients receiving chemotherapy has been shown to decrease toxicity to the gastrointestinal system [25], and to improve patient quality of life through decreasing nausea/vomiting and improving appetite [26]. This may be particularly important for patients who undergo repeated cycles of chemotherapy.

Cutting-edge research over the past decade has indicated that vitamin C has a role in epigenetic regulation through acting as a cofactor for enzymes that modify DNA and histones [27]. Cell culture and preclinical studies indicate that vitamin C regulates hematopoietic cell function and blocks leukemia progression through epigenetic mechanisms [28,29]. Recent research has indicated that supplementation of myeloid cancer patients with 500 mg/d vitamin C restored vitamin C concentrations to the normal range and was associated with epigenetic alterations in myeloid cells [30]. Preliminary evidence has also indicated that administration of high-dose vitamin C to patients with leukemia may improve mortality via epigenetic mechanisms [31,32]. Thus, vitamin C exhibits pleiotropic roles in hematological cancer therapy, decreasing chemotherapy-related toxicity and side effects, and potentially improving survival via epigenetic mechanisms.

5. Conclusions

Our study showed profound depletion of vitamin C in HSCT recipients. The nadir of vitamin C status corresponded with febrile neutropenia and elevated inflammation and oxidative stress. Clinical trials are currently underway to assess the potential effects of vitamin C administration in these patients.

Author Contributions: Conceptualization: A.C.C., S.T.C., S.M.; methodology: A.C.C., S.T.C., S.M., N.M.; investigation: E.S., N.M., A.D., C.L.; formal analysis: A.C.C.; writing—original draft preparation: A.C.C.; writing—review and editing: E.S., N.M., A.D., C.L., S.M., S.T.C.; project administration: A.C.C., N.M. All authors have read and agreed to the published version of the manuscript.

Funding: This research received no external funding.

Acknowledgments: A.C.C. is the recipient of the Sir Charles Hercus Health Research Fellowship from the Health Research Council of New Zealand. A.D. has been supported by a grant from the Bone Marrow Cancer Research Trust. We thank the participants who contributed to this study.

Conflicts of Interest: The authors declare no conflict of interest.

References

1. Nivison-Smith, I.; Bradstock, K.F.; Dodds, A.J.; Hawkins, P.A.; Szer, J. Haemopoietic stem cell transplantation in Australia and New Zealand, 1992-2001: Progress report from the Australasian Bone Marrow Transplant Recipient Registry. *Intern. Med. J.* **2005**, *35*, 18–27. [CrossRef] [PubMed]
2. Carr, A.C.; Maggini, S. Vitamin C and immune function. *Nutrients* **2017**, *9*, E1211. [CrossRef] [PubMed]
3. Waldo, A.L.; Zipf, R.E. Ascorbic acid level in leukemic patients. *Cancer* **1955**, *8*, 187–190. [CrossRef]
4. Barkhan, P.; Howard, A.N. Distribution of ascorbic acid in normal and leukaemic human blood. *Biochem. J.* **1958**, *70*, 163–168. [CrossRef]
5. Huijskens, M.J.; Wodzig, W.K.; Walczak, M.; Germeraad, W.T.; Bos, G.M. Ascorbic acid serum levels are reduced in patients with hematological malignancies. *Results Immunol.* **2016**, *6*, 8–10. [CrossRef]
6. Sharma, A.; Tripathi, M.; Satyam, A.; Kumar, L. Study of antioxidant levels in patients with multiple myeloma. *Leuk. Lymphoma* **2009**, *50*, 809–815. [CrossRef]
7. Mehdi, W.A.; Zainulabdeen, J.A.; Mehde, A.A. Investigation of the antioxidant status in multiple myeloma patients: Effects of therapy. *Asian Pac. J. Cancer Prev.* **2013**, *14*, 3663–3667. [CrossRef]
8. Hunnisett, A.; Davies, S.; McLaren-Howard, J.; Gravett, P.; Finn, M.; Gueret-Wardle, D. Lipoperoxides as an index of free radical activity in bone marrow transplant recipients. Preliminary observations. *Biol. Trace Elem. Res.* **1995**, *47*, 125–132. [CrossRef] [PubMed]
9. Rtibi, K.; Selmi, S.; Grami, D.; Amri, M.; Sebai, H.; Marzouki, L. Contribution of oxidative stress in acute intestinal mucositis induced by 5 fluorouracil (5-FU) and its pro-drug capecitabine in rats. *Toxicol. Mech. Methods* **2018**, *28*, 262–267. [CrossRef] [PubMed]
10. Jordan, K.; Pontoppidan, P.; Uhlving, H.H.; Kielsen, K.; Burrin, D.G.; Weischendorff, S.; Christensen, I.J.; Jorgensen, M.H.; Heilmann, C.; Sengelov, H.; et al. Gastrointestinal toxicity, systemic inflammation, and liver biochemistry in allogeneic hematopoietic stem cell transplantation. *Biol. Blood Marrow Transplant.* **2017**, *23*, 1170–1176. [CrossRef]
11. Goncalves, T.L.; Benvegnu, D.M.; Bonfanti, G.; Frediani, A.V.; Rocha, J.B. delta-Aminolevulinate dehydratase activity and oxidative stress during melphalan and cyclophosphamide-BCNU-etoposide (CBV) conditioning regimens in autologous bone marrow transplantation patients. *Pharmacol. Res.* **2009**, *59*, 279–284. [CrossRef] [PubMed]
12. Nannya, Y.; Shinohara, A.; Ichikawa, M.; Kurokawa, M. Serial profile of vitamins and trace elements during the acute phase of allogeneic stem cell transplantation. *Biol. Blood Marrow Transplant.* **2014**, *20*, 430–434. [CrossRef] [PubMed]
13. Rasheed, M.; Simmons, G.; Fisher, B.; Leslie, K.; Reed, J.; Roberts, C.; Natarajan, R.; Fowler, A.; Toor, A. Reduced plasma ascorbic acid levels in recipients of myeloablative conditioning & hematopoietic cell transplantation. *Eur. J. Haematol.* **2019**. [CrossRef]
14. Carr, A.C.; Spencer, E.; Dixon, L.; Chambers, S.T. Patients with community acquired pneumonia exhibit depleted vitamin C status and elevated oxidative stress. *Nutrients* **2020**, *12*, 1318. [CrossRef] [PubMed]
15. Carr, A.C.; Spencer, E.; Mackle, D.; Hunt, A.; Judd, H.; Mehrtens, J.; Parker, K.; Stockwell, Z.; Gale, C.; Beaumont, M.; et al. The effect of conservative oxygen therapy on systemic biomarkers of oxidative stress in critically ill patients. *Free Radic. Biol. Med.* **2020**, in press.
16. Carr, A.C.; Rosengrave, P.C.; Bayer, S.; Chambers, S.; Mehrtens, J.; Shaw, G.M. Hypovitaminosis C and vitamin C deficiency in critically ill patients despite recommended enteral and parenteral intakes. *Crit. Care* **2017**, *21*, 300. [CrossRef]

17. Carr, A.C.; Pullar, J.M.; Moran, S.; Vissers, M.C. Bioavailability of vitamin C from kiwifruit in non-smoking males: Determination of 'healthy' and 'optimal' intakes. *J. Nutr. Sci.* **2012**, *1*, e14. [CrossRef]
18. Buss, H.; Chan, T.P.; Sluis, K.B.; Domigan, N.M.; Winterbourn, C.C. Protein carbonyl measurement by a sensitive ELISA method. *Free Radic. Biol. Med.* **1997**, *23*, 361–366. [CrossRef]
19. Ohkawa, H.; Ohishi, N.; Yagi, K. Assay for lipid peroxides in animal tissues by thiobarbituric acid reaction. *Anal. Biochem.* **1979**, *95*, 351–358. [CrossRef]
20. Knight, J.A.; Pieper, R.K.; McClellan, L. Specificity of the thiobarbituric acid reaction: Its use in studies of lipid peroxidation. *Clin. Chem.* **1988**, *34*, 2433–2438. [CrossRef]
21. Carr, A.C.; Cook, J. Intravenous vitamin C for cancer therapy - identifying the current gaps in our knowledge. *Front. Physiol.* **2018**, *9*, 1182. [CrossRef]
22. Rubenstein, E.B.; Peterson, D.E.; Schubert, M.; Keefe, D.; McGuire, D.; Epstein, J.; Elting, L.S.; Fox, P.C.; Cooksley, C.; Sonis, S.T. Clinical practice guidelines for the prevention and treatment of cancer therapy-induced oral and gastrointestinal mucositis. *Cancer* **2004**, *100*, 2026–2046. [CrossRef] [PubMed]
23. Riley, P.; Glenny, A.M.; Worthington, H.V.; Littlewood, A.; Clarkson, J.E.; McCabe, M.G. Interventions for preventing oral mucositis in patients with cancer receiving treatment: Oral cryotherapy. *Cochrane Database Syst. Rev.* **2015**, Cd011552. [CrossRef]
24. Kletzel, M.; Powers, K.; Hayes, M. Scurvy: A new problem for patients with chronic GVHD involving mucous membranes; an easy problem to resolve. *Pediatr. Transplant.* **2014**, *18*, 524–526. [CrossRef] [PubMed]
25. Ma, Y.; Chapman, J.; Levine, M.; Polireddy, K.; Drisko, J.; Chen, Q. High-dose parenteral ascorbate enhanced chemosensitivity of ovarian cancer and reduced toxicity of chemotherapy. *Sci. Transl. Med.* **2014**, *6*, 222ra218. [CrossRef] [PubMed]
26. Carr, A.C.; Vissers, M.C.M.; Cook, J.S. The effect of intravenous vitamin C on cancer- and chemotherapy-related fatigue and quality of life. *Front. Oncol.* **2014**, *4*, 1–7. [CrossRef]
27. Young, J.I.; Zuchner, S.; Wang, G. Regulation of the epigenome by vitamin C. *Annu. Rev. Nutr.* **2015**, *35*, 545–564. [CrossRef]
28. Agathocleous, M.; Meacham, C.E.; Burgess, R.J.; Piskounova, E.; Zhao, Z.; Crane, G.M.; Cowin, B.L.; Bruner, E.; Murphy, M.M.; Chen, W.; et al. Ascorbate regulates haematopoietic stem cell function and leukaemogenesis. *Nature* **2017**. [CrossRef]
29. Cimmino, L.; Dolgalev, I.; Wang, Y.; Yoshimi, A.; Martin, G.H.; Wang, J.; Ng, V.; Xia, B.; Witkowski, M.T.; Mitchell-Flack, M.; et al. Restoration of TET2 function blocks aberrant self-renewal and leukemia progression. *Cell* **2017**, *170*, 1079–1095.e1020. [CrossRef]
30. Gillberg, L.; Orskov, A.D.; Nasif, A.; Ohtani, H.; Madaj, Z.; Hansen, J.W.; Rapin, N.; Mogensen, J.B.; Liu, M.; Dufva, I.H.; et al. Oral vitamin C supplementation to patients with myeloid cancer on azacitidine treatment: Normalization of plasma vitamin C induces epigenetic changes. *Clin. Epigenetics* **2019**, *11*, 143. [CrossRef]
31. Zhao, H.; Zhu, H.; Huang, J.; Zhu, Y.; Hong, M.; Zhu, H.; Zhang, J.; Li, S.; Yang, L.; Lian, Y.; et al. The synergy of vitamin C with decitabine activates TET2 in leukemic cells and significantly improves overall survival in elderly patients with acute myeloid leukemia. *Leuk. Res.* **2018**, *66*, 1–7. [CrossRef] [PubMed]
32. Das, A.B.; Kakadia, P.M.; Wojcik, D.; Pemberton, L.; Browett, P.J.; Bohlander, S.K.; Vissers, M.C.M. Clinical remission following ascorbate treatment in a case of acute myeloid leukemia with mutations in TET2 and WT1. *Blood Cancer J.* **2019**, *9*, 82. [CrossRef] [PubMed]

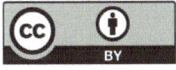

© 2020 by the authors. Licensee MDPI, Basel, Switzerland. This article is an open access article distributed under the terms and conditions of the Creative Commons Attribution (CC BY) license (http://creativecommons.org/licenses/by/4.0/).

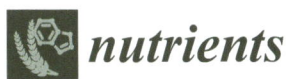

Article

Low Vitamin C Status in Patients with Cancer Is Associated with Patient and Tumor Characteristics

Rebecca White [1,†], Maria Nonis [1,†], John F. Pearson [2], Eleanor Burgess [1], Helen R. Morrin [1,3], Juliet M. Pullar [4], Emma Spencer [5], Margreet C. M. Vissers [4], Bridget A. Robinson [1,6] and Gabi U. Dachs [1,*]

1. Mackenzie Cancer Research Group, Department of Pathology and Biomedical Science, University of Otago Christchurch, Christchurch 8011, New Zealand; whire874@student.otago.ac.nz (R.W.); nonpa990@student.otago.ac.nz (M.N.); eleanor.burgess@postgrad.otago.ac.nz (E.B.); helen.morrin@otago.ac.nz (H.R.M.); bridget.robinson@cdhb.health.nz (B.A.R.)
2. Biostatistics and Computational Biology Unit, University of Otago Christchurch, Christchurch 8011, New Zealand; john.pearson@otago.ac.nz
3. Cancer Society Tissue Bank, University of Otago Christchurch, Christchurch 8011, New Zealand
4. Centre for Free Radical Research, Department of Pathology and Biomedical Science, University of Otago Christchurch, Christchurch 8011, New Zealand; juliet.pullar@otago.ac.nz (J.M.P.); margreet.vissers@otago.ac.nz (M.C.M.V.)
5. Nutrition in Medicine Research Group, Department of Pathology and Biomedical Science, University of Otago Christchurch, Christchurch 8011, New Zealand; emma.spencer@otago.ac.nz
6. Canterbury Regional Cancer and Hematology Service, Canterbury District Health Board, and Department of Medicine, University of Otago Christchurch, Christchurch 8011, New Zealand
* Correspondence: gabi.dachs@otago.ac.nz; Tel.: +64-3-3640544
† These authors contributed equally to this work.

Received: 7 July 2020; Accepted: 3 August 2020; Published: 5 August 2020

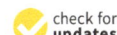

Abstract: Vitamin C (ascorbate) acts as an antioxidant and enzyme cofactor, and plays a vital role in human health. Vitamin C status can be affected by illness, with low levels being associated with disease due to accelerated turnover. However, robust data on the ascorbate status of patients with cancer are sparse. This study aimed to accurately measure ascorbate concentrations in plasma from patients with cancer, and determine associations with patient or tumor characteristics. We recruited 150 fasting patients with cancer (of 199 total recruited) from two cohorts, either prior to cancer surgery or during cancer chemo- or immunotherapy. A significant number of patients with cancer had inadequate plasma ascorbate concentrations. Low plasma status was more prevalent in patients undergoing cancer therapy. Ascorbate status was higher in women than in men, and exercising patients had higher levels than sedentary patients. Our study may prompt increased vigilance of ascorbate status in cancer patients.

Keywords: ascorbate; breast cancer; colorectal cancer; chemotherapy; immunotherapy; surgery; exercise

---

1. Introduction

The role of vitamin C (ascorbate) as an anti-cancer agent has long been debated [1,2]. There is interest in the use of ascorbate by patients with cancer, either through dietary supplementation or pharmacological infusion dosing [3,4], and isolated reports of clinical benefit have been published (reviewed in [5]). However, there are limited data available on the ascorbate status of this patient group. As humans rely solely on dietary intake for ascorbate, due to an inability to synthesize the vitamin, guidelines for intake to prevent the severe ascorbate deficiency disease scurvy have been developed [6]. Recommended daily intake (RDI) guidelines vary between countries, with Australasian standards

(RDI of 45 mg/day for both males and females [7]) being among the lowest worldwide. In comparison, the United States guidelines recommend a daily intake of 90 mg for males and 75 mg for females over the age of 19 [8], and the German Nutrition Society has calculated that healthy men required 110 mg and women 95 mg ascorbate per day [9].

The physiological effects of ascorbate are achieved through its ability to donate electrons, either as an antioxidant or as a cofactor for metal-containing enzymes [10,11]. Particularly pertinent to cancer are the 2-oxoglutarate-dependent dioxygenases, a superfamily of enzymes, for which ascorbate is an essential cofactor [11]. These ascorbate-reliant enzymes have roles in wound healing via the synthesis and stabilization of collagen, and in mood and vitality regulation via synthesis of carnitine, neurotransmitters and peptide hormones [11]. This superfamily also includes DNA and histone demethylases, that modify cancer stem cell phenotype, and hydroxylases that regulate the hypoxic response via transcription factor activation, which affects cancer progression [2,11]. Retrospective analysis of human tissue samples revealed that increased tumor ascorbate levels were associated with reduced transcription factor activity (specifically hypoxia-inducible factors) in endometrial, colorectal, thyroid, papillary renal cell and breast cancer [12–16]. Increased tumor ascorbate levels were associated with extended disease-free survival in colorectal cancer patients [13] and improved disease-specific survival in breast cancer patients [16]. These data indicate that optimal levels of ascorbate may be clinically important in cancer.

Despite this interest in ascorbate for cancer, there are limited data on the ascorbate status of patients with cancer, with many studies involving small sample sizes (median n = 50, with 27/31 studies having fewer than 100 patients) [17–22]. In addition, most used the colorimetric assay (21/24 studies) (e.g., [17–19]), which can be prone to interference by other reducing substances present in plasma [23]. Only three studies used high-performance liquid chromatography (HPLC, the gold standard for measuring ascorbate), all three containing fewer than 70 patients [20–22]. Most studies (20/31) reported inadequate plasma ascorbate levels in patients with cancer e.g., [17–22].

The aim of our study was therefore to measure the concentration of ascorbate in plasma using HPLC in a cohort of outpatients with cancer. Plasma levels of ascorbate are indicative of whole body status and correlate with tissue levels, with plasma saturation being reflective of general tissue saturation [6,24]. Of interest were newly diagnosed patients prior to the planned surgical resection of their cancer (largely treatment naïve), as well as patients undergoing cancer therapy (chemotherapy or immunotherapy). We hypothesized that certain lifestyle factors, patient characteristics or tumor characteristics would predict patients at risk of deficiency or hypovitaminosis C. We also hypothesized that therapy patients may be at particular risk of ascorbate depletion due to reduced intake or increased requirements.

2. Materials and Methods

2.1. Human Ethics and Patient Consent

Ethics approval for this study was obtained from the New Zealand Health and Disability Ethics Committee (18/STH/223). Patients were recruited between November 2018 and June 2019 at Christchurch Hospital, New Zealand, to either a pre-surgical cohort or a therapy cohort. Patients gave informed consent for a blood draw of 5 mL via venipuncture, for administration of a health questionnaire and for collection of related medical data. Patients declared their ethnicity using the New Zealand census question and were offered the option of disposal of samples by karakia (blessing).

2.2. Eligibility Criteria

Participants were aged over 18 with a confirmed diagnosis of cancer and able to provide informed consent. Participants were not required to be fasting prior to blood draw, but their food and drink consumption, and any ascorbate supplementation, on the day of blood draw was recorded.

2.3. Study Populations

Patients in the pre-surgical cohort had confirmed cancer that was to be surgically resected and were thus recruited from the surgical pre-admission clinics in Christchurch Hospital. Patients in the therapy cohort were recruited from the chemotherapy day ward at Christchurch Hospital and were partway through their treatment schedule for cancer having received at least one prior treatment (chemotherapy or immunotherapy) on the day of recruitment. All participants completed a brief health questionnaire to collect demographic variables (details below). Medical records provided clinicopathological information (cancer type, Tumor Node Metastasis (TNM) stage) and treatment details (type of chemotherapy or immunotherapy).

2.4. Blood Sample Collection and Processing

Peripheral blood was collected into 4 mL Ethylene-diamine-tetra-acetic acid (EDTA) vacutainer tubes (Becton Dickinson, Auckland, New Zealand), immediately placed on ice and processed within 60 min. Samples were centrifuged at 4 °C to pellet cells, and plasma was collected for the extraction of ascorbate. Plasma was mixed at a ratio of 1:1 with ice-cold 0.54 M perchloric acid (PCA) solution containing 100 µM of the metal chelator di-ethylenetriamine penta-acetic acid (DTPA) to precipitate protein (chemicals from Sigma-Aldrich, St Louis, MO, USA). Cleared plasma was stored at −80 °C until analysis.

2.5. Ascorbate Measurement in Plasma

Total ascorbate content of plasma was analyzed using reverse-phase HPLC with electrochemical detection, as described previously [25]. Samples were reduced with 10 mg/mL tris-(2-carboxyethyl)-phosphine (TCEP) at a 1:10 ratio for 3 h at 4 °C, and diluted 1:1 in 77 mM perchloric acid containing DTPA (100 µM). Samples were separated on a Synergi 4 µ Hydro-RP 80A 150 × 4.6 mm column (Phenomenex NZ Ltd., Auckland, New Zealand) using a Dionex Ultimate 3000 HPLC unit with a refrigerated autosampler and an Ultimate 3000 ECD–3000RS electrochemical detector and a Model 6011RS coulometric analytical cell (+200 mV electrode potential). The mobile phase comprised 80 mM sodium acetate buffer, pH 4.8, containing DTPA (0.54 mM) and freshly added paired-ion reagent n-octylamine (1 µM), delivered at a flow rate of 1.2 mL/min. A standard curve of sodium-L-ascorbate (1.25–40 µM), standardized spectrophotometrically, was freshly prepared for each HPLC run in 77 mM perchloric acid containing 100 µmol/L DTPA. All chemicals were from Sigma-Aldrich (St Louis, MO, USA). Plasma ascorbate concentrations are expressed as µM and patients were classified according to international clinical guidelines as follows: deficient < 11 µM, marginal 11 ≤ 23 µM, inadequate 23–50 µM or adequate >50 µM [25]; >70 µM is deemed saturating.

2.6. Health Data and Dietary Intake Assessment

Health questionnaires provided age, gender, height and weight; height and weight were used to calculate BMI (kg/m^2). Frequency of physical activity was recorded to be <60 min/week, 60–150 min/week or >150 min/week, according to Ministry of Health NZ guidelines [26]). Smoking habits were recorded as: never smoked; ex-smoker or current smoker. Patient's diet on the day prior to sampling (24-hour dietary recall) was used to estimate ascorbate intake using the US Department of Agriculture database [27]. In addition, reported intake on the morning of blood draw enabled patients to be separated into fasting and non-fasting groups. Those patients who had consumed less than 45 mg ascorbate and who had not taken any ascorbate supplements on the day of blood draw, were defined as being fasting, with respect to ascorbate intake. Information on the use of ascorbate supplements and high dose ascorbate injections was collected.

2.7. Statistical Analyses

Clinical and demographic characteristics between cohorts were compared with t-tests with Satterthwaite's adjustment for unequal variance or Fisher's exact test for continuous and categorical measurements, respectively. Categorical variables were compared with analysis of variance (ANOVA) followed by Tukey's post-hoc tests and relationships between continuous variables were described by locally weighted regression smoothers and Pearson's correlation coefficient. All continuous variables had no linear effect on plasma ascorbate ($p > 0.022$) so were appropriately categorized for regression analyses. Effect of demographics (age, gender, ethnicity), health (smoking, exercise, body mass index (BMI)), plasma intake and supplementation on plasma concentrations (continuous) were compared with simple linear regression. There was sufficient power to fit multiple linear regression models with 2-way interactions. Variables which did not improve fit were sequentially removed and the final model was graphically assessed for goodness of fit. Data were analyzed in R version 3.6.4 (R Foundation for Statistical Computing, Vienna, Austria), all p values are two-tailed, unpaired and with statistical significance set at $p < 0.05$.

3. Results

3.1. Characteristics of the Two Cohorts of Patients with Cancer

The pre-surgical cohort comprised of 99 patients with 81 deemed fasting (<45 mg ascorbate intake on day of blood draw), and the therapy cohort comprised of 100 patients receiving chemotherapy or immunotherapy with 69 fasting (Table S1). Breast and colorectal cancer were the two most frequent cancer types in both cohorts (Table S1). Most patients in the therapy cohort received chemotherapy (including adjuvant, neoadjuvant and palliative therapy), and 17 received immunotherapy (14 pembrolizumab and 3 nivolumab, all melanoma).

A comparison was made between fasting, non-fasting and all patients (combined fasting with non-fasting) in the two cohorts (Table S1). As patients were recruited at their clinic visits, many had already eaten on the day of the blood test. Fasting status was therefore determined following an assessment of the ascorbate content of food consumed prior to the blood sampling, with an upper limit of 45 mg vitamin C consumed in the previous 6 h for the fasting group. Mean dietary ascorbate intake in patients from the pre-surgical cohort, according to 24-hour recall, was similar in fasting, non-fasting and all patients (61.0 ± 6.2, 67.3 ± 14.9 and 61.5 ± 5.7 mg ascorbate, respectively).

In patients from the therapy cohort, fasting patients had lower levels compared to non-fasting and all therapy patients (61.9 ± 6.7, 129.5 ± 43.6 and 82.8 ± 14.4 mg ascorbate, respectively). In the pre-surgical cohort, non-fasting patients had predominantly (82%) saturating plasma ascorbate levels (14/17), whereas only 55% of the non-fasting patients in the therapy cohort had saturating levels (17/31). Three-quarters of the pre-surgical cohort reported recent or regular supplement use (13/17), compared to 61% (19/31) of the treatment cohort. Although supplement use was common in both cohorts, high dose ascorbate infusions were rare (one in pre-surgical and four in treatment cohorts, Table S1). Plasma ascorbate levels were higher in the pre-surgical cohort compared to therapy cohort in fasting, non-fasting and all patients (pre-surgical 57.2 ± 2.7, 104.8 ± 6.5 and 65.4 ± 3.1 µM and therapy 46.8 ± 3.2, 73.8 ± 5.5 and 55.1 ± 3.0 µM ascorbate, respectively, Table S1). It is noteworthy that although ascorbate intake was generally higher in the therapy cohort compared to the pre-surgical cohort, plasma ascorbate levels were lower.

Recent ascorbate intake temporarily increases plasma concentrations [28,29], with plasma levels increasing by at least 20 µM from 1–6 h following intake of 200 mg ascorbate from a food source or supplement [28]. Hence, fasting measurements are a more reliable indicator of body status, and subsequent ascorbate data is presented only for those who had ascorbate intake below 45 mg on the day of blood draw—defined as fasting patients (Table 1).

Table 1. Comparison of characteristics of the two cohorts of fasting patients with cancer.

		Pre-Surgical Cohort $n = 81$ (%)	Therapy Cohort $n = 69$ (%)	Effect Size [95% CI]	p Value
Age (years)	Mean (±SD)	63.88 (±12.08)	58.71 (±13.76)	5.17 [0.95,9.38]	**0.017**
Gender	Female	49 (60)	39 (57)		
	Male	32 (40)	30 (43)	1.18 [0.61,2.26]	0.740
Ethnicity	European	72 (89)	63 (91)		
	Māori/Pacifica	9 (11)	6 (9)	0.76 [0.26,2.26]	0.786
BMI (kg/m^2)	Mean (±SD)	30.50 (±7.17)	28.62 (±7.13)	1.88 [−0.45,4.20]	0.112
Smoking	never	42 (52)	35 (51)		
	ex	35 (43)	25 (36)	0.86 [0.43,1.69]	0.730
	current	4 (5)	9 (13)	2.70 [0.77,9.52]	0.140
Exercise (min/week)	>150	35 (43)	26 (38)		
	60–150	27 (33)	22 (32)	1.10 [0.51,2.34]	0.848
	<60	19 (23)	20 (29)	1.42 [0.63,3.18]	0.418
Stage	TNM 1–3	67 (83)	30 (43)		
	TNM 4, recurrence	12 (15)	39 (57)	7.26 [3.34,15.79]	1.30×10^{-7}
Ascorbate intake (mg/day)	<45	42 (52)	34 (49)		
	45–90	19 (23)	15 (22)	0.98 [0.43,2.20]	1.000
	≥90	20 (25)	20 (29)	1.24 [0.57,2.66]	0.696
Supplement	No	66 (81)	56 (81)		
	Yes	15 (19)	13 (19)	1.02 [0.45,2.33]	1.000

Age and body mass index (BMI) show mean (±standard deviation) and are compared with t-tests with Satterthwaites adjustment for unequal variance. Effect is difference [95% Confidence Interval]. Categories show counts (%) and are compared with Fisher's exact test with effect shown as odds ratio [95% confidence interval (CI)]. There is 1 participant who received therapy with no exercise record, and 2 pre-surgical patients with no stage information. TNM stage, tumor node, metastasis stage. Significant p-values are shown in bold.

Most fasting patients in both cohorts were female, non-Māori/non-Pacifica with a BMI >25 (Table 1). Patients on therapy were, on average, 5 years younger than those in the pre-surgical group ($p = 0.017$). Current smokers represented 13% of patients in the therapy cohort, compared to 5% in the pre-surgical cohort ($p > 0.05$), and approximately one quarter of patients in both cohorts reported doing less than one hour of exercise per week. As expected, most patients in the pre-surgical cohort had localized disease (TNM stage 1–3), whereas patients in the therapy cohort had a majority of disseminated disease or recurrence ($p = 1.30 \times 10^{-7}$). There were no other significant differences in patient characteristics or behavior between the two cohorts.

3.2. Ascorbate Intake versus Plasma Ascorbate Status of Fasting Patients with Cancer

Reported ascorbate intake was on average 60–62 mg/day and was similar between the two cohorts that met fasting criteria (Table S1, Figure 1A). Similarly, intake divided into categories of below NZ RDI (<45 mg/day), between NZ and US RDI (45–90 mg/day), and above US RDI (>90 mg/day), did not differ between the two cohorts (Table 1). Almost 1/5 of patients reported regular supplement use (Table 1).

Mean fasting plasma ascorbate concentrations in the pre-surgical cohort were significantly higher than levels in the therapy cohort ($p = 0.013$, Figure 1B). Mean fasting plasma concentrations in the pre-surgical cohort were 57.2 ± 2.7 µM, compared to 46.8 ± 3.2 µM in the treatment cohort. Patients in the pre-surgical cohort who consumed above NZ RDI ascorbate had significantly higher plasma ascorbate concentrations than those consuming below ($p < 0.01$, Figure 1C). However, patients in the therapy cohort did not show this benefit, and had significantly lower plasma concentrations than patients in the pre-surgical cohort even when consuming above NZ RDI ($p < 0.05$, Figure 1C).

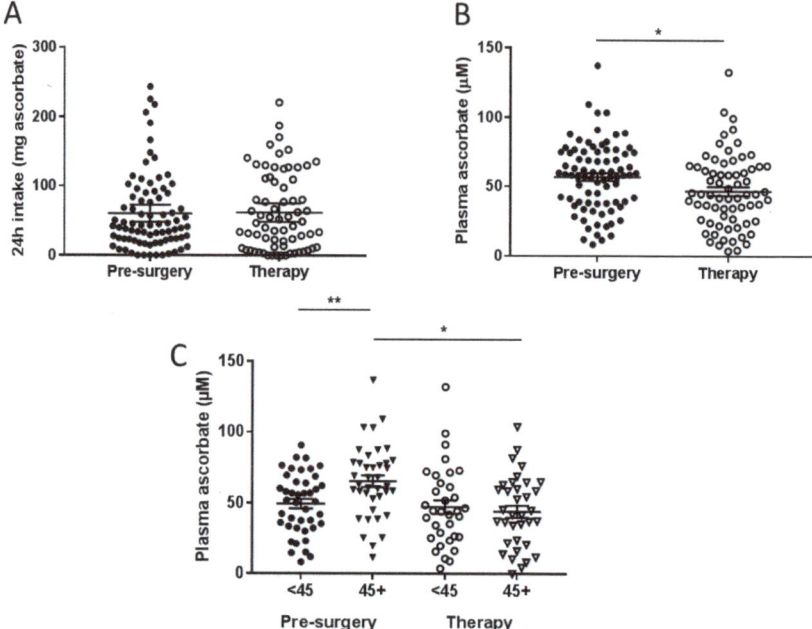

Figure 1. Ascorbate intake (**A**) and plasma ascorbate concentrations (**B**) in fasting patients from the pre-surgical and therapy cohorts. (**C**) Plasma ascorbate levels according to reported intake dicotemized at NZ recommended daily intake (RDI) of 45 mg/day. Pre-surgical cohort $n = 81$; therapy cohort $n = 69$. * $p < 0.05$, ** $p < 0.01$, unpaired t-test; mean ± standard error of the mean (SEM).

Fewer patients in the pre-surgical cohort were ascorbate deficient (<11 µM, 1 vs. 7) or were marginally deficient (11–23 µM, 7 vs. 8), compared to the therapy cohort ($p = 0.027$, Table 2). About one quarter of the pre-surgical cohort had inadequate plasma ascorbate levels (23–50 µM) compared to more than one third of the therapy cohort ($p = 0.026$). These data indicate that undergoing therapy is associated with odds of 2.4 of having inadequate (23–50 µM) plasma ascorbate, and 3.2 of having low (<23 µM) plasma ascorbate levels (Table 2).

Table 2. Comparison of fasting cancer patient cohorts according to categories of plasma ascorbate.

Plasma Ascorbate	Pre-Surgical Cohort	Therapy Cohort	OR [95% CI]	p-Value
	$n = 81$ (%)	$n = 69$ (%)		
>50 µM	53 (65.4)	29 (42.0)	1	
23–50 µM	20 (24.7)	26 (37.7)	2.38 [1.14, 4.97]	**0.026**
<23 µM	8 (9.9)	14 (20.3)	3.20 [1.20, 8.52]	**0.027**

OR odds ratio, CI confidence interval, p value from Fisher exact test relative to >50µM plasma ascorbate level. Significant p-values are shown in bold.

A weak association was evident between reported ascorbate intake (24-hour recall) and measured fasting plasma concentrations in patients with cancer. The 'smoother' graph in the pre-surgical cohort showed a linear relationship for ascorbate intake below 90 mg ($r = 0.42$, $p = 0.0007$), which is lost at ascorbate intake above 90 mg (Figure 2). The therapy cohort showed a linear but less steep incline of plasma ascorbate with increasing intake up to ~60 mg, which again is lost at higher estimated ascorbate intake; neither are significant for the entire cohort (Figure 2).

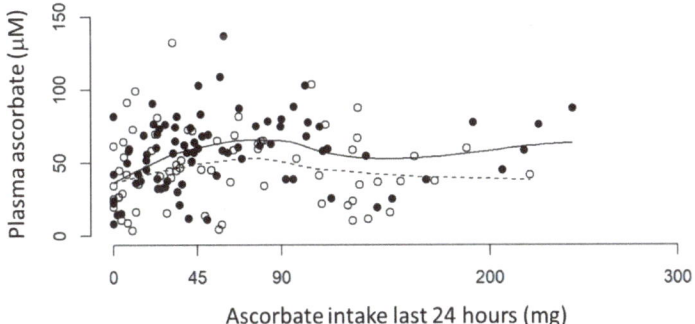

Figure 2. Ascorbate intake vs. plasma ascorbate levels in fasting patients with cancer. Pre-surgical (•) and therapy (°) cohorts are shown with lines locally weighted 'smooths' for each group. Solid line shows pre-surgical cohort, dotted line shows therapy cohort. Plasma concentrations are from fasting patients (<45 mg ascorbate on day of blood draw) and ascorbate intake is from 24-hour dietary recall. Pre-surgical cohort $n = 81$, therapy cohort $n = 69$.

3.3. Associations between Plasma Concentrations of Ascorbate and Patient Characteristics

Fasting plasma ascorbate levels were significantly lower in men compared to women in the pre-surgical cohort ($p = 0.005$), with a similar trend seen in the therapy cohort ($p = 0.08$) (Figure 3A,B). This was seen despite there being no difference in intake of ascorbate by gender (Figure 3C,D). When both cohorts were combined, women consuming above NZ RDI had higher plasma ascorbate levels than women who consumed lesser amounts, and also higher levels than men who consumed above NZ RDI (Figure 3E). Similarly, women consuming below NZ RDI had higher plasma ascorbate levels than men consuming below NZ RDI (Figure 3E).

Patients in the pre-surgical cohort doing less than 60 min exercise per week had significantly lower fasting plasma ascorbate concentrations than those doing more exercise each week ($p = 0.004$, Figure 4A). A similar trend was seen in patients from the therapy cohort, but this did not reach significance ($p = 0.11$, Figure 4B). Post-hoc tests on the pre-surgical cohort showed no significant difference between exercise at 60–150 min or >150 min ($p = 0.96$) so exercise was collapsed to two levels at 60 min for subsequent analyses (Figure 4C). In both cohorts combined, patients who consumed below NZ RDI and did less than 60 min exercise per week had significantly lower plasma ascorbate levels than those doing more exercise, regardless of their ascorbate intake ($p < 0.001$, Figure 4C).

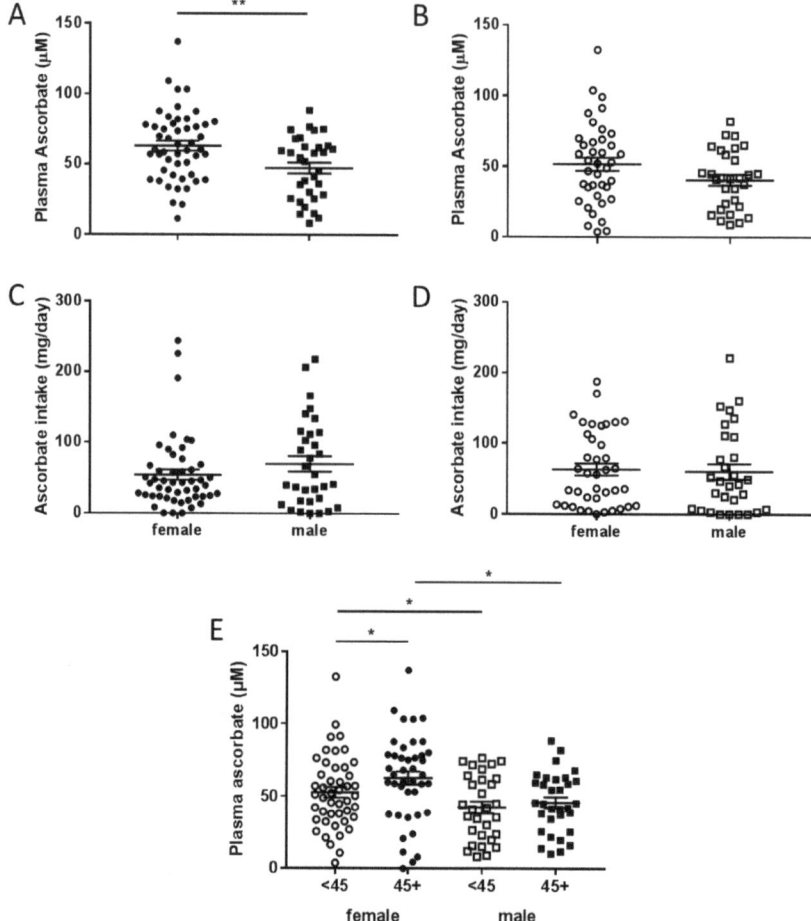

Figure 3. Plasma ascorbate levels and intake according to gender in fasting patients. Plasma data is compared between female and male patients from the pre-surgical (**A**) and therapy cohorts (**B**), intake data (24-hour dietary recall) from the pre-surgical (**C**) and therapy cohorts (**D**). (**E**) Association of plasma ascorbate and gender with intake dicotemized at NZ RDI of 45 mg/day. Unpaired t-test, * $p < 0.05$, ** $p < 0.01$, pre-surgical cohort $n = 81$, therapy cohort $n = 69$, mean ± SEM.

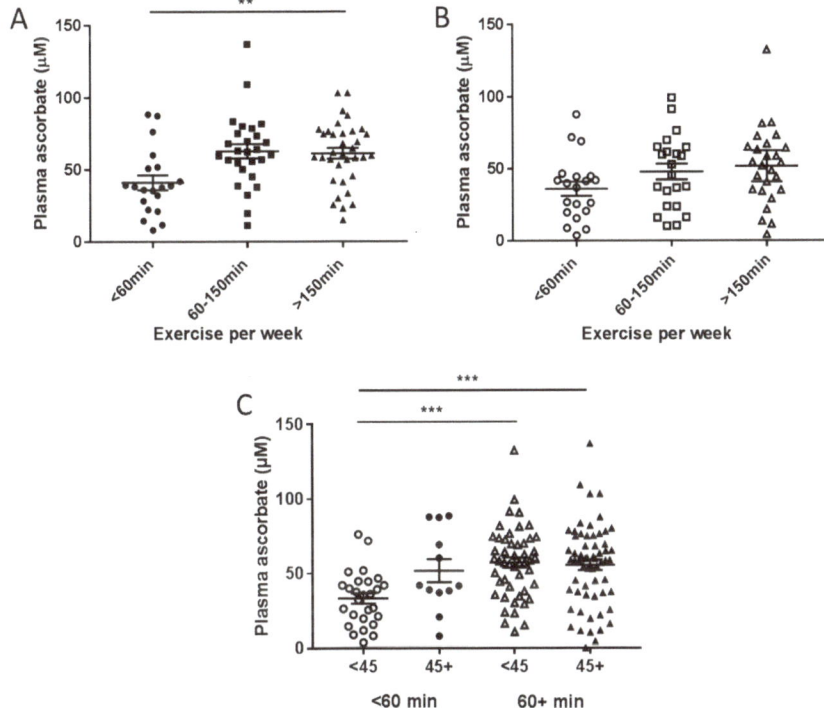

Figure 4. Fasting plasma ascorbate levels according to reported exercise levels in patients from the pre-surgical (**A**) and treatment cohorts (**B**). (**C**) Association of plasma ascorbate and exercise with intake dicotemized at NZ RDI of 45 mg/day and exercise dicotemized at 60 min/week. Pre-surgical cohort $n = 81$, therapy cohort $n = 69$. ** $p = 0.004$ one-way analysis of variance (ANOVA), *** $p < 0.001$ unpaired t-test, mean ± SEM.

3.4. Modeling of Associations with Plasma Ascorbate

The effect of patient characteristics on ascorbate status was further explored in all fasting patients combined using univariate analysis (Table 3). Male gender, low ascorbate intake (<45 mg/day), low exercise (<60 min/week) and being in the treatment cohort were associated with lower plasma ascorbate levels, whereas regular supplement use was associated with higher plasma ascorbate levels (all $p < 0.05$). Higher cancer stage was weakly associated with lower plasma ascorbate ($p = 0.084$), whereas age, BMI, smoking status, and ethnicity were not associated with ascorbate status (Table 3). Note, cancer stage and treatment were interdependent; most patients receiving therapy had high stage disease, and most patients in the pre-surgical cohort had lower stage disease (Table 1).

Multiple linear regression (Table 4) demonstrated that male gender was associated with lower plasma ascorbate. Daily ascorbate intake >45 mg was associated with higher plasma ascorbate, but this was significantly reduced in the cohort receiving treatment. Exercising more than 60 min per week was associated with a significant increase in plasma ascorbate, but only in those with ascorbate intake less than 45 mg. Together all predictors explained 26% of the variability (multiple R^2), however age, BMI, ethnicity and smoking were not significant.

Table 3. Univariate effects of patient characteristics on plasma ascorbate.

		Estimate	95% CI	p-Value
Age	50–70	3.39	[−7.41,14.19]	0.415
	70+	−3.21	[−15.49,9.07]	
Gender	Male	−13.97	[−22.14,−5.79]	**0.001**
BMI	30–40	2.63	[−6.68,11.93]	0.719
	<18.5 or >40	−3.57	[−18.71,11.56]	
Smoking	ex	−5.69	[−14.46,3.07]	0.272
	current	−9.90	[−25.16,5.37]	
Ethnicity	Māori/Pacifica	3.19	[−10.73,17.11]	0.651
Exercise	60–150	−1.09	[−10.37,8.20]	**0.001**
	<60	−18.24	[−28.15,−8.32]	
Ascorbate Intake	45–90	9.76	[−1.96,21.47]	**0.049**
	<45	−3.10	[−13.01,6.81]	
Supplementation	yes	12.32	[1.79,22.86]	**0.022**
Tumor Stage	TNM 1–3	−7.16	[−18.29,3.97]	0.084
	TNM 4, recurrent	−10.42	[−19.83,−1.00]	
Cohort	Treatment	−10.43	[−18.64,−2.22]	**0.013**

Estimates, 95% confidence intervals and p values from univariate linear regression on plasma ascorbate. Combined cohorts of fasting patients n = 150, age (years) vs. <50, BMI, body mass index (kg/m2) vs. 18.5–30, ethnicity Māori/Pacifica vs. other, exercise (min/week) vs. >150, ascorbate intake (mg/day) vs. >90, tumor stage TNM (tumor node metastasis) local vs. metastatic or recurrent disease. Significant p-values are shown in bold.

Table 4. Multiple linear regression of plasma ascorbate in fasting patients with cancer.

Predictor	Level	Effect	95% CI	p-Value
Gender	Male	−12.31	[−19.73,−4.89]	**0.0013**
Ascorbate Intake	>45 mg	29.74	[12.47,47.01]	**0.0009**
Exercise	>60 min	22.08	[11.40,32.77]	**0.0001**
Ascorbate Intake × Exercise	>45 mg and >60 min	−19.93	[−37.62,−2.25]	**0.0275**
Cohort	Therapy	0.02	[−10.24,10.28]	0.9968
Ascorbate Intake × Cohort	>45 mg and Therapy	−20.83	[−35.47,−6.18]	**0.0056**

Linear effect, 95% confidence interval and p-value from linear regression of plasma ascorbate on gender, ascorbate intake, exercise by ascorbate intake and cohort by ascorbate intake on combined cohorts of fasting patients n = 150. Significant p-values are shown in bold.

4. Discussion

Our study demonstrated that a significant proportion of patients with cancer had inadequate plasma ascorbate levels, consumed below NZ RDI for ascorbate (<45 mg/day) and exercised less than recommended (<60 min/week). Patients in the therapy cohort had significantly lower plasma ascorbate levels compared to those in the pre-surgical cohort. Men had lower ascorbate status than women, and patients who exercised for less than one hour per week had lower ascorbate levels than those doing more than one hour per week.

Average plasma ascorbate levels in patients with more advanced disease and who were receiving chemo- or immunotherapy were 10 µM lower than levels measured in the pre-surgical cohort. This discrepancy could not be explained by reduced ascorbate intake (e.g., due to treatment-induced nausea) in the therapy cohort. Indeed, our data showed that ascorbate intake was similar or higher in patients in the therapy cohort compared to those prior to surgery, yet plasma ascorbate levels were lower. This is an interesting observation and may be due to increased requirements of ascorbate in patients with advanced cancer. Only about half of non-fasting therapy patients had saturating plasma ascorbate levels compared to 82% of the non-fasting pre-surgical cohort. These combined data support the notion that patients currently undergoing cancer therapy are at increased risk of low ascorbate status.

Our analysis indicates a more complex relationship between ascorbate in the blood and dietary intake for cancer patients than has been reported in healthy individuals. For lower levels of intake, the data showed a linear increase in plasma concentrations with increasing intake, similar to what has been described in healthy volunteers [29], and levels appeared to (at best) plateau as intake reached the RDI recommended in Europe and the USA (90 mg/day). In fact, not many patients reached saturation levels. However, importantly, the patients with more advanced disease undergoing therapy appeared to require higher ascorbate intake to achieve similar plasma concentrations than those with localized disease prior to cancer surgery. Ascorbate supports many aspects of human health, including immune health and mood, and can support the health, quality of life and outcomes for cancer patients [30–34]. Independent studies are needed to confirm the relationship between treatment and ascorbate status observed in our study.

Our treatment cohort had 6/69 (8.7%) patients with ascorbate deficiency, compared to 1/81 (1.1%) in the pre-surgical cohort, and 9/369 (2.4%) in a cohort of healthy 50-year old's [25]; with an additional 11.6% with marginal deficiency, a total of 1/5. Low plasma ascorbate levels have also been reported in patients receiving intensive chemotherapy [35]. This may have serious clinical implications, including poor wound healing, depression, poor response to therapy and risk of cancer death [30]. A previous study reported deficiency in 30% (15/50) of patients with advanced cancer and found that deficient patients had significantly shorter mean survival (29 versus 121 days, $p = 0.001$) [22]. Health can also be impaired in those patients with marginal ascorbate deficiency or inadequate levels. In a cohort of 598 kidney transplant recipients, low plasma ascorbate status was associated with risk of death from cancer [36]. Kidney transplant recipients are known to be at increased risk of several cancer types due to ongoing immune-suppression [37], and there is growing evidence of the importance of ascorbate in immune cell function [31].

We showed an association between low activity levels and low ascorbate levels in patients with cancer. Similar findings were reported for healthy elderly Japanese women ($n = 655$), where plasma ascorbate was correlated with handgrip strength, balance and walking speed [38]. Support was also recently published from the European Prospective Investigation into Cancer (EPIC)-Norfolk study [39]. This population-based cross-sectional study in England ($n = 22,474$ of largely healthy adults) showed an association between ascorbate deficiency and reduced reported physical activity [39]. Likewise, in cohorts of pre-diabetic and diabetic individuals ($n = 89$), plasma ascorbate and physical activity were related [40]. A small intervention trial in healthy men ($n = 28$) showed a slight improvement in physical activity with ascorbate supplementation [41]. These studies in healthy adults support our findings in patients with cancer, although it remains to be shown whether low activity levels are a reflection of poor health and diet, or whether low ascorbate, via its requirement as enzyme cofactor associated with energy metabolism and vitality [11], directly affects activity levels.

Male gender was associated with lower ascorbate in our study and others [39]. This does not appear to depend on ascorbate intake, and a higher requirement for ascorbate in males has previously been reported in healthy individuals [6,42]. Accordingly, the RDI for males is often higher for men than for women [43]. The reasons for increased requirement for males may indicate increased average body size, or an increased requirement for the vitamin, but this remains unclear.

We saw no associations between plasma ascorbate and age, BMI or smoking, which contrasts with reports from individuals without cancer [39,40]. The importance of these differences is not yet clear, but may be due to low numbers or may reflect the impact of cancer burden in our study.

The strength of our study is the reasonable size of the cohort which has statistical power to assess ascorbate in relationship to numerous health risk factors (only one other study contained more than 150 patients with cancer [44]). Other strengths are robust measurements (HPLC) of ascorbate, and sampling at different stages of the cancer continuum. Limitations are that fasting ascorbate data was only available for 150 of the 199 patients, dietary intake was estimated from a single survey time point, and exercise was assessed from a simple survey. Additional factors that potentially affect ascorbate status, such as systemic inflammation, were not assessed.

5. Conclusions

Our data demonstrates that plasma ascorbate levels in cancer patients are driven by more than ascorbate intake or any single health risk factor. Modeling showed male gender, sedentary behavior and current cancer treatment to be predictive of risk of low ascorbate status. Based on the present study findings, it appears that patients with advanced cancer currently undergoing chemo- or immunotherapy may be at particular risk of ascorbate depletion associated with increased requirements, and not necessarily due to reduced intake. As ascorbate deficiency is a severe health risk, this information is valuable for clinicians when advising their patients on health and dietary choices, including consideration of supplement use. It is of note that the vast majority of people with cancer will never have their plasma ascorbate measured, and this report may prompt increased vigilance of ascorbate status in cancer patients.

Supplementary Materials: The following are available online at http://www.mdpi.com/2072-6643/12/8/2338/s1: Table S1: Characteristics of the two cohorts of patients with cancer.

Author Contributions: Conceptualization, M.C.M.V. and G.U.D.; Formal analysis, J.F.P.; Funding acquisition, B.A.R. and G.U.D.; Investigation, R.W., M.N., E.B., J.M.P. and E.S.; Resources, H.R.M.; Supervision, B.A.R. and G.U.D.; Writing—original draft, R.W. and M.N.; Writing—review and editing, M.C.M.V., B.A.R. and G.U.D. All authors have read and agreed to the published version of the manuscript.

Funding: This research was funded by the Mackenzie Charitable Foundation (GUD), Vitamin C for Cancer Trust (EB), Canterbury Medical Research Foundation (RW) and Cancer Society of New Zealand, Canterbury/West Coast Division (MN).

Acknowledgments: We would like to thank the nurses and staff at Christchurch Hospital Preadmission and Oncology Services for their help and phlebotomy services. We are especially grateful to the patients who have consented to be part of this study. We also like to thank Karen Keelan for consulting with us on Māori responsiveness.

Conflicts of Interest: The authors declare no conflict of interest. The funders had no role in the design of the study; in the collection, analyses, or interpretation of data; in the writing of the manuscript, or in the decision to publish the results.

References

1. Wilson, M.K.; Baguley, B.C.; Wall, C.; Jameson, M.B.; Findlay, M.P. Review of high-dose intravenous vitamin C as an anticancer agent. *Asia Pac. J. Clin. Oncol.* **2014**, *10*, 22–37. [CrossRef] [PubMed]
2. Ngo, B.; Van Riper, J.M.; Cantley, L.C.; Yun, J. Targeting cancer vulnerabilities with high-dose vitamin C. *Nat. Rev. Cancer* **2019**, *19*, 271–282. [CrossRef] [PubMed]
3. Padayatty, S.J.; Sun, A.Y.; Chen, Q.; Espey, M.G.; Drisko, J.; Levine, M. Vitamin C: Intravenous use by complementary and alternative medicine practitioners and adverse effects. *PLoS ONE* **2010**, *5*, e11414. [CrossRef] [PubMed]
4. Dachs, G.U.; Munn, D.G.; Carr, A.C.; Vissers, M.C.; Robinson, B.A. Consumption of vitamin C is below recommended daily intake in many cancer patients and healthy volunteers in Christchurch. *N. Z. Med. J.* **2014**, *127*, 73–76. [PubMed]
5. van Gorkom, G.N.Y.; Lookermans, E.L.; Van Elssen, C.H.M.J.; Bos, G.M.J. The Effect of Vitamin C (Ascorbic Acid) in the Treatment of Patients with Cancer: A Systematic Review. *Nutrients* **2019**, *11*, 977. [CrossRef] [PubMed]
6. Levine, M.; Conry-Cantilena, C.; Wang, Y.; Welch, R.W.; Washko, P.W.; Dhariwal, K.R.; Park, J.B.; Lazarev, A.; Graumlich, J.F.; King, J.; et al. Vitamin C pharmacokinetics in healthy volunteers: Evidence for a recommended dietary allowance. *Proc. Natl. Acad. Sci. USA* **1996**, *93*, 3704–3709. [CrossRef]
7. Nutrient Reference Values for Australia and New Zealand. Available online: https://www.nrv.gov.au/nutrients/vitamin-c (accessed on 2 July 2020).
8. Institute of Medicine (US) Panel on Dietary Antioxidants and Related Compounds. *Dietary Reference Intakes for Vitamin C, Vitamin E, Selenium, and Carotenoids*; National Academies Press: Washington, DC, USA, 2000. Available online: https://www.ncbi.nlm.nih.gov/books/NBK225480/ (accessed on 2 July 2020).
9. German Nutrition Society (DGE): New Reference Values for Vitamin C Intake. *Ann. Nutr. Metab.* **2015**, *67*, 13–20. [CrossRef]

10. Smirnoff, N. Ascorbic acid metabolism and functions: A comparison of plants and mammals. *Free Radic. Biol. Med.* **2018**, *122*, 116–129. [CrossRef]
11. Vissers, M.C.; Kuiper, C.; Dachs, G.U. Regulation of the 2-oxoglutarate-dependent dioxygenases and implications for cancer. *Biochem. Soc. Trans.* **2014**, *42*, 945–951. [CrossRef]
12. Kuiper, C.; Molenaar, I.G.; Dachs, G.U.; Currie, M.J.; Sykes, P.H.; Vissers, M.C. Low ascorbate levels are associated with increased hypoxia-inducible factor-1 activity and an aggressive tumor phenotype in endometrial cancer. *Cancer Res.* **2010**, *70*, 5749–5758. [CrossRef]
13. Kuiper, C.; Dachs, G.U.; Munn, D.; Currie, M.J.; Robinson, B.A.; Pearson, J.F.; Vissers, M.C. Increased tumor ascorbate is associated with extended disease-free survival and decreased hypoxia-inducible factor-1 activation in human colorectal cancer. *Front. Oncol.* **2014**, *4*, 10. [CrossRef] [PubMed]
14. Jóźwiak, P.; Ciesielski, P.; Zaczek, A.; Lipińska, A.; Pomorski, L.; Wieczorek, M.; Bryś, M.; Forma, E.; Krześlak, A. Expression of hypoxia inducible factor 1α and 2α and its association with vitamin C level in thyroid lesions. *J. Biomed. Sci.* **2017**, *24*, 83. [CrossRef] [PubMed]
15. Wohlrab, C.; Vissers, M.C.M.; Phillips, E.; Morrin, H.; Robinson, B.A.; Dachs, G.U. The association between ascorbate and the hypoxia-inducible factors in human renal cell carcinoma requires a functional von Hippel-Lindau protein. *Front. Oncol.* **2018**, *8*, 574. [CrossRef] [PubMed]
16. Campbell, E.J.; Dachs, G.U.; Morrin, H.R.; Davey, V.C.; Robinson, B.A.; Vissers, M.C.M. Activation of the hypoxia pathway in breast cancer tissue and patient survival are inversely associated with tumor ascorbate levels. *BMC Cancer* **2019**, *19*, 307. [CrossRef] [PubMed]
17. Marcus, S.L.; Dutcher, J.P.; Paietta, E.; Ciobanu, N.; Strauman, J.; Wiernik, P.H.; Hutner, S.H.; Frank, O.; Baker, H. Severe hypovitaminosis C occurring as the result of adoptive immunotherapy with high-dose interleukin 2 and lymphokine-activated killer cells. *Cancer Res.* **1987**, *47*, 4208–4212. [PubMed]
18. Khanzode, S.S.; Khanzode, S.D.; Dakhale, G.N. Serum and plasma concentration of oxidant and antioxidants in patients of *Helicobacter pylori* gastritis and its correlation with gastric cancer. *Cancer Lett.* **2003**, *195*, 27–31. [CrossRef]
19. Marakala, V.; Malathi, M.; Shivashankara, A.R. Lipid peroxidation and antioxidant vitamin status in oral cavity and oropharyngeal cancer patients. *Asian Pac. J. Cancer Prev.* **2012**, *13*, 5763–5765. [CrossRef]
20. Mayland, C.; Allen, K.R.; Degg, T.J.; Bennet, M. Micronutrient concentrations in patients with malignant disease: Effect of the inflammatory response. *Ann. Clin. Biochem.* **2004**, *41 Pt 2*, 138–141. [CrossRef]
21. Gackowski, D.; Kowalewski, J.; Siomek, A.; Olinski, R. Oxidative DNA damage and antioxidant vitamin level: Comparison among lung cancer patients, healthy smokers and nonsmokers. *Int. J. Cancer* **2005**, *114*, 153–156. [CrossRef]
22. Mayland, C.R.; Bennett, M.I.; Allan, K. Vitamin C deficiency in cancer patients. *Palliat. Med.* **2005**, *19*, 17–20. [CrossRef]
23. Levine, M.; Wang, Y.; Rumsey, S.C. Analysis of ascorbic acid and dehydroascorbic acid in biological samples. *Methods Enzymol.* **1999**, *299*, 65–76. [CrossRef]
24. Lykkesfeldt, J.; Tveden-Nyborg, P. The Pharmacokinetics of Vitamin C. *Nutrients* **2019**, *11*, 2412. [CrossRef] [PubMed]
25. Pearson, J.F.; Pullar, J.M.; Wilson, R.; Spittlehouse, J.K.; Vissers, M.C.M.; Skidmore, P.M.L.; Willis, J.; Cameron, V.A.; Carr, A.C. Vitamin C status correlates with markers of metabolic and cognitive health in 50-year-olds: Findings of the CHALICE cohort study. *Nutrients* **2017**, *9*, 831. [CrossRef] [PubMed]
26. Eating and Activity Guidelines. Available online: https://www.health.govt.nz/our-work/eating-and-activity-guidelines (accessed on 2 July 2020).
27. Food Data Central, U.S. Department of Agriculture. Available online: https://fdc.nal.usda.gov (accessed on 2 July 2020).
28. Carr, A.C.; Bozonet, S.M.; Vissers, M.C. A randomised cross-over pharmacokinetic bioavailability study of synthetic versus kiwifruit-derived vitamin C. *Nutrients* **2013**, *5*, 4451–4461. [CrossRef] [PubMed]
29. Levine, M.; Padayatty, S.J.; Espey, M.G. Vitamin C: A concentration-function approach yields pharmacology and therapeutic discoveries. *Adv. Nutr.* **2011**, *2*, 78–88. [CrossRef]
30. Aune, D.; Keum, N.; Giovannucci, E.; Fadnes, L.T.; Boffetta, P.; Greenwood, D.C.; Tonstad, S.; Vatten, L.J.; Riboli, E.; Norat, T. Dietary intake and blood concentrations of antioxidants and the risk of cardiovascular disease, total cancer, and all-cause mortality: A systematic review and dose-response meta-analysis of prospective studies. *Am. J. Clin. Nutr.* **2018**, *108*, 1069–1091. [CrossRef]

31. Ang, A.; Pullar, J.M.; Currie, M.J.; Vissers, M.C.M. Vitamin C and immune cell function in inflammation and cancer. *Biochem. Soc. Trans.* **2018**, *46*, 1147–1159. [CrossRef]
32. Zhang, M.; Robitaille, L.; Eintracht, S.; Hoffer, L.J. Vitamin C provision improves mood in acutely hospitalized patients. *Nutrition* **2011**, *27*, 530–533. [CrossRef]
33. Nechuta, S.; Lu, W.; Chen, Z.; Zheng, Y.; Gu, K.; Cai, H.; Zheng, W.; Shu, X.O. Vitamin supplement use during breast cancer treatment and survival: A prospective cohort study. *Cancer Epidemiol. Biomarkers Prev.* **2011**, *20*, 262–271. [CrossRef]
34. Poole, E.M.; Shu, X.; Caan, B.J.; Flatt, S.W.; Holmes, M.D.; Lu, W.; Kwan, M.L.; Nechuta, S.J.; Pierce, J.P.; Chen, W.Y. Postdiagnosis supplement use and breast cancer prognosis in the After Breast Cancer Pooling Project. *Breast Cancer Res. Treat* **2013**, *139*, 529–537. [CrossRef]
35. Huijskens, M.J.; Wodzig, W.K.; Walczak, M.; Germeraad, W.T.; Bos, G.M. Ascorbic acid serum levels are reduced in patients with hematological malignancies. *Results Immunol.* **2016**, *6*, 8–10. [CrossRef] [PubMed]
36. Gacitúa, T.A.; Sotomayor, C.G.; Groothof, D.; Eisenga, M.F.; Pol, R.A.; Borst, M.H.; Gans, R.O.B.; Berger, S.P.; Rodrigo, R.; Navis, G.J.; et al. Plasma Vitamin C and cancer mortality in kidney transplant recipients. *J. Clin. Med.* **2019**, *8*, 2064. [CrossRef] [PubMed]
37. Mackenzie, K.A.; Miller, A.P.; Hock, B.D.; Gardner, J.; Simcock, J.W.; Roake, J.A.; Dachs, G.U.; Robinson, B.A.; Currie, M.J. Angiogenesis and host immune response contribute to the aggressive character of non-melanoma skin cancers in renal transplant recipients. *Histopathology* **2011**, *58*, 875–885. [CrossRef] [PubMed]
38. Saito, K.; Yokoyama, T.; Yoshida, H.; Kim, H.; Shimada, H.; Yoshida, Y.; Iwasa, H.; Shimizu, Y.; Kondo, Y.; Handa, S.; et al. A significant relationship between plasma vitamin C concentration and physical performance among Japanese elderly women. *J. Gerontol. A Biol. Sci. Med. Sci.* **2012**, *67*, 295–301. [CrossRef]
39. McCall, S.J.; Clark, A.B.; Luben, R.N.; Wareham, N.J.; Khaw, K.T.; Myint, P.K. Plasma Vitamin C levels: Risk factors for deficiency and association with self-reported functional health in the European Prospective Investigation into Cancer-Norfolk. *Nutrients* **2019**, *11*, 1552. [CrossRef]
40. Wilson, R.; Willis, J.; Gearry, R.; Skidmore, P.; Fleming, E.; Frampton, C.; Carr, A. Inadequate vitamin C status in prediabetes and type 2 diabetes mellitus: Associations with glycaemic control, obesity, and smoking. *Nutrients* **2017**, *9*, 997. [CrossRef]
41. Johnston, C.S.; Barkyoumb, G.M.; Schumacher, S.S. Vitamin C supplementation slightly improves physical activity levels and reduces cold incidence in men with marginal vitamin C status: A randomized controlled trial. *Nutrients* **2014**, *6*, 2572–2583. [CrossRef]
42. Levine, M.; Wang, Y.; Padayatty, S.J.; Morrow, J. A new recommended dietary allowance of vitamin C for healthy young women. *Proc. Natl. Acad. Sci. USA* **2001**, *98*, 9842–9846. [CrossRef]
43. Carr, A.C.; Frei, B. Toward a new recommended dietary allowance for vitamin C based on antioxidant and health effects in humans. *Am. J. Clin. Nutr.* **1999**, *69*, 1086–1107. [CrossRef]
44. Kapil, U.; Singh, P.; Bahadur, S.; Shukla, N.K.; Dwivedi, S.; Pathak, P.; Singh, R. Association of vitamin A, vitamin C and zinc with laryngeal cancer. *Indian J. Cancer* **2003**, *40*, 67–70.

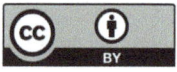

© 2020 by the authors. Licensee MDPI, Basel, Switzerland. This article is an open access article distributed under the terms and conditions of the Creative Commons Attribution (CC BY) license (http://creativecommons.org/licenses/by/4.0/).

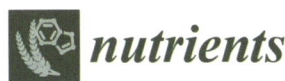

Review

Vitamin C for Cardiac Protection during Percutaneous Coronary Intervention: A Systematic Review of Randomized Controlled Trials

Sher Ali Khan [1], Sandipan Bhattacharjee [1], Muhammad Owais Abdul Ghani [2], Rachel Walden [3] and Qin M. Chen [1,*]

1. Department of Pharmacy Practice and Science, College of Pharmacy, University of Arizona, 1295 N. Martin Ave, Tucson, AZ 85721, USA; sheralikhan6161@gmail.com (S.A.K.); bhattacharjee@pharmacy.arizona.edu (S.B.)
2. Department of Cardiac Surgery, Vanderbilt University, Nashville, TN 37203, USA; owais.a.gh@gmail.com
3. Annette and Irwin Eskind Family Biomedical Library, Jean & Alexander Heard Libraries, Vanderbilt University, Nashville, TN 37203, USA; Rachel.l.walden@vanderbilt.edu
* Correspondence: qchen1@pharmacy.arizona.edu; Tel.: +1-(520)626-9126

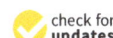

Received: 27 June 2020; Accepted: 21 July 2020; Published: 23 July 2020

Abstract: Percutaneous coronary intervention (PCI) is the preferred treatment for acute coronary syndrome (ACS) secondary to atherosclerotic coronary artery disease. This nonsurgical procedure is also used for selective patients with stable angina. Although the procedure is essential for restoring blood flow, reperfusion can increase oxidative stress as a side effect. We address whether intravenous infusion of vitamin C (VC) prior to PCI provides a benefit for cardioprotection. A total of eight randomized controlled trials (RCT) reported in the literature were selected from 371 publications through systematic literature searches in six electronic databases. The data of VC effect on cardiac injury biomarkers and cardiac function were extracted from these trials adding up to a total of 1185 patients. VC administration reduced cardiac injury as measured by troponin and CK-MB elevations, along with increased antioxidant reservoir, reduced reactive oxygen species (ROS) and decreased inflammatory markers. Improvement of the left ventricular ejection fraction (LVEF) and telediastolic left ventricular volume (TLVV) showed a trend but inconclusive association with VC. Intravenous infusion of VC before PCI may serve as an effective method for cardioprotection against reperfusion injury.

Keywords: Vitamin C (VC); periprocedural myocardial injury (PMI); troponin; CK-MB; left ventricular ejection fraction (LVEF); reactive oxygen species (ROS)

1. Introduction

Cardiovascular disease (CVD) is the number one cause of death worldwide [1]. CVD claimed 859,125 lives in 2017 in the United States [2] or 17.9 million in 2016 worldwide [1]. Among all forms of CVD, acute coronary syndrome (ACS) accounts for 40–50% of CVD deaths and is a leading cause of mortality and morbidity [3,4]. Common presentations of ACS include unstable angina, ST-elevation myocardial infarction (STEMI), and non-ST elevation myocardial infarction (NSTEMI) [5,6]. The advancement of medical science has led to effective management of ACS, mostly with percutaneous coronary intervention (PCI) and adjuvant pharmacological therapy [6–12]. About 90% of STEMI patients or 50% of NSTEMI patients are treated with PCI [13]. Despite the improvement in PCI technology, there is a possibility that patients can suffer from complications, including a bleeding event, hematoma, re-infarction, cardiogenic shock, heart failure, and death in the worst-case scenario [14–18].

The PCI procedure results in a periprocedural myocardial injury (PMI) in 5–30% of the patients [11,19,20]. Such injury is measurable by biomarkers of myocardial cell death, i.e., elevation of cardiac troponin I (cTnI) and creatinine phosphokinase MB isoenzyme (CK-MB) in the circulation [19,21]. While myocardial revascularization is essential for relieving symptoms and preventing death, reperfusion can cause escalation of oxidative stress on top of ischemia and is estimated to account for 40% of the final infarct size [22,23]. Reperfusion injury can lead to fatal arrhythmias and re-infarction [3,24]. Reactive oxygen species (ROS) are detectable in the blood circulation in higher levels within the first few minutes of reperfusion [25–31]. ROS produced during reperfusion are believed to be an important cause of cell death and procedure-related complications [23,32].

Clinical studies have confirmed that antioxidant supplements are indeed effective in reducing ROS measured in the serum [33,34]. Vitamin C (ascorbic acid or ascorbate, VC) is a water soluble molecule that can be administered orally or via an intravenous route [35]. VC is a classic antioxidant that has a proven record for scavenging ROS, but whether it plays a role in reducing reperfusion injury has been a matter of debate [36–43]. In studies with experimental animals, administration of antioxidant agents significantly reduces ROS, appears to lower apoptotic load, and improves the outcome of reperfusion [28]. The biologic plausibility of the cardioprotective effect of VC has been shown in clinical trials where VC reduced ROS when administered prior to PCI [33,34,42,43]. However, the outcomes are conflicting, with some studies showing reduction of the biomarkers of myocardial injury cTnI and CK-MB [39,41], whereas others fail to show a benefit [29,44]. Given these inconsistences, it is prudent to address the question whether or not VC administration is benefits following PCI.

Here we address whether addition of VC to the standard PCI protocol offers protection against reperfusion related myocardial injury using a systematic review approach. Three systematic reviews and meta-analysis have determined the effect of VC following cardiac surgery, but none have been summarized the effect following PCI [45–48]. Given the fact that PCI is increasingly common for the treatment of ACS, and in selective patients for the treatment of stable angina, a systematic review of VC treatment for PCI patients can provide needed information to guide its use during clinical practice. Our primary measures include biomarkers of myocardial injury, cardiac function, and vascular perfusion indices. The potential benefit was traced to the effect of VC on the levels of reactive oxygen species (ROS) and inflammatory mediators.

2. Materials and Methods

The Preferred Reporting Items for Systematic Reviews (PRISMA) guideline [49] was followed for this systematic literature review using an a-priori inclusion and exclusion criteria.

2.1. Inclusion and Exclusion Criteria

The a priori inclusion criteria were: (1) randomized controlled trials (RCTs) assessing the effect of VC in patients greater than 18 years old who underwent PCI. (2) VC was administered within 24 h before or during PCI, (3) the control group received either placebo or standard care, (4) published and unpublished RCTs, (5) RCTs published in any language, (6) RCTs published from inception of respective databases to 18 February 2020. The excluded reports did not meet the inclusion criteria. We considered the following endpoints: myocardial injury (troponin, CK-MB), cardiac contractility (left ventricular ejection fraction, LVEF and telediastolic left ventricular volume, TLVV), restenosis of the treated coronary artery, reactive oxygen species (ROS), inflammatory mediators or markers, and vascular endothelial dysfunction.

2.2. Literature Search

The PRISMA flowchart summary is shown in Figure 1. The librarian of Vanderbilt University (Rachel Walden) was involved in developing the literature search strategies for the different electronic databases. Search for the appropriate electronic databases by primary (Sher Ali Khan) or secondary reviewer (Muhammad Owais Abdul Ghani) was performed independently in the first stage and with the input from the librarian in the second phase. No major discrepancy was noted among the two independent reviewers in shortlisted trials and quality assessment. Minor discrepancy was noted in extracted data, which was resolved with discussion reaching mutual agreement.

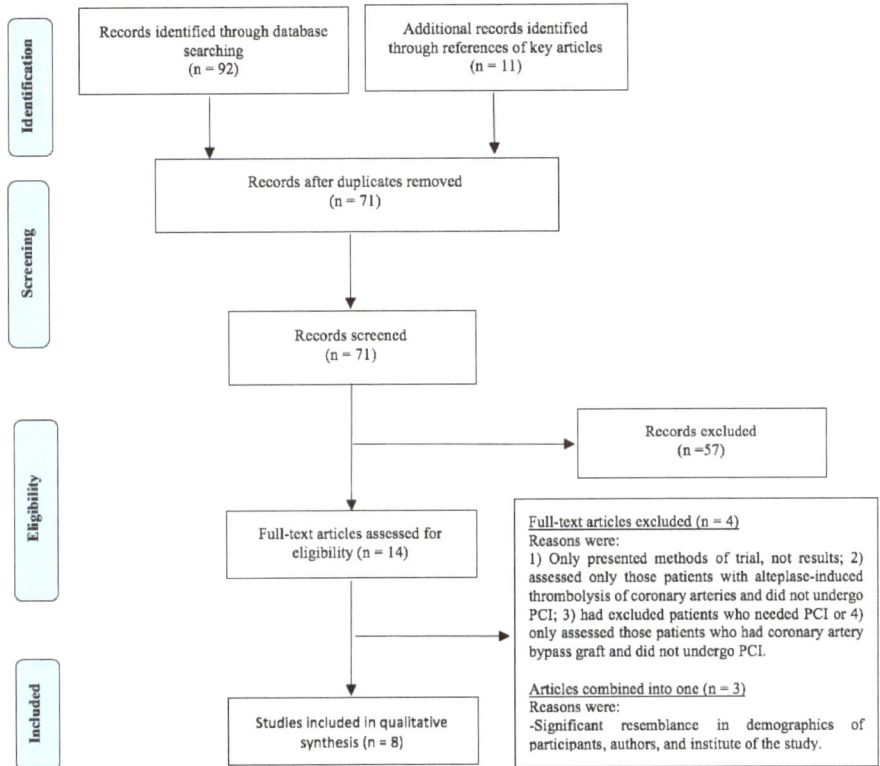

Figure 1. Preferred Reporting Items for Systematic Reviews and Meta-Analyses (PRISMA) Flow Diagram. The numbers document the literature search results.

The search strategy used a combination of keywords and subject headings to find studies discussing the use of VC in percutaneous coronary intervention. The following terms were used to create the search strategy: ascorbic acid, ascorbicum, l-ascorbic acid, hybrin, ascorbate, vitamin C, magnorbin, angioplasty, percutaneous coronary intervention, percutaneous coronary revascularization, myocardial and coronary reperfusion, and myocardial reperfusion injury (see Supplementary Material, which presents full search strategies). Search strategy was created for PubMed using both keywords and medical subject headings and then translated to use in Embase (Ovid), Web of Science (Clarivate Analytics), Cumulative Index to Nursing and Allied Health Literature (CINAHL), Cochrane Library (Wiley) and Clinicaltrials.gov from the inception of the database till 18th February 2020. The resulting reports were screened using Raayan web application. A manual search of full content of key references was also performed. The duplicate records were removed electronically followed by careful checking.

2.3. Quality Assessment of Included Trials

The revised Cochrane risk of bias tool for randomized trials (RoB2) was applied to assess the risk of bias for each included trial [50]. The following domains were evaluated: random sequence generation, allocation concealment, blinding of patients and personnel, blinding of outcome assessment and incomplete outcome data. Each domain was assigned with a low, unclear or high risk of bias score.

3. Results

3.1. Characteristics of the Trials

In total 103 publications were found in which 92 were revealed with electronic search of databases and 11 were revealed with manual search of key references. After removing duplicates, 71 publications were screened and 14 relevant trials were shortlisted. Four trials were excluded due to the fact that only the protocol was reported [51], focused on alteplase induced thrombolysis [52], did not include a PCI procedure [53], or only reported the patients who received coronary artery bypass grafting instead of PCI [54]. Among the 10 remaining trials, 3 had significant resemblance in demographics of participants, authors, and institute where they were conducted [34,42,43]. Authors of these three trials were contacted multiple times to confirm if they are conducted on the same patient cohort. The consensus was to combine and weight them as one trial and to only consider those outcomes from each article which are not common among the them. Hence, only 8 trials were included in this review as shown in the flow of search strategy (Figure 1).

Geographically, the reported trials were carried out in five countries: Iran (one), Chile (two), Japan (one), China (one), Italy (two) and Canada (one) (Table 1). Total sample size of adding ten trials together was 1297 patients, a number which is derived from the subject number in the final statistics of each included trial. The mean age of the patients ranged from 56 to 68 years among nine trials with one trial not reporting the age distribution [33]. The gender ratio showed 60% to 95% male in the included ten trials. VC was administered via intravenous (i.v.) infusion in 9 trials and the oral route in one trial [55]. One trial had VC given through both i.v. infusion and intra coronary injection [39]. The dose of VC in most trials was 1 to 3 g (Table 1), with an exception of two trials from the same institute [40,44] where patients received 960 mL of 320 mmol/L of VC, equivalent to 54 g.

All trials administered VC within 12 h prior to PCI. VC was the only antioxidant regimen in all trials except 4 with additional supplements: vitamin E and beta-carotene before PCI [55], oral vitamin E [40,44] or vitamin A plus vitamin E after PCI [33] (Table 1). In one of the included trials, all patients received 325 mg of aspirin daily for entire study period [55]. Five trials enrolled patients who had ACS and underwent urgent PCI, whereas the remaining five trials included participants who had stable angina and underwent elective PCI. One trial contained patients who had either ACS or stable angina and underwent urgent or elective PCI respectively [29]. In this trial authors had assessed the outcomes of three groups: ACS patients received VC, ACS patients without VC, and stable angina patients not treated with VC. We only considered ACS patients who either or not received VC.

Table 1. Demographics of 10 Randomized Clinical Trials Meeting the Inclusion and Exclusion Criteria.

	Trial	Country	Diag	Sample Size (Ctr, VC)	Age (Mean (±SD) Years)		Sex (Male) n (%)		Vitamin C			Additional Therapy to VC Group (Yes/No)
					Ctr	VC	Ctr	VC	Route	Dose (g)	Time before PCI (min)	
1	Shafaei et al. (2019) [39]	Iran	ACS	252 (126,126)	57.18 ± 10.4	58.64 ± 10.41	97 (76.9)	104 (82.5)	IV, IC	3	0	No
2	Ramos et al. (2017) [a] [44]	Chile	ACS	67 (41,26)	56.16 ± 8.51	59.2 ± 11.98	NA	NA	IV	56	30	Yes [e]
3	Valls et al. (2016) [a] [40]	Chile	ACS	43 (21,22)	57.1 ± 7.2	59.8 ± 13.3	19 (95.2)	20 (90.9)	IV	56	60	Yes [e]
4	Wang et al. (2014) [41]	China	SA	532 (267,265)	58.0 ± 10.1	57.9 ± 10.4	182 (68.1)	192 (72)	IV	3	360	No
5	Basili et al. (2010–2011) [c]	Italy	SA	56 (28,28)	68 ± 9	66 ± 8	23 (82)	24 (86)	IV	1	60	No
6	Gasparetto et al. (2005) [33]	Italy	ACS	98 (49,49)	40–86 years		74.4% Males		IV	1	60	Yes [f]
7	Guan et al. (1999) [d] [29]	Japan	ACS	21 (11,10)	68 ± 4	68 ± 4	8(72)	6 (60)	IV	2	0	No
8	Tardif et al. (1997) [b] [55]	Canada	SA	116 (62,54)	60.3 ± 8.4	57.7 ± 11.1	61 (77)	66 (84)	PO	1	720	Yes [g]

The trial did not have a funding source unless indicated by "a" or "b". "a" indicates funding source of Chile National Fund for Scientific and Technological Development (FONDECYT), "b" indicates funding source of the Medical Research Council of Canada. "c" indicates that three articles were combined to represent one trial, they were Basili et al., 2010 [43], Pignatelli et al., 2011 [42] and Basili et al., 2011 [34]. The trial was placebo controlled unless indicated by "d". "d" indicates control group received standard treatment. "e" indicates that an oral dose of vitamin E (alpha Tocopherol) 800 IU administered before PCI, oral doses of vitamin C 500 mg/12 h and vitamin E (alpha Tocopherol) 400 IU/d administered after PCI for 84 days. "f" indicates that oral doses of vitamin C 1 g, vitamin A 50 U and vitamin E 300 mg were administered after PCI daily for one month. "g" indicates that oral doses of vitamin C 500 mg, vitamin E (alpha Tocopherol) 700 IU and beta-carotene 30,000 IU twice daily for one month before PCI and for five to seven months after PCI, plus an extra dose of Vitamin E (alpha Tocopherol) 2000 IU 12 h before PCI. SA: stable angina; ACS: acute coronary syndrome; Diag: diagnosis; Ctr: control group; VC: vitamin C group; Tx: Treatment; IV: intravenous; IC: Intra-coronary; NA: not available despite the effort of contacting the correspondent authors.

3.2. Risk of Bias Analysis

The results of the risk of bias analysis are indicated in Figure 2. Most trials had generated random sequences for assigning intervention versus control groups. Two trials did not report randomization strategy, one of which is represented by three articles (i.e., Basili et al., 2011, Pignatelli et al., 2011 and Basili et al., 2010) [29,34,42,43], for which their corresponding authors were contacted via emails in an effort to find the details of randomization. However, we did not receive any replies. The concern about randomization did not affect the outcome values. As there was no significant difference in baseline characteristics between comparison groups, the overall risk of bias of these studies is judged as low.

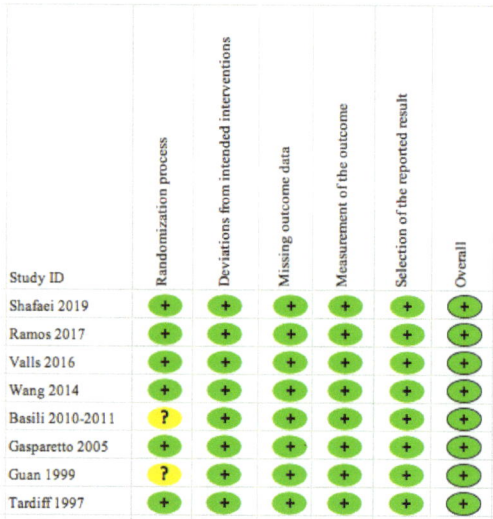

Figure 2. Risk of Bias of 8 Included Trials. The plus sign in green (+) shows "low risk" for bias and the question mark in yellow (?) shows "some concerns" for bias. None of the trials show "high risk" for bias.

3.3. Effect of VC Administration on Myocardial Injury

3.3.1. Elevation of Troponin

An elevated level of cardiac troponins in the circulation is considered a hallmark of cardiac injury [5]. Three trials in four articles reported the blood levels of cardiac troponins within 24 h of PCI [39,41–43] (Table 2). Three trials analyzed cTnI using a traditional assay, whereas one trial reported the results from a high sensitivity cardiac troponin T (hs-cTnT) assay [39]. Two of the included articles had published results from same trials [42,43]. We considered the values from only one assay [43]. As a result, the findings from three trials are reported here [39,41,43].

Table 2. Cardiac Injury and Functional Outcomes of Vitamin C Administration.

Trial [Ref]	Troponin < 24 h			CK-MB < 24 h			LVEF < 15 Days or 3 mo			Infarct Size < 15 Days or 3 mo			TLVV (mL), 7 or 30 Days		
	Ctr	VC	p	Ctr	VC	p	Ctr	VC	p	Ctr	VC	p	Ctr	VC	p
Shafaei et al. (2019) [39]	7.5 ng/L [a,b]	7.1 ng/L [a,b]	0.003	3.98 ng/L [b]	3.52 ng/L [b]	0.00									
Ramos et al. (2017) [44]				387 u/L (189.0–725.0)	335 u/L (134.0–478.0)	0.66	49.1% [c] (41.0–59.4) 47.5% [d] (38.0–61.7)	47.3% [c] (40.0–56.4) 54.6% [d] (39.9–64.8)	0.54 0.41	21.5% [c] (17.0–34.2) 19.0% [d] (14.0–34.0)	17.0% [c] (13.0–36.0) 21.0% [d] (14.0–34.0)	0.66 0.96			
Valls et al. (2016) [40]				NA [g]	NA [g]	NS [g]	48.0% [c,b] (56.6–33.3) 44% [d,b] (34.0–56.0)	56% [c,b] (44.0–58.6) 63% [d,b] (50.0–68.0)	NS [g] 0.05						
Wang et al. (2014) [41]	0.04 ng/mL (0.02–1.12)	0.03 ng/mL (0.03–0.06)	0.02	6.1 ng/mL (4.4–6.4)	4.9 ng/mL (4.1–5.7)	0.001									
Pignatelli et al. [h] (2011) [42]							54.1 ± 4.7%	58.3 ± 2.9%	0.03						
Basili et al. [h] (2010) [43]	Δ 0.027 ng/mL (0.05 to 0.032)	Δ 0.008 ng/mL (0.02 to 0.013)	0.08												
Gasparetto et al. (2005) [33]													125.12 ± 29.8 [e] 132.0 ± 33.5 [f]	119.4 ± 29.4 [e] 123.4 ± 21.6 [f]	0.05 0.05

All numbers represent means unless they are italicized, which indicate median. The data were extracted from numeric numbers from the publication unless indicated with "b", which was derived from graphs in the publication. "a" indicates high sensitivity troponin T (hs-TnT) test results. Ctr: control group; VC: vitamin C group; TLVV: telediastolic left ventricular volume. NS: non-significant; "c" or "d" indicates that LVEF or infarct size was measured within 15 days or at 3 months after PCI, respectively. "e" or "f" indicates that TLVV was measured at 7 or 30 days after PCI, respectively. "g" indicates number not available despite the effort of contacting the correspondent author; NA: not available; "h" indicates that the articles represent the same trial. Δ indicates change from baseline value.

Two trials, with a sample size of 252 and 532 respectively, showed significantly less elevation of cardiac troponins following PCI in the VC group as compared to controls [39,41] (Table 2). An additional trial with a total of 56 enrolled patients showed a trend for troponin reduction by VC treatment ($p = 0.08$) [43]. Procedure related myocardial infarction (PMI) was defined as elevation of myocardial injury marker cTnI or hs-TnT five-fold above the upper limit of normal (5xULN). The incidence of 5xULN was significantly less frequent in the VC group compared to controls (91.5% vs. 93.8%, $p = 0.009$; and 10.9% vs. 18.4%, $p = 0.016$) [39,41]. Multivariable logistic regression analysis revealed that VC treatment before PCI was an independent predictor of lower frequency of PMI (odds ratio 0.56; 95% confidence interval, 0.33–0.97; $p = 0.037$) [41]. Overall, there is evidence that administration of VC before or after PCI is associated with a decrease in blood levels of troponin and a lower frequency of PMI.

3.3.2. Elevation of CK-MB

Circulating CK-MB serves as an additional biomarker of cardiac injury. Four trials presented CK-MB data as measured within 24 h after PCI [39–41,44]. The two trials with enrollment of 252 or 532 patients showed significantly less CK-MB elevation in the VC group compared with controls [39,41] (Table 2). One trial with a sample size of 27 patients in the VC group showed a decrease in the mean value but the statistics did not show significant difference ($p = 0.66$) [44]. Another trial did not provide the values for CK-MB, however, these investigators stated that no significant difference was noted with VC treatment [40]. The corresponding author was contacted via email twice ten days apart for retrieving the values of CK-MB without success.

The two trials that reported positive outcomes for VC reducing CK-MB levels also showed that 5xUNL of CK-MB was significantly less frequent in the VC group compared with the control group (60.8% vs. 69.9%, $p = 0.03$; and 4.2% vs. 8.6%, $p = 0.035$) [39,41]. Again, multivariable logistic regression analysis showed that administration of VC before PCI independently predicted a lower frequency of PMI as defined by CK-MB elevation (odds ratio, 0.37; 95% confidence interval, 0.14–0.99; $p = 0.048$) [41]. Consistent with the data from troponins, VC administration prior to PCI was associated with significant inhibition of CK-MB release and a lower frequency of PMI.

3.4. Effect of VC on Cardiac Contractility

Cardiac contractile function was measured by LVEF and TLVV. Three trials measured LVEF at 6 to 15 days after PCI [40,42,44], while one trial measured TLVV [33] (Table 2). One trial used echocardiography to assess LVEF [42], while two trials used cardiac resonance imaging (CMR) [40,44]. Two of these trials did second measurements of LVEF with CMR at 3 months after PCI with a smaller sample size (i.e., 21 and 40, respectively) than originally randomized to the treatment (i.e., 43 and 67, respectively) [40,44]. The reasons for the lower than original sample size included refusal from participants, lost to follow up, contraindication to contrast-based imaging (such as renal impairment), and death.

An improvement in LVEF due to VC, when measured at 6 to 15 days following PCI was reported in one trial [42]. The second trial showing a significant improvement in the median value for LVEF in the VC group at three months following PCI, but not at day 6 [40]. The third trial did not find any significant improvement in LVEF at 7–15 days or at three months [44]. An independent trial measured TLVV at one week or one month after PCI and found significantly lowered TLVV in the VC group, indicating better preservation of cardiac function [33]. Overall the evidence was inconclusive for the effect of VC on cardiac contractility.

3.5. Effect of VC on Infarct Size and Coronary Artery Restenosis

One trial used CMR to determine infarct size at two weeks for 67 participants and at three months for 43 follow-up participants [44] (Table 2). The measurements did not yield significant differences between the control and VC groups at either time point. One trial administered two pills of multivitamins to the intervention group daily for 30 days before PCI; each pill contains 250 mg of VC, 15,000 IU of beta carotene and 350 IU of vitamin E [55]. This trial assessed coronary artery restenosis at six months after PCI with coronary angiography and did not show any significant difference between the control and VC groups (38.9% vs. 40.3%, $p = 0.89$). This trial had two more intervention groups, Procubol ($n = 58$) or Procubol plus multivitamins ($n = 56$). The combination did not provide additional benefit compared to Procubol alone.

Overall the results are inconclusive for reducing infarct size, TLVV, and coronary artery restenosis, due to the fact that each of these endpoints was reported by only one study with limited numbers of patients enrolled.

3.6. Effect of VC on Total Antioxidant Status (TAS)

Three trials evaluated antioxidant reservoirs after PCI [33,40,44] (Table 3). The levels of ascorbate in serum, reduced glutathione (GSH) in erythrocytes, and ferric reducing ability of plasma (FRAP) were measured immediately after PCI or at 6–8 h following PCI in two trials [40,44]. Both trials showed significantly elevated ascorbate and FRAP levels at either time point in the VC group. At the time of hospital discharge (with no specific timeline provided), there was no significant difference between the comparison groups [40,44].

GSH levels were significantly higher in the VC group than in the control group immediately after PCI in one trial [44] or at 6–8 h after in two trials [40,44]. There was no significant difference between the comparison groups at the time of hospital discharge [40,44]. The third trial [33] measured total antioxidant status at 48 h and 1 month after PCI. They found significantly higher levels at 48 h ($p < 0.01$) but not 1 month following VC administration. Overall, administration of VC was associated with increased antioxidant reservoirs within 48 h after PCI.

3.7. Effect of VC on Reactive Oxidation Species (ROS)

Five trials in seven published articles had evaluated the impact of VC administration on ROS, measured as 8-hydroxy-2-deoxyguanosine (8-OHdG), 8-iso-prostaglandin F2a (8-iso-PGF2a), F2-isoprostanes (F2-IPs) and 8-isoprostane [29,33,34,40–43] (Table 4). The results of one trial is published in three articles [34,42,43]. Most of the trials measured blood levels of these markers except for one trial, which quantified 8-epi prostaglandin in the urine [29]. Significant reduction of 8-OHdG in the VC group was observed immediately, at 1 h [42], or 6 h after PCI [41]. Lower levels of 8-iso-PGF2a were reported due to VC at 6–8 h after PCI [43]. A similar time frame for reduction of plasma 8-isoprostane ($p < 0.01$) was also observed [40].

Table 3. Effect of Vitamin C on Antioxidant Reservoir.

Trial [Ref]	Measure		Baseline	0 h	6–8 h	48 h	1 Month	Discharge
Ramos et al. (2017) [44]	Vit C (mmol/L)	ctr	0.02 (0.02–0.050)	0.02 (0.01–0.03)	0.02 (0.01–0.04)			0.03 (0.01–0.05)
		VC	0.04 (0.02–0.09)	9.63 (6.25–11.64)	0.72 (0.23–2.43)			0.02 (0.01–0.05)
		p	NS	<0.0001	<0.0001			NS
	FRAP (umol/L)	ctr	304.1 (213.0–429.6)	310.3 (227.7–400.0)	287 (250.2–391.2)			352.2 (220.0–371.8)
		VC	271.7 (200.2–396.4)	8050 (50275.0–11418.0)	1080 (699.9–2062.0)			378.2 (257.9–464.3)
		p	NS	<0.0001	<0.0001			NS
	GSH (mmol/L)	ctr	3.59 (3.21–4.54)	3.92 (3.26–5.28)	4.13 (3.48–5.06)			4.02 (3.34–4.43)
		VC	4.11 (3.61–6.56)	3.71 (1.75–4.60)	2.59 (1.61–4.15)			3.87 (3.55–4.86)
		p	NS	0.0149	0.0198			NS
Valls et al. (2016) [40]	Vit C (mmol/L)	ctr	0.03 ± 0.02	0.03 ± 0.04	0.03 ± 0.03			0.02 ± 0.01
		VC	0.1 ± 0.20	9.79 ± 3.87	1.79 ± 1.51			0.06 ± 0.06
		p	NS	<0.01	<0.01			NS
	FRAP (umol/L)	ctr	NA	1×	1×			NA
		VC	NA	29×	4.8×			NA
		p	NS	<0.01	<0.01			NS
	GSH [b] (mmol/L)	ctr	4.2 ± 1.54	4.7 ± 2.2	4.9 ± 2.4			4.4 ± 2.0
		VC	5 ± 2.29	3 ± 2.1	2.4 ± 1.76			3.8 ± 0.7
		p	NS	NS	<0.01			NS
Gasparetto et al. (2005) [33]	TAS (umol/L)	ctr	419.79 ± 34.26			526.47 ± 44.24	598.47 ± 54.99	
		VC	401.95 ± 19.02			737.65 ± 51.15	647.38 ± 54.33	
		p	NS			<0.01	NS	

All numbers represent means unless they are italicized, which indicate median. Ctr: control group; VC: vitamin C group; FRAP: ferric reducing ability of plasma; TAS: Total antioxidant status; NA: not available despite the effort of contacting the correspondent authors; NS: p value not significant. Baseline shows the value before PCI and 0 h values were samples taken immediately after PCI. "b" indicates the number was derived from graphs in the publication.

Table 4. Effect of Vitamin C on ROS and Inflammatory Biomarkers.

Trial [Ref]	Measure		Baseline	0–1 h	1–2 h	6–8 h	48 h	1 Month
Valls et al. (2016) [40]	8-isoprotane [b] (pg/mL)	ctr	24.0 ± 16.0	28.0 ± 18.0		17.1 ± 7.0		
		VC	24.0 ± 10.4	47 ± 23.0		26 ± 13.0		
		p	NS	<0.05		NS		
Wang et al. (2014) [41]	8-OHdG (ng/mL)	ctr	3.8 ± 1.2			2.4 ± 1.0		
		VC	3.6 ± 1.2			4.1 ± 1.1		
		p	NS			<0.001		
Basili et al. (2011) [c] [34]	TxB2 [b] (ng/mL)	ctr	23 ± 2.0	26 ± 1.1	26.5 ± 4.0			
		VC	24 ± 3.5	21 ± 3.3	23 ± 3.5			
		p	NS	<0.05	<0.05			
	sNOX2-dp [b] (pg/mL)	ctr	19 ± 1.0	21.8 ± 0.2	22 ± 1.8			
		VC	21.4 ± 1.2	18.4 ± 1.4	19 ± 2.3			
		p	NS	0.05	<0.05			
	8-OHdG (ng/mL)	ctr	3.7 ± 1.3	4.2 ± 1.1	4.6 ± 1.0			
		VC	3.7 ± 1.1	2.6 ± 1.1	2.7 ± 0.87			
		p	NS	<0.0001	<0.0001			
	hs-crp (mg/L)	ctr	1.25 (0.80–2.00)	1.3 (0.75–2.0)	1.25 (0.95–2.10)			
		VC	1.0 (0.71–1.90)	1 (0.67–1.60)	1.37 (1.0–2.0)			
		p	0.451	NS	NS			
Pignatelli et al. [c] (2011) [42]	TNFα (pg/mL)	ctr	40 (40.0–50.0)	40 (40.0–50.0)	46.5 (40.0–58.0)			
		VC	42.5 (35.0–50.0)	45 (40.0–60.0)	43.5 (36.5–58.5)			
		p	0.735	NS	NS			
	sCD40L (ng/mL)	ctr	2.3 ± 1.2	3.2 ± 1.5	3.4 ± 1.7			
		VC	2.3 ± 1.4	2.2 ± 1.1	2.4 ± 1.0			
		p	0.95	0.0057	0.016			
	CD40L (MF)	ctr	4.3 ± 0.78	5.1 ± 1.3	5.4 ± 1.2			
		VC	4.2 ± 0.88	3.8 ± 1.3	3.8 ± 1.1			
		p	0.0724	0.0008	0.0001			
Basili et al. [c] (2010) [43]	8-iso-PGF2a (pg/mL)	ctr	126 (85.0 to 170.0)	50 (20.7 to 102.5)				
		VC	142.5 (85.5 to 187.5)	161.5 (117.5 to 190.0)				
		p	NS	<0.0001				
Gasparetto et al. (2005) [33]	ROM (U.CARR)	ctr	295.4 ± 36.30				335.6 ± 35.8	377.3 ± 39.0
		VC	308.6 ± 40.30				307.5 ± 47.1	369.1 ± 42.3
		p	NS				<0.05	<NS

All numbers represent means unless they are italicized, which indicate median. "b" indicates that the values extracted from graphs in the publication; "c": indicates that the articles represent the same trial. 8-OHdG: 8-hydroxy-2-deoxyguanosine; TxB2: thromboxane B2; sNOX2-dp: soluble NOX2 derived peptide; hs-crp: high sensitivity C-reactive protein; sCD40L: soluble CD40L; 8-iso-PGF2a: 8-iso-prostaglandin F2 alpha; ROMs: reactive oxygen metabolites in Carratelli Units (U.CARR). 1 U.CARR = 0.08 mg % oxygen peroxide. Ctr: control group; VC: vitamin C group; NS: p value not significant. Baseline shows the value before PCI and 0 h values were samples taken immediately after PCI.

An assay measuring hydroperoxydes as a reflection of ROS levels in the blood showed benefit for VC ($p < 0.05$) at 48 h but not at 1 month after PCI [33]. Lack of VC association was reported by Guan et al. [29] with a urinary levels of ROS byproduct 8-epi-PGF2a (ng/mmol creatinine) measured at 0 to 150 min after PCI. The values for control group were 60 ± 8 at baseline, 81 ± 15 at 0–30 min, 93 ± 13 at 30–60 min, 122 ± 16 at 60–90 min and 82 ± 8 at 120–150 min after PCI. The values for VC group were 72 ± 12 at baseline, 98 ± 26 at 0–30 min, 104 ± 13 at 30–60 min, 123 ± 15 at 60–90 min and decreased to baseline levels at 120 to 150 min after PCI. Overall, four out of five trials showed significant association of VC with lower levels of ROS, especially when ROS products were measured in the blood within 48 h of PCI.

3.8. Effect of VC on Inflammation Mediators/Markers

One trial in three published articles had evaluated the effect of VC on serum levels of inflammatory markers or mediators [34,42,43] (Table 5). The inflammatory mediators or markers measured included thromboxane B2 (TxB2), soluble NOX2 derived peptide (sNOX2-dp), soluble CD40L (sCD40L), platelet CD40L, high sensitivity C-reactive protein (hs-CRP), and tumor necrosis factor alpha (TNFa).

Table 5. Effect of Vitamin C on Reperfusion Indices and Vascular Endothelial Dysfunction.

Trial	Measure		Baseline	0 h	48 h	1 Month
Valls et al. (2016) [40]	TIMI (TMPG of 2–3)	ctr		79%		
		VC		95%		
		p		<0.01		
	TIMI (TMPG of 0–1)	ctr		21%		
		VC		5%		
		p		<0.01		
Basili et al. (2010) [43]	%Δ cTFC (frames/s)	ctr	40.2	−23%		
		VC	36.1	−41%		
		p	NS	<0.0001		
	TIMI (TMPG < 2)	ctr	89%	32%		
		VC	86%	4%		
		p	NS	<0.01		
	TIMI (TMPG = 3)	ctr		39%		
		VC		79%		
		p		<0.01		
Gasparetto et al. (2005) [33]	sVCAM-1	ctr	1.44 ± 0.7		2.03 ± 0.5	2.13 ± 0.8
	(ug/mL)	VC	1.53 ± 0.6		1.63 ± 0.7	1.86 ± 0.9
		p	NS		<0.01	NS

All numbers represent means unless they are italicized, which indicate median. TIMI: Thrombolysis in Myocardial Infarction; TMPG: TIMI Myocardial Perfusion Grade; cTFC: TIMI Frame Counts; %Δ cTFC: % changes of cTFC; sVCAM-1: soluble vascular adhesion molecule 1. Baseline shows the value before PCI and 0 h values were samples taken immediately after PCI.

TxB2 and sNOX2 were significantly lower in the VC group compared with the control group (Table 5) immediately or at 1 h after PCI in one trial [34]. VC administration resulted in decreases in sCD40L and platelet CD40L at these time points [42]. However, VC did not affect the level of circulating hs-CRP and TNFa as measured immediately or at 1 h after PCI [42]. Therefore, VC administration is associated with lower levels TxB2, sNOX2-dp, sCD40L, platelet CD40L, but not hs-CRP and TNFa when measured within a short time frame after PCI.

3.9. Effect of VC on Reperfusion Indices and Vascular Endothelial Dysfunction

Three trials determined the effect of VC on coronary reperfusion indices and vascular endothelial dysfunction [33,40,43] (Table 5). The reperfusion indices were corrected Thrombolysis in Myocardial Infarction (TIMI) Frame Counts (cTFC) and TIMI Myocardial Perfusion Grades (TMPG), both reflecting blood flow in the coronary arteries. The higher values of TMPG and lower values of cTFC indicate a better perfusion outcome. The perfusion indices (TMPG and cTFC) were surveyed immediately after PCI. TMPG 2–3 was more frequent and TMPG 0–1 was less frequent in the VC group compared with controls [40]. Similar findings were reported independently [43] with TMPG = 3 which was more frequent and TMPG < 2 which was less frequent in the VC group. The scores of cTFC were significantly reduced in the VC group [43]. These data indicate better perfusion in VC groups compared with controls.

The biomarker for endothelial dysfunction was the soluble vascular adhesion molecule (sVCAM-l). The level of sVCAM was reduced in the VC group ($p < 0.01$) at 48 h after PCI, with no significant difference noted at one month after PCI [33]. This suggests that improvement in coronary perfusion in the VC group and inhibition of endothelial dysfunction is short term.

3.10. Overall Results

A summary of overall results is shown in Table 6. Among the eight included trials, six trials reported positive results of VC judged by various measurements to reflect the outcomes of myocardial injury, cardiac contractility, antioxidant level, ROS, inflammation, reperfusion efficiency and endothelial dysfunction. These add to a total of 18 positive outcomes (Table 6). Among these six trials, four trials also reported certain measurements showed no statistically significant improvement with VC, including CK-MB, LVEF, infarct size, crp and TNFa. Two trials showed only negative data, with urinary oxidant measurement or coronary artery restenosis.

In total, nine types of outcomes were evaluated in the included trials seeking to evaluate possible benefit from VC administration prior to PCI. Six types of outcomes (myocardial injury, antioxidant reservoir, ROS, inflammatory mediators, coronary perfusion index, endothelial dysfunction) showed statistically significant improvement, while three types of outcomes showed inconclusive associations (infarct size, coronary artery restenosis and cardiac contractility as assessed by LVEF). By adding up the sample sizes based on significant or inconclusive associations, it was noted that 1048 participants were in the groups showing significant benefit from VC while 303 participants were in the groups with inconclusive associations.

Table 6. Summary of All Outcomes.

	Studies	Trial Enrollment (Ctr, VC)	Measure	Positive Outcomes					Negative Outcomes		
				Outcome Types	Outcome Count	Enrollment	Measure	Outcome Types	Outcome Count	Enrollment
1	Shafaei et al. (2019) [39]	252 (126,126)	Troponin, CK-MB	Myocardial injury	1	252				0
2	Ramos et al. (2017) [44]	67 (41,26)	VC, FRAP, GSH	Antioxidants	1	67	CK-MB, LVEF, Infarct size	Myocardial injury, Cardiac contractility, Infarct size	3	67
3	Valls et al. (2016) [40]	43 (21,22)	LVEF, VC, FRAP, GSH, 8-isoprotane, TIMI	Cardiac contractility, Antioxidants, ROS, Reperfusion	4	43	CK-MB, LVEF	Myocardial injury, Cardiac contractility	2	43
4	Wang et al. (2014) [41]	532 (267,265)	Troponin, CK-MB, 8-OHdG	Myocardial injury, ROS	2	532				0
5	Basili et al. (2010–2011) [a]	56 (28,28)	TxB2, sNOX2-dp, LVEF, 8-OHdG, sCD40L, 8-oxo-PGF2a, cTFC, TIMI	Inflammation, Cardiac contractility, ROS, ROS, Reperfusion	6	56	hs-crp, TNFa, Troponin,	Inflammation, Myocardial injury	2	56
6	Gasparetto et al. (2005) [33]	98 (49,49)	TLVV, TAS, ROS, sVCAM-1	Cardiac contractility, Antioxidant, ROS, Endothelial dysfunction	4	98				0
7	Guan et al. (1999) [29]	21 (11,10)			0		8-epi-PGF2a in urine	ROS	1	21
8	Tardif et al. (1997) [55]	116 (62,54)			0		Coronary artery restenosis	Coronary artery restenosis	1	116
	Total	1185 (605, 580)			18	1048			9	303

The positive outcomes denote those showing significantly improvement in association with administration of vitamin C. The negative outcomes denote the count of those types of outcomes which are not showing significant improvement due to administration of vitamin C. "a": indicates that three articles were combined to represent one trial, they were Basili et al., 2010 [43], Pignatelli et al. 2011 [42] and Basili et al., 2011 [34].

4. Discussion

Significantly improved features due to intravenous (iv) administration of VC prior to PCI included lower levels of myocardial injury biomarkers (troponin, CK-MB), increased antioxidant reservoir (ascorbate, FRAP, GSH), reduced ROS (8-OHdG, 8-iso-PGF2a and 8-isoprostane), decreased inflammatory mediators (TxB2, sNOX2-dp, CD40L, and sCD40L), inhibition of vascular endothelial dysfunction (sVCAM-l) and improvement of coronary reperfusion (TMPG and cTFC). However, data is inconclusive with regard to the benefit of VC for improving cardiac function as measured by LVEF and TLVV, and reducing infarct size or coronary restenosis. The measures of LVEF from three trials showed a trend of improvement, however the statistical evidence is absent. One trial measured TLVV and showed an improvement, whereas infarct size and coronary restenosis, measured in one trial each, failed to show an effect of VC. Overall there are more trials, more outcomes and larger sample size showed the benefit of VC than that showed the lack of effect.

Half of the included trials enrolled patients with ACS whereas the other half had participants with stable angina. The trials for ACS patients administered higher doses of VC compared to those trials for stable angina patients. Both patient populations had shown significant improvements in antioxidant status, reduction of ROS, inflammatory mediators or endothelial dysfunction, and enhancement of reperfusion indices. This leads to the hypothesis that ACS may be associated with more reperfusion related oxidative and inflammatory injury compared to stable angina, and therefore requires higher doses of VC for salvage. Compared to ACS, chronic coronary syndromes such as stable angina may produce lower levels of ROS, which can be reduced by the infusion of lower doses of VC. The limitation of the included trials in cardiac injury biomarkers, such as troponin, CK-MB and LVEF, pointing to the need of future trials to demonstrate the hypothesis. A strategy for enhancing the benefit of VC is to continue administering VC for weeks to months before and after PCI procedure. Such strategy to some extent has been adopted in four of the included trials (Table 1), where the participants had either ACS or stable angina. This continuing dosing strategy may provide additional benefit in addition to the bolus dose of VC during PCI as it presumably reduces the baseline ROS and offers prolonged antioxidant protection against ROS and inflammation secondary to reperfusion injury.

The overall findings here are consistent with the data on the cardioprotective effect of VC from clinical trials of coronary reperfusion surgery patients. Two of these clinical trials showed that administration of VC before coronary artery bypass grafting (CABG) surgery significantly improved LVEF [56,57]. Similar to the PCI trials presented here, VC was given via iv infusion before CABG and was found to reduce cardiac injury [56,57]. Three systematic reviews with meta-analysis have summarized the benefit of VC for CABG and cardiac surgery patients [45–48]. The finding of improved endothelial function was documented in two reports focusing on the effect of high doses of VC on endothelial function [58,59].

4.1. Insights into Mechanisms

The trials showing significant benefit have used iv infusion of VC. The bioavailability following iv infusion is higher than seen with oral administration, bypassing gastrointestinal absorption and first pass metabolism. In the circulation and at the site of coronary artery, VC is readily available as a reductant, thereby reducing ROS and retarding neutrophil activation, which can produce bursts of ROS [60]. This may explain the observed reductions of ROS or inflammatory mediators. Since ROS and inflammation can cause cell death, protection against myocardial cell death is shown by decreases in PCI procedurally related troponin release.

VC might exhibit a benefit beyond reduction of ROS. Upon entering into cells, ascorbate serves as an enzyme cofactor for Fe- or Cu-oxygenases. These enzymes are important for a variety of biological functions, among which are hydroxylases for hydroxylation of proline and lysine. These reactions are not only essential for collagen synthesis but also for activation of hypoxia-induced factor-1 alpha (HIF-1a). While collagen synthesis contributes to wound repair, HIF-1a turns on many genes involved in energy metabolism, angiogenesis, and tolerance [60]. Importantly HIF-1a through coordinating gene expression attenuates proinflammatory responses [61]. These features could benefit the recovery from tissue injury due to ischemic reperfusion.

VC may also preserve the endothelial function of coronary arteries and thereby protect the myocardium. It has been shown that VC protects against endothelial damage during MI [62]. Specific actions of VC in this regard include reducing nitric oxide in the plasma, increasing vasopressor sensitivity, promoting vasodilation, and increasing micro-perfusion [63]. Ashor et al. [64] has summarized the positive effects of VC on endothelial function. Added together, VC would seem to offer cardioprotection through a combination of biological reactions, from suppressing ROS or inflammatory mediators, preserving endothelial integrity, to enhancing wound repair via collagen synthesis, and HIF-1a mediated transcriptional events.

4.2. Strengths and Limitations

The included trials were conducted in different geographical locations, i.e., Asia, Europe, South America and North America. Such geographical distributions provide multiethnicity in overall samples and facilitate the generalization of conclusions. The trials were either unfunded or were supported through grants from government or academic centers. None of the trials was funded by for-profit agencies, thereby reducing monetary bias. The overall risk of bias assessed with the Cochrane tool was low.

Findings from this systematic literature review have certain limitations. Four included trials had administered additional doses of VC plus alternative antioxidants, and one trial also administered aspirin to all participants for several months, all of which can potentially confound the effect of VC. The number of trials were limited and the sample sizes in most trials were small. The dose response study of VC with the desired outcomes was lacking. The studied population was relatively young with a mean age range 56 to 68 years, prohibiting extrapolation to geriatric population. There were significant heterogeneities among the reported outcomes, including the data output as means versus median, as well as discrepancies in units of measurements and distinctions in assay sensitivity. As a result, there was insufficient data for meta-analysis.

Ischemic heart disease is the number one cause of heart failure in the USA. Post MI development of heart failure is a chronic event that can take years to develop. Reduced ROS and inflammatory mediators, and improvement in coronary reperfusion efficiency in theory contribute to delay or prevention of chronic heart failure. However, the long-term course of heart failure development prohibits effective measurement of the benefit of an isolated bolus treatment with VC.

5. Conclusions

The qualitative synthesis of the included studies suggests that iv infusion of VC should be considered as an adjuvant therapy for PCI for prevention against reperfusion injury. Given the fact that none of the trials reviewed here has reported a detrimental effect of VC, further clinical trials with a larger enrollment could address the beneficial effects of VC, and define the therapeutic dose range of this molecule for incorporation into standard MI treatment protocols.

Supplementary Materials: The following are available online at http://www.mdpi.com/2072-6643/12/8/2199/s1: Search Strategies for multiple databases.

Author Contributions: S.A.K. design of study, acquisition of data, analysis and interpretation of data, drafting the manuscript; S.B. supervision, design of study, interpretation of data, revising the manuscript critically for important intellectual content; M.O.A.G. acquisition of data; R.W. building search strategy for 6 electronic databases; Q.M.C. project initiation, supervising, conception of study, writing and revising the manuscript. All authors have read and agreed to the published version of the manuscript.

Funding: This research received no external funding.

Acknowledgments: Authors would like to express sincere thanks to Joseph S. Alpert for in depth discussions, providing clinic guidance and editing the manuscript. Research works under Qin M. Chen's direction are supported by NIH R01 GM125212, R01 GM126165, Holsclaw Endowment, and University of Arizona College of Pharmacy start-up fund.

Conflicts of Interest: The authors declare that they have no conflict of interest.

References

1. World Health Organization. Cardiovascular Diseases (CVDs). Available online: https://www.who.int/en/news-room/fact-sheets/detail/cardiovascular-diseases-(cvds) (accessed on 17 May 2017).
2. Virani, S.S.; Alonso, A.; Benjamin, E.J.; Bittencourt, M.S.; Callaway, C.W.; Carson, A.P.; Chamberlain, A.M.; Chang, A.R.; Cheng, S.; Delling, F.N.; et al. Heart Disease and Stroke Statistics-2020 Update: A Report from the American Heart Association. *Circulation* **2020**, *141*, e139–e596. [CrossRef] [PubMed]
3. Neri, M.; Riezzo, I.; Pascale, N.; Pomara, C.; Turillazzi, E. Ischemia/Reperfusion Injury following Acute Myocardial Infarction: A Critical Issue for Clinicians and Forensic Pathologists. *Mediat. Inflamm.* **2017**, *2017*, 1–14. [CrossRef] [PubMed]
4. Mozaffarian, D.; Benjamin, E.J.; Go, A.S.; Arnett, D.K.; Blaha, M.J.; Cushman, M.; De Ferranti, S.; Després, J.P.; Fullerton, H.J.; Howard, V.J.; et al. Heart Disease and Stroke Statistics-2015 Update: A Report From the American Heart Association. *Circulation* **2016**, *133*, E417. [CrossRef] [PubMed]
5. Thygesen, K.; Alpert, J.S.; Jaffe, A.S.; Chaitman, B.R.; Bax, J.J.; Morrow, D.A.; White, H.D. Fourth Universal Definition of Myocardial Infarction. *J. Am. Coll. Cardiol.* **2018**, *72*, 2231–2264. [CrossRef]
6. Anderson, J.L.; Morrow, D.A. Acute Myocardial Infarction. *N. Engl. J. Med.* **2017**, *376*, 2053–2064. [CrossRef]
7. O'Gara, P.T.; Kushner, F.G.; Ascheim, D.D.; Casey, D.E.; Chung, M.K.; de Lemos, J.A.; Ettinger, S.M.; Fang, J.C.; Fesmire, F.M.; Franklin, B.A.; et al. 2013 ACCF/AHA guideline for the management of ST-elevation myocardial infarction: A report of the American College of Cardiology Foundation/American Heart Association Task Force on Practice Guidelines. *J. Am. Coll. Cardiol.* **2013**, *61*, e78. [CrossRef]
8. Keeley, E.C.; Boura, J.A.; Grines, C.L. Primary angioplasty versus intravenous thrombolytic therapy for acute myocardial infarction: A quantitative review of 23 randomised trials. *Lancet* **2003**, *361*, 13–20. [CrossRef]
9. Harold, J.G.; Bass, T.A.; Bashore, T.M.; Brindis, R.G.; Brush, J.E.; Burke, J.A.; Dehmer, G.J.; Deychak, Y.A.; Jneid, H.; Jollis, J.G.; et al. ACCF/AHA/SCAI 2013 update of the clinical competence statement on coronary artery interventional procedures: A report of the American College of Cardiology Foundation/American Heart Association/American College of Physicians Task Force on Clinical Competence and Training (Writing Committee to Revise the 2007 Clinical Competence Statement on Cardiac Interventional Procedures). *J. Am. Coll. Cardiol.* **2013**, *62*, 357.
10. Nallamothu, B.K.; Bradley, E.H.; Krumholz, H.M. Time to Treatment in Primary Percutaneous Coronary Intervention. *N. Engl. J. Med.* **2007**, *357*, 1631–1638. [CrossRef]
11. Hayato, H.; Yasuhide, A.; Teruo, N.; Yoshiaki, M.; Yu, K.; Fumiyuki, O.; Kazuhiro, N.; Masashi, F.; Toshiyuki, N.; Michikazu, N.; et al. Three-dimensional assessment of coronary high-intensity plaques with T1-weighted cardiovascular magnetic resonance imaging to predict periprocedural myocardial injury after elective percutaneous coronary intervention. *J. Cardiovasc. Magn. Reson.* **2020**, *22*, 1–11.
12. Langabeer, J.R.; Henry, T.D.; Kereiakes, D.J.; Dellifraine, J.; Emert, J.; Wang, Z.; Stuart, L.; King, R.; Segrest, W.; Moyer, P.; et al. Growth in percutaneous coronary intervention capacity relative to population and disease prevalence. *J. Am. Heart Assoc.* **2013**, *2*, e000370. [CrossRef] [PubMed]
13. Masoudi, F.A.; Ponirakis, A.; de Lemos, J.A.; Jollis, J.G.; Kremers, M.; Messenger, J.C.; Moore, J.W.M.; Moussa, I.; Oetgen, W.J.; Varosy, P.D.; et al. Trends in U.S. Cardiovascular Care: 2016 Report from 4 ACC National Cardiovascular Data Registries. *J. Am. Coll. Cardiol.* **2017**, *69*, 1427–1450. [CrossRef] [PubMed]
14. Tzlil, G.; Tamir, B.; Yoav, H.; Abid, A.; Hana, V.A.; Ran, K.; Alon, E. Temporal Trends of the Management and Outcome of Patients with Myocardial Infarction According to the Risk for Recurrent Cardiovascular Events. *Am. J. Med.* **2020**, *133*, 839–847.
15. Hess, C.N.; Clare, R.M.; Neely, M.L.; Tricoci, P.; Mahaffey, K.W.; James, S.K.; Alexander, J.H.; Held, C.; Lopes, R.D.; Fox, K.A.A.; et al. Differential occurrence, profile, and impact of first recurrent cardiovascular events after an acute coronary syndrome. *Am. Heart J.* **2017**, *187*, 194–203. [CrossRef]
16. Goldberg, R.J.; Currie, K.; White, K.; Brieger, D.; Steg, P.G.; Goodman, S.G.; Dabbous, O.; Fox, K.A.A.; Gore, J.M. Six-month outcomes in a multinational registry of patients hospitalized with an acute coronary syndrome (The Global Registry of Acute Coronary Events [GRACE]). *Am. J. Cardiol.* **2004**, *93*, 288–293. [CrossRef]

17. Steg, P.G.; Bhatt, D.L.; Wilson, P.W.F.; D'Agostino, R.; Ohman, E.M.; Röther, J.; Liau, C.-S.; Hirsch, A.T.; Mas, J.-L.; Ikeda, Y.; et al. One-Year Cardiovascular Event Rates in Outpatients With Atherothrombosis. *JAMA* **2007**, *297*, 1197–1206. [CrossRef]
18. Morrow, D.A. Cardiovascular Risk Prediction in Patients With Stable and Unstable Coronary Heart Disease. *Circulation* **2010**, *121*, 2681–2691. [CrossRef]
19. Prasad, A.; Singh, M.; Lerman, A.; Lennon, R.J.; Holmes, D.R.; Rihal, C.S. Isolated Elevation in Troponin T After Percutaneous Coronary Intervention Is Associated With Higher Long-Term Mortality. *J. Am. Coll. Cardiol.* **2006**, *48*, 1765–1770. [CrossRef]
20. Prasad, A.; Herrmann, J. Myocardial Infarction Due to Percutaneous Coronary Intervention. *N. Engl. J. Med.* **2011**, *364*, 453–464. [CrossRef]
21. Zeitouni, M.; Silvain, J.; Guedeney, P.; Kerneis, M.; Yan, Y.; Overtchouk, P.; Barthelemy, O.; Hauguel-Moreau, M.; Choussat, R.; Helft, G.; et al. Periprocedural myocardial infarction and injury in elective coronary stenting. *Eur. Heart J.* **2018**, *39*, 1100–1109. [CrossRef]
22. Yellon, D.M.; Hausenloy, D.J. Myocardial reperfusion injury. *N. Engl. J. Med.* **2007**, *357*, 1121–1135. [CrossRef] [PubMed]
23. Otani, H. Ischemic preconditioning: From molecular mechanisms to therapeutic opportunities. *Antioxid. Redox Signal.* **2008**, *10*, 207–247. [CrossRef] [PubMed]
24. Bonnemeier, H.; Wiegand, U.K.H.; Giannitsis, E.; Schulenburg, S.; Hartmann, F.; Kurowski, V.; Bode, F.; Tölg, R.; Katus, H.A.; Richardt, G. Temporal repolarization inhomogeneity and reperfusion arrhythmias in patients undergoing successful primary percutaneous coronary intervention for acute ST-segment elevation myocardial infarction: Impact of admission troponin T. *Am. Heart J.* **2003**, *145*, 484–492. [CrossRef]
25. Zweier, J.L.; Talukder, M.A. The role of oxidants and free radicals in reperfusion injury. *Cardiovasc. Res.* **2006**, *70*, 181–190. [CrossRef] [PubMed]
26. Zhao, Z.-Q. Oxidative stress-elicited myocardial apoptosis during reperfusion. *Curr. Opin. Pharmacol.* **2004**, *4*, 159–165. [CrossRef] [PubMed]
27. Duilio, C.; Ambrosio, G.; Kuppusamy, P.; Dipaula, A.; Becker, L.C.; Zweier, J. Neutrophils are primary source of O-2 radicals during reperfusion after prolonged myocardial ischemia. *Am. J. Physiol. Heart Circul. Physiol.* **2001**, *280*, H2649–H2657. [CrossRef]
28. Galang, N.; Sasaki, H.; Maulik, N. Apoptotic cell death during ischemia/reperfusion and its attenuation by antioxidant therapy. *Toxicology* **2000**, *148*, 111–118. [CrossRef]
29. Guan, W.; Osanai, T.; Kamada, T.; Ishizaka, H.; Hanada, H.; Okumura, K. Time course of free radical production after primary coronary angioplasty for acute myocardial infarction and the effect of vitamin C. *Jpn. Circ. J.* **1999**, *63*, 924–928. [CrossRef]
30. Kasap, S.; Gönenç, A.; Sener, D.E.; Hisar, I. Serum cardiac markers in patients with acute myocardial infarction: Oxidative stress, C-reactive protein and N-terminal probrain natriuretic Peptide. *J. Clin. Biochem. Nutr.* **2007**, *41*, 50–57. [CrossRef]
31. Muzáková, V.; Kandár, R.; Vojtísek, P.; Skalický, J.; Cervinková, Z. Selective antioxidant enzymes during ischemia/reperfusion in myocardial infarction. *Physiol. Res.* **2000**, *49*, 315–322.
32. Li, C.; Jackson, R.M. Reactive species mechanisms of cellular hypoxia-reoxygenation injury. *Am. J. Physiol. Cell Physiol.* **2002**, *282*, C227–C241. [CrossRef]
33. Gasparetto, C.; Malinverno, A.; Culacciati, D.; Gritti, D.; Prosperini, P.G.; Specchia, G.; Ricevuti, G. Antioxidant vitamins reduce oxidative stress and ventricular remodeling in patients with acute myocardial infarction. *Int. J. Immunopathol. Pharmacol.* **2005**, *18*, 487–496. [CrossRef]
34. Basili, S.; Pignatelli, P.; Tanzilli, G.; Mangieri, E.; Carnevale, R.; Nocella, C.; Di Santo, S.; Pastori, D.; Ferroni, P.; Violi, F. Anoxia-reoxygenation enhances platelet thromboxane A2 production via reactive oxygen species-generated NOX2: Effect in patients undergoing elective percutaneous coronary intervention. *Arterioscler. Thromb. Vasc. Biol.* **2011**, *31*, 1766–1771. [CrossRef] [PubMed]
35. Lykkesfeldt, J.; Tveden-Nyborg, P. The Pharmacokinetics of Vitamin C. *Nutrients* **2019**, *11*, 2412. [CrossRef] [PubMed]
36. Tribble, D.L. AHA Science Advisory. Antioxidant consumption and risk of coronary heart disease: Emphasison vitamin C, vitamin E, and beta-carotene: A statement for healthcare professionals from the American Heart Association. *Circulation* **1999**, *99*, 591–595. [CrossRef] [PubMed]

37. Bailey, D.M.; Raman, S.; McEneny, J.; Young, I.S.; Parham, K.L.; Hullin, D.A.; Davies, B.; McKeeman, G.; McCord, J.M.; Lewis, M.H. Vitamin C prophylaxis promotes oxidative lipid damage during surgical ischemia-reperfusion. *Free Radic. Biol. Med.* **2006**, *40*, 591–600. [CrossRef]
38. Rodrigo, R.; Prieto, J.; Castillo, R. Cardioprotection against ischaemia/reperfusion by vitamins C and E plus n-3 fatty acids: Molecular mechanisms and potential clinical applications. *Clin. Sci.* **2013**, *124*, 1–15. [CrossRef]
39. Shafaei-Bajestani, N.; Talasaz, A.; Salarifar, M.; Pourhosseini, H.; Sadri, F.; Jalali, A. Potential role of Vitamin C intracoronary administration in preventing cardiac injury after primary percutaneous coronary intervention in patients with ST-elevation myocardial infarction. *J. Res. Pharm. Pract.* **2019**, *8*, 75–82.
40. Valls, N.; Gormaz, J.G.; Aguayo, R.; Gonzalez, J.; Brito, R.; Hasson, D.; Libuy, M.; Ramos, C.; Carrasco, R.; Prieto, J.C.; et al. Amelioration of persistent left ventricular function impairment through increased plasma ascorbate levels following myocardial infarction. *Redox Rep.* **2016**, *21*, 75–83.
41. Wang, Z.J.; Hu, W.K.; Liu, Y.Y.; Shi, D.M.; Cheng, W.J.; Guo, Y.H.; Yang, Q.; Zhao, Y.X.; Zhou, Y.J. The effect of intravenous vitamin C infusion on periprocedural myocardial injury for patients undergoing elective percutaneous coronary intervention. *Can. J. Cardiol.* **2014**, *30*, 96–101. [CrossRef]
42. Pignatelli, P.; Tanzilli, G.; Carnevale, R.; Di Santo, S.; Loffredo, L.; Celestini, A.; Proietti, M.; Tovaglia, P.; Mangieri, E.; Basili, S.; et al. Ascorbic acid infusion blunts CD40L upregulation in patients undergoing coronary stent. *Cardiovasc. Ther.* **2011**, *29*, 385–394. [CrossRef]
43. Basili, S.; Tanzilli, G.; Mangieri, E.; Raparelli, V.; Di Santo, S.; Pignatelli, P.; Violi, F. Intravenous ascorbic acid infusion improves myocardial perfusion grade during elective percutaneous coronary intervention: Relationship with oxidative stress markers. *JACC Cardiovasc. Interv.* **2010**, *3*, 221–229. [CrossRef]
44. Ramos, C.; Brito, R.; Gonzalez-Montero, J.; Valls, N.; Gormaz, J.G.; Prieto, J.C.; Aguayo, R.; Puentes, A.; Noriega, V.; Pereira, G.; et al. Effects of a novel ascorbate-based protocol on infarct size and ventricle function in acute myocardial infarction patients undergoing percutaneous coronary angioplasty. *Arch. Med. Sci.* **2017**, *13*, 558–567. [CrossRef]
45. Hu, X.; Yuan, L.; Wang, H.; Li, C.; Cai, J.; Hu, Y.; Ma, C. Efficacy and safety of vitamin C for atrial fibrillation after cardiac surgery: A meta-analysis with trial sequential analysis of randomized controlled trials. *Int. J. Surg.* **2017**, *37*, 58–64. [CrossRef]
46. Shi, R.; Li, Z.H.; Chen, D.; Wu, Q.C.; Zhou, X.L.; Tie, H.T. Sole and combined vitamin C supplementation can prevent postoperative atrial fibrillation after cardiac surgery: A systematic review and meta-analysis of randomized controlled trials. *Clin. Cardiol.* **2018**, *41*, 871–878. [CrossRef]
47. Ali-Hassan-Sayegh, S.; Mirhosseini, S.J.; Rezaeisadrabadi, M.; Dehghan, H.R.; Sedaghat-Hamedani, F.; Kayvanpour, E.; Popov, A.-F.; Liakopoulos, O.J. Antioxidant supplementations for prevention of atrial fibrillation after cardiac surgery: An. updated comprehensive systematic review and meta-analysis of 23 randomized controlled trials. *Interact. Cardiovasc. Thorac. Surg.* **2014**, *18*, 646–654. [CrossRef]
48. Baker, L.W.; Coleman, I.C. Meta-analysis of ascorbic acid for prevention of postoperative atrial fibrillation after cardiac surgery. *Am. J. Health-Syst. Pharm.* **2016**, *73*, 2056–2066. [CrossRef] [PubMed]
49. Moher, D.; Liberati, A.; Tetzlaff, J.; Altman, D.G.; The PRISMA Group. Preferred Reporting Items for Systematic Reviews and Meta-Analyses: The PRISMA Statement. *Ann. Intern. Med.* **2009**, *151*, 264–269. [CrossRef]
50. Cochrane.org. Cochrane Methods Bias. Available online: https://methods.cochrane.org/bias/resources/rob-2-revised-cochrane-risk-bias-tool-randomized-trials (accessed on 18 February 2020).
51. Rodrigo, R.; Hasson, D.; Prieto, J.C.; Dussaillant, G.; Ramos, C.; Leon, L.; Garate, J.; Valls, N.; Gormaz, J.G. The effectiveness of antioxidant vitamins C and E in reducing myocardial infarct size in patients subjected to percutaneous coronary angioplasty (PREVEC Trial): Study protocol for a pilot randomized double-blind controlled trial. *Trials* **2014**, *15*, 192. [CrossRef]
52. Hicks, J.J.; Montes-Cortes, D.H.; Cruz-Dominguez, M.P.; Medina-Santillan, R.; Olivares-Corichi, I.M. Antioxidants decrease reperfusion induced arrhythmias in myocardial infarction with ST-elevation. *Front. Biosci.* **2007**, *12*, 2029–2037. [CrossRef]
53. Jaxa-Chamiec, T.; Bednarz, B.; Drozdowska, D.; Gessek, J.; Gniot, J.; Janik, K.; Kawka-Urbanek, T.; Maciejewski, P.; Ogorek, M.; Szpajer, M. Antioxidant effects of combined vitamins C and E in acute myocardial infarction. The randomized, double-blind, placebo controlled, multicenter pilot Myocardial Infarction and VITamins (MIVIT) trial. *Kardiol. Pol.* **2005**, *62*, 344–350.

54. Panczenko-Kresowska, B.; Ziemlanski, S.; Rudnicki, S.; Wojtulewicz, L.; Przepiorka, M. The influence of vitamin C and e or beta-carotene on peroxidative processes in persons with myocardial ischemia. *Pol. Merkur. Lek.* **1998**, *4*, 12–15.
55. Tardif, J.C.; Cote, G.; Lesperance, J.; Bourassa, M.; Lambert, J.; Doucet, S.; Bilodeau, L.; Nattel, S.; de Guise, P. Probucol and multivitamins in the prevention of restenosis after coronary angioplasty. Multivitamins and Probucol Study Group. *N. Engl. J. Med.* **1997**, *337*, 365–372. [CrossRef]
56. Safaei, N.; Babaei, H.; Azarfarin, R.; Jodati, A.R.; Yaghoubi, A.; Sheikhalizadeh, M.A. Comparative effect of grape seed extract. *Ann Card. Anaesth.* **2017**, *20*, 45–51.
57. Emadi, N.; Nemati, M.H.; Ghorbani, M.; Allahyari, E. The Effect of High.-Dose Vitamin C on Biochemical Markers of Myocardial Injury in Coronary Artery Bypass Surgery. *Braz. J. Cardiovasc. Surg.* **2019**, *34*, 517–524. [CrossRef]
58. Sherman, D.L.; Keaney, J.F.; Biegelsen, E.S.; Duffy, S.J.; Coffman, J.D.; Vita, J.A. Pharmacological concentrations of ascorbic acid are required for the beneficial effect on endothelial vasomotor function in hypertension. *Hypertension* **2000**, *35*, 936–941. [CrossRef]
59. Taddei, S.; Virdis, A.; Ghiadoni, L.; Magagna, A.; Salvetti, A. Vitamin C improves endothelium-dependent vasodilation by restoring nitric oxide activity in essential hypertension. *Circulation* **1998**, *97*, 2222–2229. [CrossRef]
60. Ang, A.; Pullar, J.M.; Currie, M.J.; Vissers, M.C.M. Vitamin C and immune cell function in inflammation and cancer. *Biochem. Soc. Trans.* **2018**, *46*, 1147–1159. [CrossRef]
61. Ockaili, R.; Natarajan, R.; Salloum, F.; Fisher, B.J.; Jones, D.; Fowler, A.A., 3rd; Kukreja, R.C. HIF-1 activation attenuates postischemic myocardial injury: Role for heme oxygenase-1 in modulating microvascular chemokine generation. *Am. J. Physiol. Heart Circ. Physiol.* **2005**, *289*, H542–H548. [CrossRef]
62. Morel, O.; Jesel, L.; Hugel, B.; Douchet, M.P.; Zupan, M.; Chauvin, M.; Freyssinet, J.M.; Toti, F. Protective effects of vitamin C on endothelium damage and platelet activation during myocardial infarction in patients with sustained generation of circulating microparticles. *J. Thromb. Haemost.* **2003**, *1*, 171–177. [CrossRef]
63. Hill, A.; Wendt, S.; Benstoem, C.; Neubauer, C.; Meybohm, P.; Langlois, P.; Adhikari, N.K.; Heyland, D.K.; Stoppe, C. Vitamin C to Improve Organ. Dysfunction in Cardiac Surgery Patients-Review and Pragmatic Approach. *Nutrients* **2018**, *10*, 974. [CrossRef] [PubMed]
64. Ashor, A.W.; Lara, J.; Mathers, J.C.; Siervo, M. Effect of vitamin C on endothelial function in health and disease: A systematic review and meta-analysis of randomised controlled trials. *Atherosclerosis* **2014**, *235*, 9–20. [CrossRef] [PubMed]

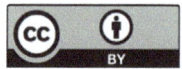

© 2020 by the authors. Licensee MDPI, Basel, Switzerland. This article is an open access article distributed under the terms and conditions of the Creative Commons Attribution (CC BY) license (http://creativecommons.org/licenses/by/4.0/).

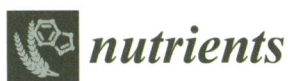

Review

The Effect of Perioperative Vitamin C on Postoperative Analgesic Consumption: A Meta-Analysis of Randomized Controlled Trials

Kuo-Chuan Hung [1,2], Yao-Tsung Lin [1,3], Kee-Hsin Chen [4,5,6,7], Li-Kai Wang [1,2], Jen-Yin Chen [1,8], Ying-Jen Chang [1,9], Shao-Chun Wu [10], Min-Hsien Chiang [10,*] and Cheuk-Kwan Sun [11,12,*]

1. Department of Anesthesiology, Chi Mei Medical Center, Tainan City 71004, Taiwan; ed102605@gmail.com (K.-C.H.); anekevin@hotmail.com (Y.-T.L.); anesth@gmail.com (L.-K.W.); chenjenyin@gmail.com (J.-Y.C.); 0201day@yahoo.com.tw (Y.-J.C.)
2. Department of Health and Nutrition, Chia Nan University of Pharmacy and Science, Tainan City 71710, Taiwan
3. Center of General Education, Chia Nan University of Pharmacy and Science, Tainan City 71710, Taiwan
4. Post-Baccalaureate Program in Nursing, College of Nursing, Taipei Medical University, Taipei City 11042, Taiwan; keehsin@gmail.com
5. Cochrane Taiwan, Taipei Medical University, Taipei City 11042, Taiwan
6. Center for Nursing and Healthcare Research in Clinical Practice Application, Wan Fang Hospital, Taipei Medical University, Taipei City 11042, Taiwan
7. Evidence-Based Knowledge Translation Center, Wan Fang Hospital, Taipei Medical University, Taipei City 11042, Taiwan
8. Department of the Senior Citizen Service Management, Chia Nan University of Pharmacy and Science, Tainan City 71710, Taiwan
9. College of Health Sciences, Chang Jung Christian University, Tainan City 71101, Taiwan
10. Department of Anesthesiology, Kaohsiung Chang Gung Memorial Hospital, Chang Gung University College of Medicine, Kaohsiung City 83301, Taiwan; shaochunwu@gmail.com
11. Department of Emergency Medicine, E-Da Hospital, Kaohsiung City 82445, Taiwan
12. College of Medicine, I-Shou University, Kaohsiung City 82445, Taiwan
* Correspondence: ducky0421@gmail.com (M.-H.C.); lawrence.c.k.sun@gmail.com; (C.-K.S.); Tel.: +886-7-6150011 (ext. 1007) (C.-K.S.)

Received: 9 September 2020; Accepted: 1 October 2020; Published: 12 October 2020

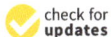

Abstract: Because the analgesic effect of vitamin C against acute pain remains poorly addressed, this meta-analysis aimed at investigating its effectiveness against acute postoperative pain. A total of seven randomized controlled trials with placebo/normal controls were identified from PubMed, Cochrane Library, Medline, Google Scholar, and Embase databases. Pooled analysis showed a lower pain score (standardized mean difference (SMD) = −0.68, 95% CI: −1.01 to −0.36, $p < 0.0001$; $I^2 = 57\%$) and a lower morphine consumption (weighted mean difference (WMD) = −2.44 mg, 95% CI: −4.03 to −0.86, $p = 0.003$; $I^2 = 52\%$) in the vitamin group than that in the placebo group within postoperative 1–2 h. At postoperative 24 h, a lower pain score (SMD = −0.65, 95% CI: −1.11 to −0.19, $p = 0.005$; $I^2 = 81\%$) and lower morphine consumption (WMD = −6.74 mg, 95% CI: −9.63 to −3.84, $p < 0.00001$; $I^2 = 85\%$) were also noted in the vitamin group. Subgroup analyses demonstrated significant reductions in pain severity and morphine requirement immediately (1–2 h) and 24 h after surgery for patients receiving intravenous vitamin C but not in the oral subgroup. These findings showed significant reductions in pain score and opioid requirement up to postoperative 24 h, respectively, suggesting the effectiveness of perioperative vitamin C use. Further large-scale trials are warranted to elucidate its optimal intravenous dosage and effectiveness against chronic pain in the postoperative pain control setting.

Keywords: vitamin C; analgesic requirement; surgery; anesthesia

---

1. Introduction

Postoperative pain, which is present in up to 80% of patients undergoing surgery [1], not only impairs the patients' quality of life such as sleep quality and level of activity [2] but also contributes to chronic postoperative pain [3]. However, a previous study has shown that less than half of the postoperative patients reported satisfactory pain control [1]. The commonly used postoperative analgesic agents including opioids and non-steroid anti-inflammatory drugs (NSAIDs) are associated with untoward side-effects including respiratory suppression and other relatively minor complications such as nausea or vomiting [4]. In addition, NSAIDs, which are usual adjuvants to opioid-based regimens, are known to contribute to adverse gastrointestinal and nephrotic side-effects. Inadequate pain control is a common tradeoff between optimal postoperative analgesia and drug-associated side-effects [5]. In an attempt to maximize the degree of analgesia while minimizing untoward side-effects, modern practice guidelines recommend a multimodal intervention for postoperative pain control that involves a combination of different analgesics with nonpharmacological approaches [4].

Vitamin C, the L-enantiomer of ascorbate also known as ascorbic acid, is widely known as a water-soluble antioxidant ubiquitously present in a variety of fruits and vegetables. The importance of vitamin C in wound healing and hemostasis was first realized more than 260 years ago when it was found to be a cure for scurvy, a disease characterized by spontaneous bleeding, anemia, and gum ulceration. Besides its role in hemostasis, vitamin C is also known to exhibit analgesic functions. Recent evidence has attributed the antinociceptive action of vitamin C to its antioxidant [6], neuroprotective, and neuromodulatory properties [7,8]. Indeed, vitamin C has been shown to reduce acute pain and the prevalence of complex regional pain syndromes with its antinociceptive effect [9–11].

Although the antinociceptive effect of vitamin C against chronic pain has been well documented [10], its effectiveness against acute pain remains poorly addressed. There was only one meta-analytic study attempting to investigate the effectiveness of vitamin C for acute pain [12]. However, most studies included in that analysis [12] focused on other analgesics, with vitamin C being used as a placebo [13–16]. Another report investigated the analgesic effect of vitamin C in patients undergoing ocular surgeries through local administration and the results could not be extrapolated to other major surgeries and the administration of vitamin C through the systemic routes [17]. Therefore, the present meta-analysis attempted to shed light on the effectiveness of vitamin C against acute postoperative pain by systematically reviewing all the available clinical trials.

2. Materials and Methods

The present meta-analysis was conducted according to Preferred Reporting Items Systematic Reviews and Meta-Analysis (PRISMA) guidelines [18] and was registered on the International Prospective Register of Systematic Reviews (CRD42020202592).

2.1. Search Strategy

We searched the databases of Medline, Embase, Google Scholar, PubMed, and the Cochrane controlled trials register, and the U.S. National Library of Medicine clinical trial register (www.clinicaltrials.gov) to obtain a list of all published or unpublished eligible randomized controlled trials (RCTs) comparing the postoperative pain outcomes with or without perioperative use of vitamin C in patients requiring surgery using the keywords "vitamin C", "ascorbic acid", "antioxidant", "pain", "analgesia", "opioid", "morphine", "pain score", "anesthesia", "postoperative", "perioperative", "surgery", "patient-controlled analgesia", and "RCT" from inception to August 10, 2020. References from relevant studies were searched to find additional studies. No publication date or language restriction was applied.

2.2. Study Selection Criteria

Two reviewers (K.-H.C., Y.-T.L.) independently examined the abstracts of the acquired articles to identify potentially eligible studies. The PICO criteria for eligibility of randomized controlled trials for the current study included: (1) Population: adult surgical patients, age above or equal to 18 years old; (2) Intervention: vitamin C was given as an intervention rather than a control through oral or intravenous route; (3) Comparison: placebo or no therapy; and (4) Outcome: analgesic consumption and/or severity of pain within postoperative 48 h. There were no restrictions on dose or timing of administration. The exclusion criteria were (1) studies that focused on dental or ocular surgeries and/or pediatric population because of the relatively low severity of pain and the difficulty in pain assessment, respectively, (2) those in which information regarding dosage of vitamin C or acute pain outcomes was unavailable, and (3) those that adopted vitamin C as a placebo. Two authors (K.-C.H., J.-Y.C.) independently investigated the selected trials for the final analysis. If disagreements arose, a third author (C.-K.S.) was involved until a consensus was reached.

2.3. Data Extraction

Three authors (L.-K.W., S.-C.W., and J.-Y.C.) extracted relevant data from each selected trial and entered them into predefined databases. Divergences were resolved by discussion. If the included studies did not report data on primary or secondary outcomes, the corresponding authors were contacted for further information. The following data were extracted from each trial: author, publication year, study setting, patient characteristics, sample size, surgical procedure, dosage of vitamin C, blood loss, postoperative analgesic technique, postoperative opioid consumption, postoperative pain score (e.g., numerical rating scale (NRS)), and adverse events. All opioid consumption was converted into parenteral morphine equivalents (i.e., 0.1 mg parenteral fentanyl = 10 mg parenteral morphine; 75 mg parenteral meperidine = 10 mg parenteral morphine) [19].

2.4. Primary Outcome, Secondary Outcomes, and Definitions

Acute pain outcomes of the present meta-analysis were defined as the severity of pain or opioid consumption within postoperative 48 h. The primary endpoint was postoperative opioid consumption at postoperative 24 h, while the secondary outcomes included the severity of pain, postoperative opioid consumption at postoperative 1–2 h or at 48 h, postoperative circulating vitamin C concentration after vitamin C supplementation as well as the risks of postoperative nausea and vomiting (PONV). The severity of pain was defined according to the pain score of each study.

2.5. Assessment of Risk of Bias for Included Studies

Two authors (M.-H.C. and Y.-J.C.) assessed the risk of bias for each trial using the criteria outlined in the *Cochrane Handbook for Systematic Reviews of Interventions* [20]. Disagreements were solved by discussion. The overall risk of bias of all included studies and the risk of bias of individual studies were analyzed. We rated the potential risk of bias by applying a rating of "low", "high," or "unclear" to each trial.

2.6. Statistical Analysis

For dichotomous outcomes, a random effects model was used to calculate the risk ratios (RRs) with 95% confidence intervals (CIs). The Mantel–Haenszel (MH) method was used to pool dichotomous data and to compute pooled RRs with 95% CIs. For continuous outcome, the selected effect size was the weighted mean difference (WMD) for analgesic dosage or standardized mean difference (SMD) for pain severity. The WMD is a standard statistic that measures the absolute difference between the mean value in two groups, while SMD is used as a summary statistic when the studies all assess the same outcome but measure it in a variety of ways (e.g., comparison of pain severity using two different pain scores). We assessed the morphine-sparing effect of vitamin C by using the method proposed by a previous meta-analysis [21] that calculated the effect with the equation: Morphine-sparing effect = (WMD/median of the average cumulative morphine in placebo group) × 100% (where WMD was the reduction in morphine dosage in the study group). The I^2 statistic was applied for heterogeneity assessment (low: 0% to 50%; moderate: 50% to 75%; high: 75% to 100%). Sources of heterogeneity were explored by prespecified subgroup analyses on the routes of administration (i.e., oral or intravenous). Sensitivity analyses were performed to explore the potential influence of a single trial on the overall findings by omitting the studies from the meta-analysis one at a time. We examined the funnel plots when we identified 10 or more studies reporting on a particular outcome to investigate the potentials of reporting and publication bias. The significance level was set at 0.05 for all analyses. Cochrane Review Manager (RevMan 5.4; Copenhagen: The Nordic Cochrane Center, The Cochrane Collaboration, 2014) was used for data synthesis.

3. Results

3.1. Study Selection

Figure 1 is the Preferred Reporting Items for Systematic Reviews and Meta-Analyses (PRISMA) flow diagram that summarizes the reasons for study exclusion. Of a total of 227 potentially eligible reports retrieved from the database search, 146 were removed as they were duplicates. We then excluded 53 records after the initial review of the titles and abstracts. Of the 53 excluded studies, 39 did not mention vitamin C, seven did not involve surgery, five did not provide outcome on pain assessment, one focused on the pediatric population, and one was an animal study (Table S1). Overall, 28 studies were considered relevant and the full text was read. Another 21 articles were excluded because of the involvement of dental or ocular surgeries (n = 3), the use of vitamin C as a placebo intervention (n = 6), no information on acute pain outcomes (n = 13), a before-and-after study design (n = 1), availability of only an abstract (n = 1), and lack of data on standard deviation (n = 1). Finally, a total of seven randomized trials were included in the current meta-analysis (Figure 1).

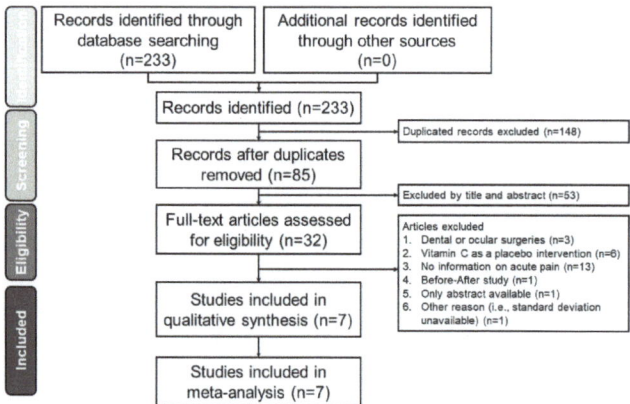

Figure 1. Preferred Reporting Items Systematic Reviews and Meta-Analysis (PRISMA) flowchart for selecting eligible studies.

3.2. Characteristics of Included Studies

Seven RCTs (n = 519 participants) published between 2012 to 2020 were analyzed. The study characteristics are described in Table 1. Vitamin C was given perioperatively in six trials [5,22–26], and was administered twice a day for three days in another trial [27]. The routes of administration included intravenous in five trials [5,22,23,26,27] and oral in two trials [24,25]. Patient-controlled analgesia (PCA) was used for postoperative pain control in five trials [23–27], while one study used boluses of analgesics [5] and the other [22] did not specify the intervention strategies. The follow-up time was 24 h in five trials [5,22–25], 48 h in one trial [26], and 72 h in the other trial [27]. All procedures were elective and most (i.e., five out of seven) were laparoscopic [22–24,26,27]. Two pain scores were adopted for pain severity assessment across the seven studies included, namely, the visual analog scale (VAS) [5,22,25] and the verbal numeric rating scale (NRS) [23,24,26,27]. The cumulative morphine consumption of the included studies at postoperative 24 h and the respective pain scores are summarized in Supplemental Table S2. Placebos used in the seven included studies were normal saline [5,22,23,26,27], carbonated orange beverage [24], and oral placebo tablet [25]. Dropout rates, which were mentioned in three studies [23,24,26], ranged from 2% to 3% in the vitamin group and from 4% to 9.1% in the placebo group.

3.3. Risk of Bias Assessment

The risks of bias of individual studies and the overall risk of bias are summarized in Figures 2 and 3, respectively. Most included studies were found to give sufficient details about randomization and assigned a low risk of allocation bias [23–27]. Several studies were able to adopt methods to keep both the investigators unaware of the administration of vitamin C (e.g., the syringes were covered with black plastic sheets), the risk of performance bias of those trials was considered low [23–26]. Other risks of bias including attrition bias, measurement bias, reporting bias, and overall bias were also considered to be low in all studies. Detailed information on bias assessment of the included studies is shown in Supplemental Table S3.

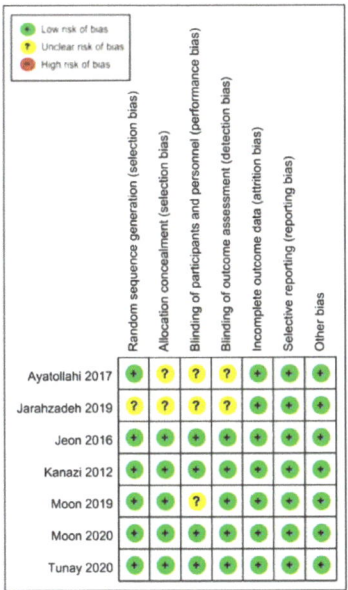

Figure 2. Risks of bias of individual studies.

Table 1. Characteristics of the included studies.

Author/Year	Vitamin C Dosage	Time of Administration	Route	Analgesia Methods	Surgical Procedures	Surgical Time (V vs. P)	Patient Number /Age	Follow-Up Time
Ayatollahi 2017 [5]	3 g	30 min after the BOS	i.v.	Pethidine bolus ‡	Uvulopalatopharyngoplasty and tonsillectomy	111.8 ± 20.8 vs. 113.7 ± 20.9 min	n = 40; 25–50 years	24 h
Jarahzadeh 2019 [21]	2 g	30 min after the AI	i.v.	NA	Laparoscopic surgery	NA	n = 70; 20–60 years	24 h
Jeon 2016 [22]	50 mg/kg	Immediately after AI	i.v.	PCA with morphine	Laparoscopic colectomy	160.2 ± 39.3 vs. 160.7 ± 46.0 min	n = 97; 20–75 years	24 h
Kanazi 2012 [23]	2 g	60 min before AI	oral	PCA with morphine	Laparoscopic cholecystectomy	98.8 ± 33.6 vs. 91.3 ± 31.3 min	n = 80; 18–75 years	24 h
Tunay 2020 [24]	2 g	60 min before BOS	oral	PCA with morphine	Major abdominal surgery	84.5 ± 23.9 vs. 94.5 ± 27.5 min	n = 110, 18–65 years	24 h
Moon 2019 [26]	0.5 g twice a day	The day of surgery to the third day after surgery	i.v.	PCA with fentanyl	Laparoscopic hysterectomy	99.0 ± 30.3 vs. 96.0 ± 19.4 min	n = 60, 20–60 years	72 h
Moon 2020 [25]	50 mg/kg	Immediately prior to AI	i.v.	PCA with fentanyl	Laparoscopic gynecologic surgery	78.4 ± 34.7 vs. 92.8 ± 30 min	n = 66, 20–60 years	48 h

AI: anesthesia induction; BOS: beginning of surgery; i.v.: intravenous; PCA: patient-controlled analgesia; ‡ 1 g paracetamol for patients with pain score <5; pethidine 0.5 mg/kg for patients with pain score ≥5; V vs. P: vitamin C vs. placebo.

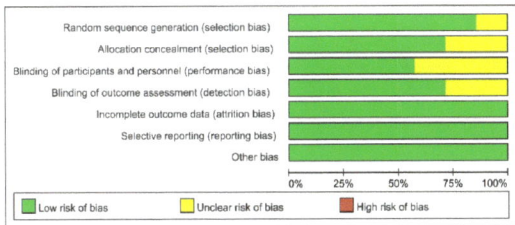

Figure 3. Overall risks of bias of the seven included studies.

3.4. Outcomes

3.4.1. Severity of Pain within 1–2 h after Surgery

Five studies with a total of 379 patients (vitamin group, n = 191 vs. placebo group, n = 188) were available for the analysis of pain score within 1–2 h after surgery [5,22,23,25,26]. Pooled analysis showed a lower pain score in the vitamin group than that in the placebo group (SMD = −0.68, 95% CI −1.01 to −0.36, $p < 0.0001$; $I^2 = 57\%$) (Figure 4). In contrast to the overall result, subgroup analysis revealed no significant reduction in pain score among patients receiving vitamin C through the oral route (Figure 4). Sensitivity analysis demonstrated no significant impact on outcome by omitting certain trials.

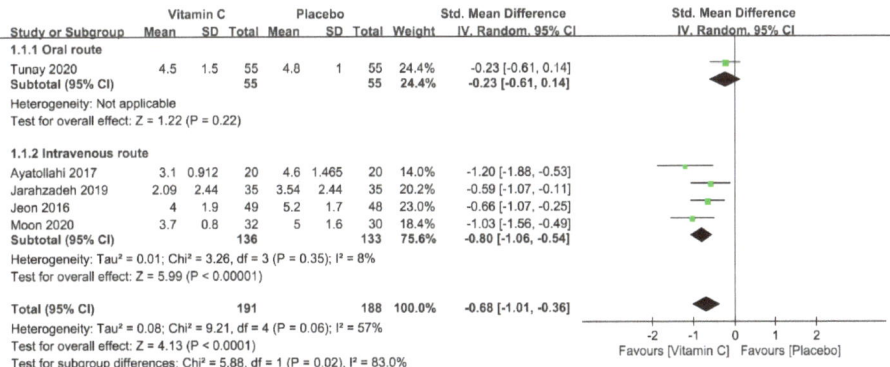

Figure 4. Forest plot for comparing the severity of pain within postoperative 1–2 h between vitamin and placebo groups. CI, confidence interval; IV, inverse variance; Std., standardized.

3.4.2. Severity of Pain 6 h after Surgery

Five studies with a total of 379 patients (vitamin group, n = 191 vs. placebo group, n = 188) were eligible for the analysis [5,22,23,25,26]. A forest plot, presented in Figure 5, demonstrated a lower mean pain score at postoperative 6 h in the vitamin group compared with that in the placebo group (SMD = −0.67, 95% CI −0.93 to −0.42, $p < 0.00001$; $I^2 = 31\%$) (Figure 5). Subgroup analysis based on the routes of administration selected (i.e., oral vs. intravenous) also showed consistent findings (Figure 5). Sensitivity analysis showed no significant impact on outcome by omitting certain trials.

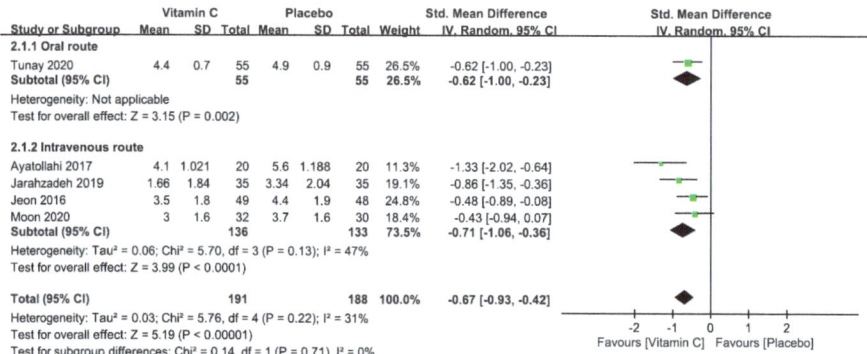

Figure 5. Forest plot for the comparison of pain severity 6 h after surgery between vitamin and placebo groups. CI, confidence interval; IV, inverse variance; Std., standardized.

3.4.3. Severity of Pain at 24 h after Surgery

The forest plot on six available studies with a total of 439 patients (vitamin group, n = 221 vs. placebo group, n = 218) [5,22,23,25–27] (shown in Figure 6) demonstrated a lower pain severity at postoperative 24 h in the vitamin group compared with that in the placebo group (SMD = −0.65, 95% CI −1.11 to −0.19, p = 0.005; I^2 = 81%) (Figure 6). Again, contrary to the overall result, subgroup analysis demonstrated that oral vitamin C supplementation was ineffective for pain alleviation (Figure 6) also showed similar findings. Sensitivity analysis found no significant impact on this outcome by omitting certain trials.

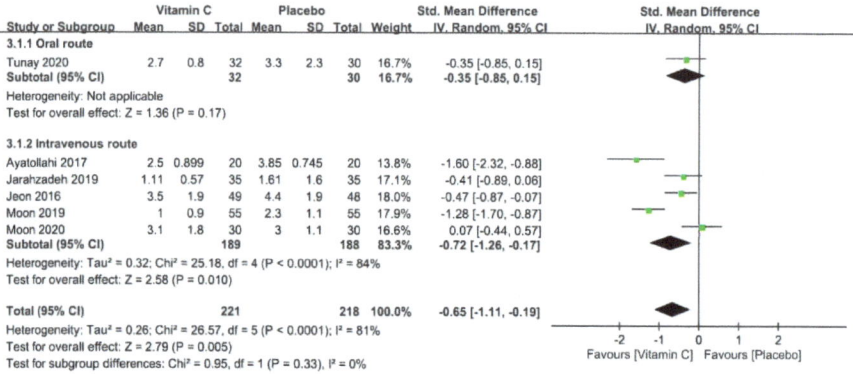

Figure 6. Forest plot for comparing the severity of pain at 24 h after surgery between vitamin and placebo groups. CI, confidence interval; IV, inverse variance; Std., standardized.

3.4.4. Opioid Consumption within 1–2 h after Surgery

Three studies with a total of 239 patients (vitamin group, n = 121 vs. placebo group, n = 118) were available for the analysis [23,24,26]. All studies used PCA for postoperative pain control. Within postoperative 1–2 h, the median of the average cumulative morphine dosages in the placebo groups was 7.9 mg (range, 5.76–16.7 mg). A forest plot, (presented in Figure 7) demonstrated a significantly lower morphine consumption in the vitamin group than that in the placebo group (WMD = −2.44 mg, 95% CI −4.03 to −0.86, p = 0.003; I^2 = 52%), suggesting a vitamin C-associated morphine-sparing effect of 30.9% (i.e., 2.44 mg/7.9 mg × 100%). Nevertheless, subgroup analysis showed no significant reduction in opioid use when the oral route was chosen for vitamin C administration.

Sensitivity analysis demonstrated no difference in morphine consumption between both groups when either the study by Jeon et al. [23] or that by Moon et al. [26] was omitted from the current meta-analysis.

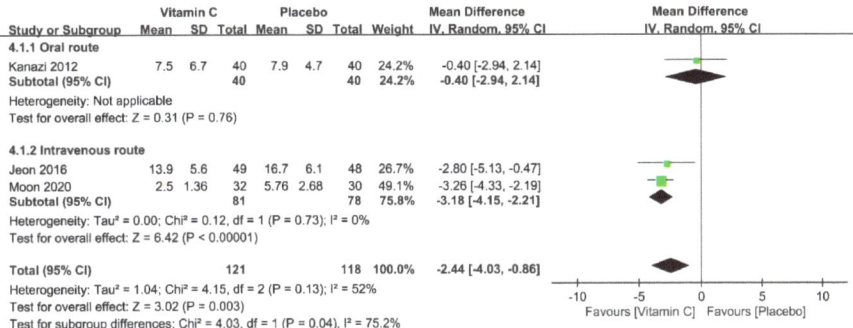

Figure 7. Forest plot for the comparison of opioid consumption (mg) within postoperative 1–2 h between vitamin and placebo groups. CI, confidence interval; IV, inverse variance; WMD, weighted mean difference.

3.4.5. Opioid Consumption within 6 h after Surgery

Two studies using PCA for postoperative pain control involving a total of 159 patients (vitamin group, n = 81 vs. placebo group, n = 78) were eligible for the analysis [23,26]. At 6 h, the median of the average cumulative morphine dosages in placebo groups was 20.6 mg (range, 18.57–22.7 mg). The forest plot demonstrated a lower morphine consumption in the vitamin group than that in the placebo group (WMD = −6.45 mg, 95% CI −11.83 to −1.08, $p = 0.02$; $I^2 = 86\%$) (Figure 8), showing a vitamin C-associated morphine-sparing effect of 31.3% (i.e., 6.45 mg/20.6 mg × 100%).

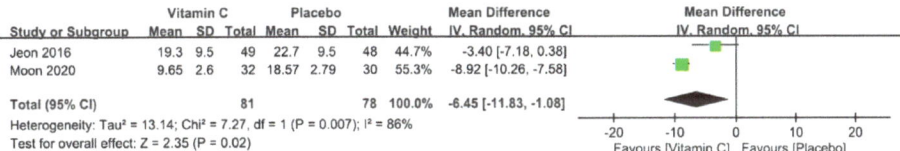

Figure 8. Forest plot for the comparing opioid consumption (mg) within 6 h after surgery between vitamin and placebo groups. CI, confidence interval; IV, inverse variance; WMD, weighted mean difference.

3.4.6. Opioid Consumption within 24 h after Surgery

Of the six studies with a total of 449 patients (vitamin group, n = 226 vs. placebo group, n = 223) available for the analysis [5,23–27], five used PCA for postoperative pain control [23–27]. At 24 h, the median of the average cumulative morphine dosages in the placebo groups was 23.7 mg (range, 6.06–37.7 mg). The forest plot demonstrated a lower morphine consumption in the vitamin group than that in the placebo group (WMD = −6.74 mg, 95% CI −9.63 to −3.84, $p < 0.00001$; $I^2 = 85\%$) (Figure 9), suggesting a vitamin C-associated morphine-sparing effect of 28.4% (i.e., 6.74 mg/23.7 mg × 100%). Despite the overall reduction in morphine use, subgroup analysis demonstrated that administration of vitamin C through the oral route only showed borderline significance in this aspect ($p = 0.05$). Sensitivity analysis demonstrated no significant impact on outcome by omitting certain trials.

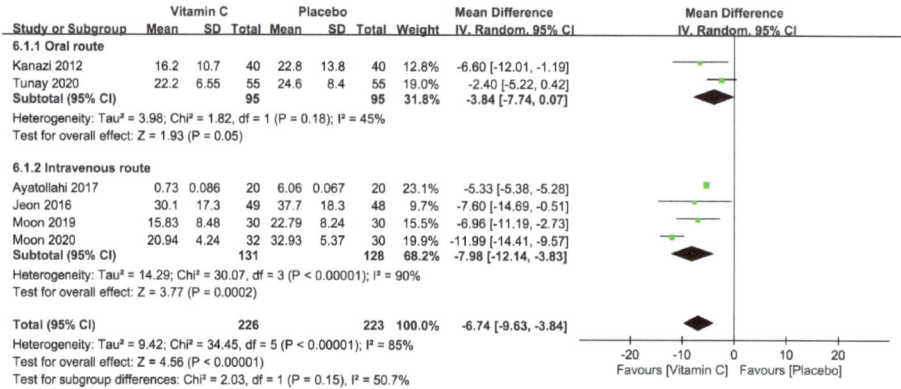

Figure 9. Forest plot for the comparison of opioid consumption (mg) within postoperative 24 h between vitamin and placebo groups. CI, confidence interval; IV, inverse variance.

3.4.7. Opioid Consumption within 48 h after Surgery

Two studies utilizing PCA for postoperative pain control in a total of 122 patients (vitamin group, n = 62 vs. placebo group, n = 60) [26,27] were available for analysis, which showed a lower level of morphine consumption in the vitamin group than that in the placebo group (WMD = −10.49 mg, 95% CI −15.69 to −5.29, $p < 0.0001$; $I^2 = 28\%$) (Figure 10), suggesting a vitamin C-associated morphine-sparing effect of 29.5% (i.e., 10.49 mg/35.55 mg × 100%).

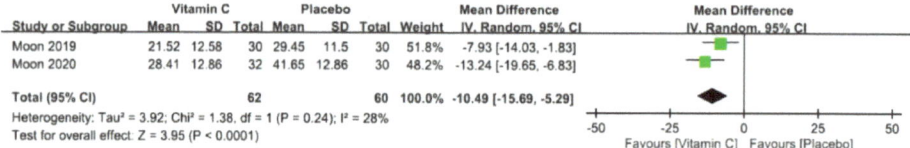

Figure 10. Forest plot for comparing opioid consumption (mg) within 48 h after surgery between vitamin and placebo groups. CI, confidence interval; IV, inverse variance.

3.4.8. Perioperative Blood Loss

Two studies investigating the intraoperative blood loss in a total of 137 patients (vitamin group, n = 69 vs. placebo group, n = 68) [5,23] eligible for analysis demonstrated no significant difference in this outcome between the vitamin group and the placebo group (WMD = 24.88 mL, 95% CI −57.36 to 107.13, $p = 0.55$; $I^2 = 76\%$) (Figure 11).

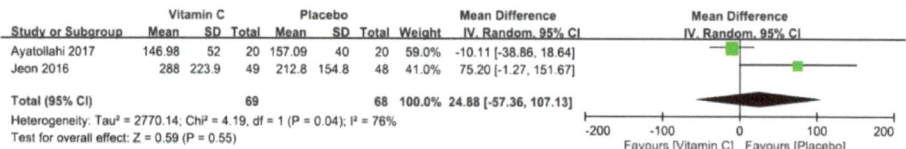

Figure 11. Forest plot for the comparison of perioperative blood loss between vitamin and placebo groups. CI, confidence interval; IV, inverse variance.

3.4.9. Postoperative Nausea and Vomiting

The pooled RRs of PONV at postoperative 1 h [22,26,27] and 24 h [22,24,26,27] were 0.42 (95% CI 0.21 to 0.86, $p = 0.02$, $I^2 = 26\%$) (Figure 12) and 0.54 (95% CI 0.17 to 1.72, $p = 0.30$, $I^2 = 60\%$) (Figure 13), respectively. The findings showed that the use of vitamin C was associated with a lower risk of PONV at postoperative 1 h. However, there was no significant difference in the risk of PONV between the two groups at postoperative 24 h.

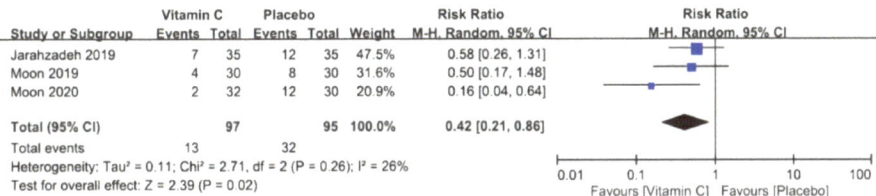

Figure 12. Forest plot for comparing the incidences of postoperative nausea or vomiting within postoperative 1–2 h between vitamin and placebo groups. CI, confidence interval; RR, risk ratio; M-H = Mantel–Haenszel.

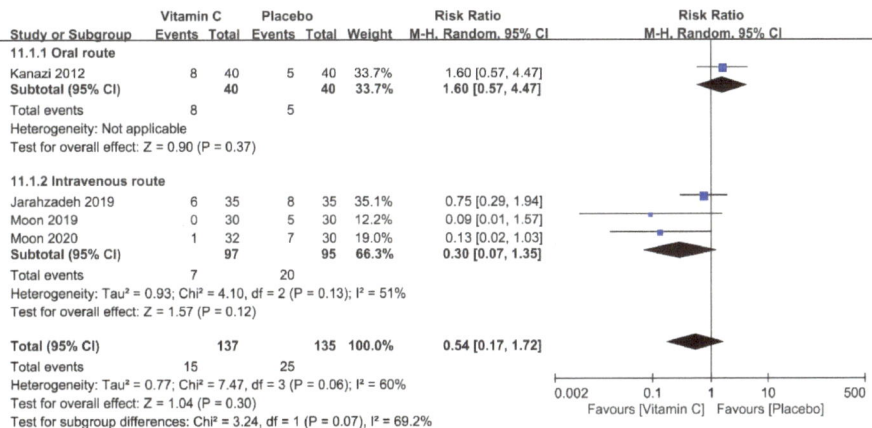

Figure 13. Forest plot for the comparison of the incidences of postoperative nausea or vomiting 24 h after surgery between vitamin and placebo groups. CI, confidence interval; RR, risk ratio; M-H = Mantel–Haenszel.

3.4.10. Postoperative Circulating Vitamin C Concentration after Vitamin C Supplementation

Two studies investigating the postoperative vitamin C blood concentration in a total of 177 patients (vitamin group, n = 89 vs. placebo group, n = 88) [23,24] were available for analysis, which demonstrated a highly significant increase in circulating vitamin C concentration in patients with perioperative vitamin C supplementation compared with that in those without (WMD = 4.91 mg/L, 95% CI 2.85 to 6.97, $p < 0.00001$; $I^2 = 65\%$) (Figure 14).

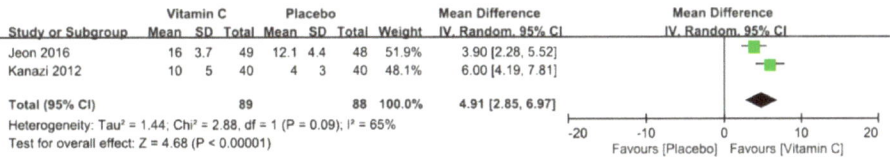

Figure 14. Forest plot for the comparison of postoperative circulating vitamin C concentration between vitamin and placebo groups. CI, confidence interval; IV, inverse variance; WMD, weighted mean difference.

4. Discussion

The current study, which is the first to systematically address the analgesic effectiveness of vitamin C against postoperative pain, had several striking clinical implications. First, our findings showed that vitamin C was associated with a reduced pain score at postoperative 1–2, 6, and 24 h as well as a decreased morphine requirement for up to postoperative 48 h. In addition, the incidence of postoperative nausea or vomiting at postoperative 1–2 h was reduced despite the lack of significant difference between the two groups at 24 h after surgery. Although a previous study reported that intraoperative administration of vitamin C was associated with a decreased operative blood loss [28], the present study demonstrated no significant difference in blood loss between the vitamin and placebo groups.

Postoperative pain control is an important concern because up to 75% of patients who experienced postoperative pain classified the severity of their pain as moderate, severe, or even extreme [29]. Even in the ambulatory surgery setting, a large-scale study on more than five thousand outpatients demonstrated significant pain sensation in up to 30% of the studied population with pain severity being moderate to severe [30]. Acute pain control is also crucial to the prevention of chronic postoperative pain [3,31]. A previous study has demonstrated a positive correlation between the intensity of acute postsurgical pain with the risk of persistent pain development [3]. Nevertheless, achieving a balance between postoperative pain management and minimization of analgesics-associated side-effects is always a challenge to clinicians. Therefore, despite the proven effectiveness of opioids and other common analgesics against postoperative pain, inadequate pain control was not uncommon because of their untoward side-effects [5]. Accordingly, modern clinical practice guidelines recommend a multimodal approach to analgesia, including the use of various analgesic medications and techniques in combination with non-pharmacological interventions [4]. One of the most common adjuvants to opioid-based analgesia are non-steroidal anti-inflammatory drugs (NSAIDs) which, however, are also associated with adverse side-effects [4,32–34]. Vitamin C, which is a water-soluble vitamin with the excesses in circulation rapidly excreted in the urine, has a remarkably low acute toxicity [35]. In this way, vitamin C may be a promising adjuvant to conventional analgesics.

To compare the morphine-sparing effect of vitamin C with that associated with other analgesics, we investigated previous meta-analytic studies that showed reductions in morphine requirement at 24 h by 14.7%, 20%, and 21% corresponding to 7.2, 9, and 10.3 mg for celecoxib (200 mg) [36], acetaminophen [37], and a single dose of NSAID [36], respectively. Therefore, a decrease by 28.4% in the current study appeared to be higher than that previously reported for other analgesics. As the above medications are popular clinical adjuvants to opioid-based regimens in the multi-modal approach to operative antinociception, the finding of the current study may imply the possibility of incorporating vitamin C into the postoperative care protocol.

Previous studies have attributed the antinociceptive effects of vitamin C to its antioxidative and neuromodulatory properties. A previous report has shown a positive association between reactive oxygen species (ROS) and neuropathic pain through the demonstration of pain alleviation by administering ROS scavengers to a rat model of single nerve ligation pain [38]. The analgesic action of vitamin C through its role as a free radical scavenger has been suggested in a previous experimental study [6]. With respect to neuromodulation, there is evidence linking the antinociceptive property of vitamin C to its action on the N-methyl-D-aspartate (NMDA) receptor. Previous investigations not only revealed that vitamin C could modulate the neurotransmission of glutamate and dopamine through altering the redox changes on the NMDA receptor [39] but also demonstrated that vitamin C exerted an antinociceptive effect in chemically induced animal pain models possibly through an inhibition of the ionotropic NMDA receptor [40]. Furthermore, vitamin C is critical for the biosynthesis of neurotransmitters known to be key components of the inhibitory pain pathway [41]. Being a substrate of the enzyme dopamine beta-hydroxylase for the conversion of dopamine to norepinephrine, vitamin C has an important role to play in this rate-limiting step in norepinephrine formation [42,43]. In addition, vitamin C participates in cholinergic and GABAergic transmission [44].

Clinically, because surgery is known to increase oxidative stress, which is associated with a reduction in postoperative plasma vitamin C level [45], a previous review has suggested an alleviation of the free radical burden among surgical patients through vitamin C supplementation to boost its circulating level [45]. This proposal is supported by two of our included studies that showed a significant elevation in plasma vitamin C level after a single bolus supplementation either through the intravenous route at a dose of 50 mg/kg [23] or orally at a dose of 2 g [24]. The antinociceptive effect of vitamin C was also evident in another study in which patients with post herpetic neuralgia, who were found to have a decreased plasma concentration of vitamin C, exhibited a reduction in spontaneous but not brush-evoked pain after the intravenous administration of vitamin C at 50 mg/kg with a maximum dose 2.5 g/day every other day for three doses [9]. An interesting finding of the current study was that despite the demonstration of a reduction in opioid dosage up to postoperative 48 h among patients with vitamin C administration compared to those without, our results showed no difference in the incidence of PONV between the two groups. The findings, therefore, suggested that PONV among the included patients may not be opioid related. Indeed, a previous meta-analysis [46] has shown that up to 50% to 75% of patients would experience PONV after laparoscopic procedures, which comprised five out of seven of our included studies. Taken together, the findings of the current meta-analysis supported the antinociceptive benefit of perioperative vitamin C supplementation without notable increase in side-effects among surgical patients [9,23,24].

Besides antinociception, another issue regarding patient safety is the association between vitamin C deficiency and surgical bleeding. Vitamin C is pivotal to platelet aggregation and prevention of platelet depletion in the process of hemostasis [47]. Spontaneous hemorrhage has been reported in patients with plasma vitamin C concentrations less than 0.6 mg/dL [48] due to impaired vascular integrity from defective collagen formation [48]. Therefore, vitamin C deficiency should be included as a differential diagnosis for surgical patients with nonspecific bleeding especially in those with severe illnesses, prolonged hospitalization, and poor dietary intake, which are known contributors to vitamin C deficiency [48]. Consistently, previous randomized controlled trials have demonstrated a significant reduction in surgical blood loss among patients undergoing abdominal myomectomy [28] and cardiopulmonary bypass surgery [47] with intraoperative vitamin C supplementation compared to those without. Nevertheless, the current study did not demonstrate a significant association between perioperative vitamin C supplementation and surgical blood loss.

One of the interesting findings of the present study was the differences in pain alleviation and morphine use between the intravenous and oral routes of vitamin C administration. While intravenous supplementation of vitamin C was found effective for decreasing pain severity at 1–2, 6, and 24 h after surgery, oral administration was associated with significant pain relief only at postoperative 6 h. Similarly, although intravenous vitamin C was significantly related to a reduction in morphine requirement immediately (1–2 h) and one day after surgery, similar therapeutic benefits were not seen for the oral route. Indeed, vitamin C administration through the intravenous route has been found to produce a 70-fold higher blood level than that when it was given orally at the maximum tolerable dose [49]. The downside of vitamin C administration through the oral route is the tightly controlled plasma concentration. In contrast, intravenous administration can attain a substantially higher blood concentration through bypassing such a tight control [49]. This may explain the enhanced effectiveness of intraoperative vitamin C administration through the intravenous route compared to that given orally in the current study.

The present study had its strengths and limitations. Because pain is a subjective feeling, analysis of morphine dosages from patient-controlled analgesia in five out of the seven included studies could reliably reflect the severity of pain for accurate assessment of the antinociceptive effect of vitamin C. In addition, we excluded patients with relatively low severity of postoperative pain including those undergoing dental and ocular surgeries as well as the pediatric population, who could not provide reliable information. Furthermore, the included studies for the present meta-analysis involved patients receiving similar procedures (i.e., laparoscopic surgeries in 5 out of 7 studies) so that variations in the severity of pain from different operations were minimized.

Nevertheless, the downside of the high homogeneity in surgical procedures also restricted the extrapolation of our findings to patients undergoing other operations. Another limitation was that the number of included studies was not large enough to analyze the publication bias. In addition, a single perioperative bolus of vitamin C in most studies (i.e., six out of seven) could not shed light on the possible additional benefits from repeated administrations for maintaining a high circulating level. Moreover, the follow-up periods of the included trials were too short (i.e., 24–48 h) to elucidate the long-term antinociceptive benefit of vitamin C as previous studies have demonstrated a reduction in chronic pain after perioperative vitamin C administration [50]. Moreover, statistically, although pooled analysis of the current study showed a lower pain score in the vitamin group compared to that in the placebo controls with substantial significance (i.e., $p < 0.0001$ within 1–2 h after surgery), the small p value only represented the unlikeliness that the observation happened by random chance [51] but did not actually reflect the efficacy of the intervention, which needs to be further investigated through large-scale clinical trials. Pharmacologically, because different analgesics were used in the included studies (e.g., fentanyl and meperidine), we used equianalgesic parenteral dosage conversion into parenteral morphine [19] for comparison. However, the accuracy of such conversions remains questionable because of a lack of professional consensus [19]. In the current study, we adopted the same conversion ratios for both vitamin and placebo groups to minimize the impact of such conversions on our outcomes. Furthermore, because the present meta-analysis aimed at investigating the impact of perioperative vitamin C administration on early postoperative opioid consumption, we did not use different keyword combinations such as "pediatric" and "vitamin C" OR "serum vitamin C concentration" and "pain" OR "long-term vitamin C supplementation" and "pain" OR "vitamin C" and "postoperative chronic pain" in our literature search so that the impacts of routine dietary vitamin C supplementation, circulating vitamin C concentration, and perioperative vitamin C administration on the incidence of chronic pain as well as the analgesic effect of vitamin C in the pediatric population remain unclear. Finally, the heterogeneity of the included studies including the differences in routes and dosages of vitamin C administration [52] may be potential a confounder of the present meta-analysis.

5. Conclusions

The results of this meta-analysis demonstrated significant postoperative reductions in opioid requirement as well as a decrease in pain severity in patients receiving perioperative vitamin C, suggesting that vitamin C may be incorporated into the multimodal approach to postoperative analgesia in surgical patients. Taking into consideration its effectiveness through intravenous administration and the low toxicity, further large-scale trials are warranted to elucidate its optimal intravenous dosage and antinociceptive role in other clinical settings.

Supplementary Materials: The following are available online at http://www.mdpi.com/2072-6643/12/10/3109/s1, Table S1: Reasons for exclusion of studies based on titles and abstracts, Table S2: Cumulative morphine consumptions at postoperative 24 h and the respective pain scores, Table S3: Risks of bias for included studies.

Author Contributions: Conceptualization, K.-C.H. and M.-H.C.; methodology, Y.-T.L.; software, K.-H.C.; validation, L.-K.W. and J.-Y.C.; formal analysis, Y.-J.C.; investigation, S.-C.W.; resources, S.-C.W.; data curation, K.-C.H.; writing—original draft preparation, K.-C.H.; writing—review and editing, K.-C.H., M.-H.C., and C.-K.S.; visualization, M.-H.C.; supervision, C.-K.S. All authors have read and agreed to the published version of the manuscript.

Funding: This research received no external funding.

Conflicts of Interest: The authors declare no conflict of interest.

References

1. Apfelbaum, J.L.; Chen, C.; Mehta, S.S.; Gan, T.J. Postoperative pain experience: Results from a national survey suggest postoperative pain continues to be undermanaged. *Anesth. Analg.* **2003**, *97*, 534–540. [CrossRef]
2. Pavlin, D.J.; Chen, C.; Penaloza, D.A.; Buckley, F.P. A survey of pain and other symptoms that affect the recovery process after discharge from an ambulatory surgery unit. *J. Clin. Anesth.* **2004**, *16*, 200–206. [CrossRef]
3. Kehlet, H.; Jensen, T.S.; Woolf, C.J. Persistent postsurgical pain: Risk factors and prevention. *Lancet (Lond. Engl.)* **2006**, *367*, 1618–1625. [CrossRef]
4. Chou, R.; Gordon, D.B.; de Leon-Casasola, O.A.; Rosenberg, J.M.; Bickler, S.; Brennan, T.; Carter, T.; Cassidy, C.L.; Chittenden, E.H.; Degenhardt, E. Management of Postoperative Pain: A clinical practice guideline from the American pain society, the American Society of Regional Anesthesia and Pain Medicine, and the American Society of Anesthesiologists' committee on regional anesthesia, executive committee, and administrative council. *J. Pain* **2016**, *17*, 131–157.
5. Ayatollahi, V.; Dehghanpour Farashah, S.; Behdad, S.; Vaziribozorg, S.; Rabbani Anari, M. Effect of intravenous vitamin C on postoperative pain in uvulopalatopharyngoplasty with tonsillectomy. *Clin. Otolaryngol.* **2017**, *42*, 139–143. [CrossRef]
6. Li, R.; Shen, L.; Yu, X.; Ma, C.; Huang, Y. Vitamin C enhances the analgesic effect of gabapentin on rats with neuropathic pain. *Life Sci.* **2016**, *157*, 25–31. [CrossRef]
7. Du, J.; Cullen, J.J.; Buettner, G.R. Ascorbic acid: Chemistry, biology and the treatment of cancer. *Biochim. Biophys. Acta* **2012**, *1826*, 443–457. [CrossRef] [PubMed]
8. Englard, S.; Seifter, S. The biochemical functions of ascorbic acid. *Annu. Rev. Nutr* **1986**, *6*, 365–406. [CrossRef]
9. Chen, J.Y.; Chang, C.Y.; Feng, P.H.; Chu, C.C.; So, E.C.; Hu, M.L. Plasma vitamin C is lower in postherpetic neuralgia patients and administration of vitamin C reduces spontaneous pain but not brush-evoked pain. *Clin. J. Pain* **2009**, *25*, 562–569. [CrossRef]
10. Shibuya, N.; Humphers, J.M.; Agarwal, M.R.; Jupiter, D.C. Efficacy and safety of high-dose vitamin C on complex regional pain syndrome in extremity trauma and surgery–systematic review and meta-analysis. *J. Foot Ankle Surg.* **2013**, *52*, 62–66. [CrossRef]
11. Rokyta, R.; Holecek, V.; Pekárkova, I.; Krejcová, J.; Racek, J.; Trefil, L.; Yamamotová, A. Free radicals after painful stimulation are influenced by antioxidants and analgesics. *Neurol. Endocrinol. Lett.* **2003**, *24*, 304–309.
12. Chen, S.; Roffey, D.M.; Dion, C.A.; Arab, A.; Wai, E.K. Effect of Perioperative Vitamin C Supplementation on Postoperative Pain and the Incidence of Chronic Regional Pain Syndrome: A Systematic Review and Meta-Analysis. *Clin. J. Pain* **2016**, *32*, 179–185. [CrossRef]
13. Ma, H.; Tang, J.; White, P.F.; Zaentz, A.; Wender, R.H.; Sloninsky, A.; Naruse, R.; Kariger, R.; Quon, R.; Wood, D.; et al. Perioperative rofecoxib improves early recovery after outpatient herniorrhaphy. *Anesth. Analg.* **2004**, *98*, 970–975. [CrossRef]
14. Watcha, M.F.; Issioui, T.; Klein, K.W.; White, P.F. Costs and effectiveness of rofecoxib, celecoxib, and acetaminophen for preventing pain after ambulatory otolaryngologic surgery. *Anesth. Analg.* **2003**, *96*, 987–994. [CrossRef]
15. Issioui, T.; Klein, K.W.; White, P.F.; Watcha, M.F.; Coloma, M.; Skrivanek, G.D.; Jones, S.B.; Thornton, K.C.; Marple, B.F. The efficacy of premedication with celecoxib and acetaminophen in preventing pain after otolaryngologic surgery. *Anesth. Analg.* **2002**, *94*, 1188–1193. [CrossRef]
16. Issioui, T.; Klein, K.W.; White, P.F.; Watcha, M.F.; Skrivanek, G.D.; Jones, S.B.; Hu, J.; Marple, B.F.; Ing, C. Cost-efficacy of rofecoxib versus acetaminophen for preventing pain after ambulatory surgery. *Anesthesiology* **2002**, *97*, 931–937. [CrossRef]
17. Alishiri, A.; Mosavi, S.A. Ascorbic acid versus placebo in postoperative lid edema postphotorefractive keratectomy: A double-masked, randomized, prospective study. *Oman. J. Ophthalmol.* **2019**, *12*, 4–9. [CrossRef]
18. Moher, D.; Liberati, A.; Tetzlaff, J.; Altman, D.G. Preferred reporting items for systematic reviews and meta-analyses: The PRISMA statement. *BMJ (Clin. Res. Ed.)* **2009**, *339*, b2535. [CrossRef]
19. Shaheen, P.E.; Walsh, D.; Lasheen, W.; Davis, M.P.; Lagman, R.L. Opioid equianalgesic tables: Are they all equally dangerous? *J. Pain Symptom Manag.* **2009**, *38*, 409–417. [CrossRef]

20. Higgins, J.P.; Altman, D.G.; Gøtzsche, P.C.; Jüni, P.; Moher, D.; Oxman, A.D.; Savovic, J.; Schulz, K.F.; Weeks, L.; Sterne, J.A. The Cochrane Collaboration's tool for assessing risk of bias in randomised trials. *BMJ (Clin. Res. Ed.)* **2011**, *343*, d5928. [CrossRef]
21. Blaudszun, G.; Lysakowski, C.; Elia, N.; Tramèr, M.R. Effect of perioperative systemic α2 agonists on postoperative morphine consumption and pain intensity: Systematic review and meta-analysis of randomized controlled trials. *Anesthesiology* **2012**, *116*, 1312–1322. [CrossRef]
22. Jarahzadeh, M.H.; Mousavi, B.M.H.; Abbasi, H.; Jafari, M.A.; Sheikhpouar, E. The efficacy of vitamin C infusion in reducing post-intubation sore throat. *Med. časopis* **2019**, *53*, 95–100. [CrossRef]
23. Jeon, Y.; Park, J.S.; Moon, S.; Yeo, J. Effect of intravenous high dose vitamin C on postoperative pain and morphine use after laparoscopic colectomy: A randomized controlled trial. *Pain Res. Manag.* **2016**, *2016*. [CrossRef]
24. Kanazi, G.E.; El-Khatib, M.F.; Yazbeck-Karam, V.G.; Hanna, J.E.; Masri, B.; Aouad, M.T. Effect of vitamin C on morphine use after laparoscopic cholecystectomy: A randomized controlled trial. *Can. J. Anaesth.* **2012**, *59*, 538–543. [CrossRef]
25. Tunay, D.L.; Ilgınel, M.T.; Ünlügenç, H.; Tunay, M.; Karacaer, F.; Biricik, E. Comparison of the effects of preoperative melatonin or vitamin C administration on postoperative analgesia. *Bosn. J. Basic Med. Sci.* **2020**, *20*, 117. [CrossRef]
26. Moon, S.; Lim, S.; Yun, J.; Lee, W.; Kim, M.; Cho, K.; Ki, S. Additional effect of magnesium sulfate and vitamin C in laparoscopic gynecologic surgery for postoperative pain management: A double-blind randomized controlled trial. *Anesth. Pain Med.* **2020**, *15*, 88–95. [CrossRef]
27. Moon, S.; Lim, S.H.; Cho, K.; Kim M-h Lee, W.; Cho, Y.H. The efficacy of vitamin C on postlaparoscopic shoulder pain: A double-blind randomized controlled trial. *Anesth. Pain Med.* **2019**, *14*, 202–207. [CrossRef]
28. Pourmatroud, E.; Hormozi, L.; Hemadi, M.; Golshahi, R. Intravenous ascorbic acid (vitamin C) administration in myomectomy: A prospective, randomized, clinical trial. *Arch. Gynecol. Obstet.* **2012**, *285*, 111–115. [CrossRef]
29. Gan, T.J.; Habib, A.S.; Miller, T.E.; White, W.; Apfelbaum, J.L. Incidence, patient satisfaction, and perceptions of post-surgical pain: Results from a US national survey. *Curr. Med. Res. Opin.* **2014**, *30*, 149–160. [CrossRef]
30. McGrath, B.; Elgendy, H.; Chung, F.; Kamming, D.; Curti, B.; King, S. Thirty percent of patients have moderate to severe pain 24 hr after ambulatory surgery: A survey of 5,703 patients. *Can. J. Anaesth.* **2004**, *51*, 886–891. [CrossRef]
31. Gjeilo, K.H.; Stenseth, R.; Klepstad, P. Risk factors and early pharmacological interventions to prevent chronic postsurgical pain following cardiac surgery. *Am. J. Cardiovasc. Drugs* **2014**, *14*, 335–342. [CrossRef] [PubMed]
32. Hyllested, M.; Jones, S.; Pedersen, J.L.; Kehlet, H. Comparative effect of paracetamol, NSAIDs or their combination in postoperative pain management: A qualitative review. *Br. J. Anaesth.* **2002**, *88*, 199–214. [CrossRef] [PubMed]
33. Gorissen, K.J.; Benning, D.; Berghmans, T.; Snoeijs, M.G.; Sosef, M.N.; Hulsewe, K.W.; Luyer, M.D. Risk of anastomotic leakage with non-steroidal anti-inflammatory drugs in colorectal surgery. *Br. J. Surg.* **2012**, *99*, 721–727. [CrossRef] [PubMed]
34. Dodwell, E.R.; Latorre, J.G.; Parisini, E.; Zwettler, E.; Chandra, D.; Mulpuri, K.; Snyder, B. NSAID exposure and risk of nonunion: A meta-analysis of case-control and cohort studies. *Calcif. Tissue Int.* **2010**, *87*, 193–202. [CrossRef] [PubMed]
35. Rivers, J.M. Safety of high-level vitamin C ingestion. *Ann. N. Y. Acad. Sci.* **1987**, *498*, 445–454. [CrossRef]
36. Elia, N.; Lysakowski, C.; Tramèr, M.R. Does multimodal analgesia with acetaminophen, nonsteroidal antiinflammatory drugs, or selective cyclooxygenase-2 inhibitors and patient-controlled analgesia morphine offer advantages over morphine alone? Meta-analyses of randomized trials. *Anesthesiology* **2005**, *103*, 1296–1304. [CrossRef]
37. Remy, C.; Marret, E.; Bonnet, F. Effects of acetaminophen on morphine side-effects and consumption after major surgery: Meta-analysis of randomized controlled trials. *Br. J. Anaesth.* **2005**, *94*, 505–513. [CrossRef]
38. Kim, H.K.; Park, S.K.; Zhou, J.L.; Taglialatela, G.; Chung, K.; Coggeshall, R.E.; Chung, J.M. Reactive oxygen species (ROS) play an important role in a rat model of neuropathic pain. *Pain* **2004**, *111*, 116–124. [CrossRef]
39. Rebec, G.V.; Pierce, R.C. A vitamin as neuromodulator: Ascorbate release into the extracellular fluid of the brain regulates dopaminergic and glutamatergic transmission. *Prog. Neurobiol.* **1994**, *43*, 537–565. [CrossRef]

40. Rosa, K.A.; Gadotti, V.M.; Rosa, A.O.; Rodrigues, A.L.; Calixto, J.B.; Santos, A.R. Evidence for the involvement of glutamatergic system in the antinociceptive effect of ascorbic acid. *Neurosci. Lett.* **2005**, *381*, 185–188. [CrossRef]
41. Willis, W.D.; Westlund, K.N. Neuroanatomy of the pain system and of the pathways that modulate pain. *J. Clin. Neurophysiol.* **1997**, *14*, 2–31. [CrossRef] [PubMed]
42. Jones, R.B.; Satterlee, D.G.; Cadd, G.G. Timidity in Japanese quail: Effects of vitamin C and divergent selection for adrenocortical response. *Physiol. Behav.* **1999**, *67*, 117–120. [CrossRef]
43. Harrison, F.E.; Yu, S.S.; Van Den Bossche, K.L.; Li, L.; May, J.M.; McDonald, M.P. Elevated oxidative stress and sensorimotor deficits but normal cognition in mice that cannot synthesize ascorbic acid. *J. Neurochem.* **2008**, *106*, 1198–1208. [CrossRef] [PubMed]
44. Rice, M.E. Ascorbate regulation and its neuroprotective role in the brain. *Trends Neurosci.* **2000**, *23*, 209–216. [CrossRef]
45. Fukushima, R.; Yamazaki, E. Vitamin C requirement in surgical patients. *Curr. Opin. Clin. Nutr. Metab. Care* **2010**, *13*, 669–676. [CrossRef]
46. Karanicolas, P.J.; Smith, S.E.; Kanbur, B.; Davies, E.; Guyatt, G.H. The impact of prophylactic dexamethasone on nausea and vomiting after laparoscopic cholecystectomy: A systematic review and meta-analysis. *Ann. Surg.* **2008**, *248*, 751–762. [CrossRef]
47. Ghorbaninezhad, K.; Bakhsha, F.; Yousefi, Z.; Halakou, S.; Mehrbakhsh, Z. Comparison Effect of Tranexamic Acid (TA) and Tranexamic Acid Combined with Vitamin C (TXC) on Drainage Volume and Atrial Fibrillation Arrhythmia in Patients Undergoing Cardiac Bypass Surgery: Randomized Clinical Trial. *Anesth. Pain Med.* **2019**, *9*, e96096. [CrossRef]
48. Blee, T.H.; Cogbill, T.H.; Lambert, P.J. Hemorrhage associated with vitamin C deficiency in surgical patients. *Surgery* **2002**, *131*, 408–412. [CrossRef]
49. Padayatty, S.J.; Sun, H.; Wang, Y.; Riordan, H.D.; Hewitt, S.M.; Katz, A.; Wesley, R.A.; Levine, M. Vitamin C pharmacokinetics: Implications for oral and intravenous use. *Ann. Intern. Med.* **2004**, *140*, 533–537. [CrossRef]
50. Jain, S.K.; Dar, M.Y.; Kumar, S.; Yadav, A.; Kearns, S.R. Role of anti-oxidant (vitamin-C) in post-operative pain relief in foot and ankle trauma surgery: A prospective randomized trial. *Foot Ankle Surg.* **2019**, *25*, 542–545. [CrossRef]
51. Dick, F.; Tevaearai, H. Significance and Limitations of the p Value. *Eur. J. Vasc. Endovasc. Surg.* **2015**, *50*, 815. [CrossRef] [PubMed]
52. Wang, L.-K.; Chuang, C.-C.; Chen, J.-Y. Relief of acute herpetic pain by intravenous vitamin C: The dosage may make a difference. *Ann. Dermatol.* **2018**, *30*, 262–264. [CrossRef] [PubMed]

© 2020 by the authors. Licensee MDPI, Basel, Switzerland. This article is an open access article distributed under the terms and conditions of the Creative Commons Attribution (CC BY) license (http://creativecommons.org/licenses/by/4.0/).

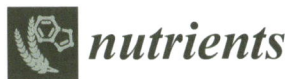

Article

Patients with Community Acquired Pneumonia Exhibit Depleted Vitamin C Status and Elevated Oxidative Stress

Anitra C. Carr [1],*, Emma Spencer [1], Liane Dixon [2] and Stephen T. Chambers [3]

1. Nutrition in Medicine Research Group, Department of Pathology and Biomedical Science, University of Otago, Christchurch 8011, New Zealand; emma.spencer@otago.ac.nz
2. Department of Infectious Diseases, Christchurch Hospital, Christchurch 8011, New Zealand; liane.dixon@cdhb.health.nz
3. The Infection Group, Department of Pathology and Biomedical Science, University of Otago, Christchurch 8011, New Zealand; steve.chambers@otago.ac.nz
* Correspondence: anitra.carr@otago.ac.nz; Tel.: +643-364-0649

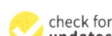

Received: 13 April 2020; Accepted: 1 May 2020; Published: 6 May 2020

Abstract: Pneumonia is a severe lower respiratory tract infection that is a common complication and a major cause of mortality of the vitamin C-deficiency disease scurvy. This suggests an important link between vitamin C status and lower respiratory tract infections. Due to the paucity of information on the vitamin C status of patients with pneumonia, we assessed the vitamin C status of 50 patients with community-acquired pneumonia and compared these with 50 healthy community controls. The pneumonia cohort comprised 44 patients recruited through the Acute Medical Assessment Unit (AMAU) and 6 patients recruited through the Intensive Care Unit (ICU); mean age 68 ± 17 years, 54% male. Clinical, microbiological and hematological parameters were recorded. Blood samples were tested for vitamin C status using HPLC with electrochemical detection and protein carbonyl concentrations, an established marker of oxidative stress, using ELISA. Patients with pneumonia had depleted vitamin C status compared with healthy controls (23 ± 14 μmol/L vs. 56 ± 24 μmol/L, $p < 0.001$). The more severe patients in the ICU had significantly lower vitamin C status than those recruited through AMAU (11 ± 3 μmol/L vs. 24 ± 14 μmol/L, $p = 0.02$). The pneumonia cohort comprised 62% with hypovitaminosis C and 22% with deficiency, compared with only 8% hypovitaminosis C and no cases of deficiency in the healthy controls. The pneumonia cohort also exhibited significantly elevated protein carbonyl concentrations compared with the healthy controls ($p < 0.001$), indicating enhanced oxidative stress in the patients. We were able to collect subsequent samples from 28% of the cohort (mean 2.7 ± 1.7 days; range 1–7 days). These showed no significant differences in vitamin C status or protein carbonyl concentrations compared with baseline values ($p = 0.6$). Overall, the depleted vitamin C status and elevated oxidative stress observed in the patients with pneumonia indicates an enhanced requirement for the vitamin during their illness. Therefore, these patients would likely benefit from additional vitamin C supplementation to restore their blood and tissue levels to optimal. This may decrease excessive oxidative stress and aid in their recovery.

Keywords: vitamin C; ascorbic acid; ascorbate; pneumonia; community acquired pneumonia; oxidative stress; protein carbonyls; hypovitaminosis C; vitamin C deficiency

1. Introduction

Pneumonia is a severe lower respiratory tract infection that can be caused by bacterial, fungal and viral pathogens, including the novel severe acute respiratory syndrome coronavirus (SARS-CoV-2) [1,2]. Lower respiratory tract infections are the leading cause of morbidity and mortality for communicable disease worldwide [3]. In 2016, lower respiratory tract infections resulted in more than 65 million hospital admissions and nearly 2.4 million deaths worldwide [4]. Mortality is particularly high for children under five and the elderly, which is of concern due to the increasingly aging population [5]. Increased incidence of community-acquired pneumonia is also associated with lower socioeconomic status and certain ethnic groups [5–7].

Pneumonia is a common complication and a major cause of mortality of the vitamin C deficiency disease scurvy, which suggests an important link between vitamin C status and lower respiratory tract infections [8]. The EPIC-Norfolk longitudinal study comprising more than 19,000 men and women has shown a 30% lower risk of pneumonia and a 39% lower mortality from pneumonia for people in the top quartile of vitamin C status (>66 µmol/L, i.e., saturating status), ascertained from a single baseline measurement at enrolment, compared with those in the bottom quartile of vitamin C status (≤41 µmol/L) [9]. Despite the known roles of vitamin C in supporting immune function through acting as an antioxidant and enzyme cofactor [10], surprisingly few studies have explored the link between vitamin C and pneumonia [11]. Two case control studies have indicated that patients with pneumonia have significantly lower vitamin C status than healthy controls, and there was an inverse correlation with the severity of the condition [12,13]. Two other studies that explored the time course indicated that up to 40% of patients with pneumonia exhibited vitamin C deficiency (i.e., plasma vitamin C concentrations <11 µmol/L) at hospital admission, and concentrations remained low for at least four weeks [14,15].

These studies indicate a higher utilization of, and potentially also a higher requirement for, vitamin C during lower respiratory tract infections. Patients with pneumonia may also have lower baseline vitamin C status, which could potentially make them more susceptible to infection. Due to the paucity of recent studies investigating the link between vitamin C and pneumonia, and the global relevance due to periodic outbreaks of SARS-related coronaviruses, we measured the vitamin C status of patients with community-acquired pneumonia who were admitted to the Acute Medical Assessment Unit or Intensive Care Unit of our public hospital. We also measured protein carbonyl concentrations, an established marker of oxidative stress. These parameters were compared with those measured in healthy controls.

2. Methods

2.1. Setting and Study Participants

Christchurch Hospital is the largest tertiary, teaching and research hospital in the South Island of New Zealand; it is located in New Zealand's second largest city and services 600,000 people in the Canterbury region. A total of 50 patients were recruited for this observational study in Christchurch Hospital; 44 patients with community-acquired pneumonia were recruited in the Acute Medical Assessment Unit and medical wards (July 2017 to February 2018) and six patients with CAP were recruited in the Intensive Care Unit (December 2015 to August 2016). Ethical approval was obtained from the New Zealand Southern Health and Disability Ethics Committee (#16STH235 and #15STH36). Radiology reports for suspected pneumonia were viewed daily to identify potential patients. Many of the patients were elderly and to ensure a correct consent process, cognition was considered, along with a supportive family, to discuss this before continuing. All patients signed informed consent documents.

2.2. Inclusion and Exclusion Criteria

Community-acquired pneumonia was defined as a pneumonia that had been acquired outside of hospitals or health care settings. Pneumonia was defined in a patient with an acute illness and new inflammatory infiltrate on a chest radiograph, or a diagnosis of community-acquired pneumonia by the treating physician and the presence of at least one of the following acute respiratory signs and symptoms: Cough, increased sputum production, dyspnoea, core body temperature of ≥38.0 °C and auscultatory findings of abnormal breathing sounds or rales [16,17]. Other inclusion criteria were age ≥ 18 years and the ability to provide informed consent. Exclusion criteria were as follows: (1) pneumonia was (a) not the primary cause for hospital admission, (b) an expected terminal event or (c) distal to bronchial obstruction; (2) patients with tuberculosis or bronchiectasis; and (3) patients who had been in hospital within the previous 14 days, or had previously been entered in the study.

2.3. Disease Severity Scores

The CURB-65 score (range 0–5) was calculated from admission records using values from the first 12 h in hospital to determine severity and predict mortality of pneumonia and was calculated for all patients. The criteria were as follows: confusion of new onset (defined as an abbreviated mental test score (AMTS) of ≤8), blood urea nitrogen > 7 mmol/L, respiratory rate ≥ 30 breaths per minute, blood pressure < 90 mmHg systolic or ≤60 mmHg diastolic and age ≥ 65 years. Each criteria scored 1 point if met [18]. ICU severity scores were recorded if the patients were admitted to the ICU. These were Acute Physiology and Chronic Health Evaluation II and III score (APACHE II and III, range 0–79 and 0–299, respectively); Simplified Acute Physiology Score II (SAPS II, range 0–163); and Sequential Organ Failure Assessment score (SOFA, range 0–24). Common comorbidities were also recorded.

2.4. Blood Sampling and Processing

A blood sample (with heparin anticoagulant) was collected within 24 h of admission and pneumonia was confirmed via chest film. Because these were acutely ill patients, the blood samples were non-fasting. A blood sample was not able to be collected from one participant so their clinical data were excluded from the analysis. A second sample was collected from a subset of the participants on day of discharge ($n = 14$). Blood samples were also collected from a cohort of non-fasting healthy community controls who were resident in Christchurch ($n = 50$, 50% female, aged 57 ± 17 years). The blood samples were placed on ice and immediately transferred to the laboratory for centrifugation to separate plasma for vitamin C and oxidative stress biomarker analysis. An aliquot of the plasma was treated with an equal volume of 0.54 M perchloric acid and 100 µmol/L of the metal chelator DTPA to precipitate protein and stabilize the vitamin C. The supernatant and spare plasma samples were stored at −80 °C until analysis.

2.5. Analysis of Blood Analytes

Routine hematological analyses were carried out at Canterbury Health Laboratories, an International Accreditation New Zealand (IANZ) laboratory. Identified organisms were recorded. The vitamin C content of the processed plasma samples was determined using HPLC with electrochemical detection, as described previously [19]. The protein carbonyl content of the plasma was determined using a sensitive ELISA method, as described previously [20].

2.6. Statistical Analysis

Data are presented as mean and SD or mean and 95% CI as indicated. Statistical analyses were carried out using Excel data analysis add-in and GraphPad Prism 8.0 software (San Diego, CA, USA). Differences between groups were determined using Student's t-test or Mann–Whitney U test for non-parametric variables. Linear regression analyses were carried out using Pearson correlations. Statistical significance was set at $p < 0.05$.

3. Results

3.1. Participant Characteristics

Participants were recruited in the Acute Medical Assessment Unit (AMAU; $n = 44$) and the Intensive Care Unit (ICU; $n = 6$). One of the AMAU patients was transferred to the ICU (for 12 days) following baseline measurements. There were 54% males in the cohort and a mean age of 68 ± 17 years (Table 1). The most common comorbidities were cardiovascular diseases, asthma and chronic heart failure. Mean CURB-65 score for the cohort was 1.9: 1.8 for the AMAU patients and 3.5 for the ICU patients (excluding two ICU patients who had transferred from other hospitals and so had lower CURB-65 scores at admission). Mean length of hospital stay (LOS) was 3 days, with a higher mean LOS of 24 days for the ICU cohort. Two of the patients in the AMAU cohort died (of cardiac complications) giving an overall mortality of 4% for the total cohort.

Table 1. Participant baseline characteristics.

Characteristic	Total Cohort (n = 50)	AMAU (n = 44)	ICU (n = 6)
Age, years [1]	68 (17)	66 (22)	58 (17)
Male sex, n (%)	27 (54)	23 (52)	4 (67)
Comorbidities, n (%)		COPD 6 (14) Asthma 11 (25) Chronic heart failure 9 (20) Cardiovascular disease 19 (43) Diabetes 5 (11) Cerebrovascular disease 6 (14) Renal disease 3 (7) Solid organ malignancy 2 (5) Hematological malignancy 1 (2) Immune suppression 2 (5)	COPD 1 (17) Cardiovascular disease 1 (17) Renal failure 1 (17) Hematological malignancy 1 (17) Immune compromised 1 (17)
Temperature, °C		38 (1.2)	
Hypothermia, n (%)		2 (4.5)	
Systolic BP	139 (38)	147 (33)	80 (11)
Diastolic BP	75 (20)	79 (18)	46 (10)
Heart rate, beats/min		106 (22)	
Respiratory rate, breaths/min			36 (11)
Radiological confirmation, n (%)		37 (84)	
CURB-65 score (0–5)	1.9 (1.3)	1.8 (1.3)	3.5 (0.6) [2]
SAPS II score (0–163)			40 (11)
APACHE II score (0–79)			20 (6)
APACHE III score (0–299)			72 (24)
SOFA score (0–24)			10 (3)
Vasopressors, n (%)		0	6 (100)
Mechanical ventilation, n (%)		0	4 (67)
FiO$_2$			0.38 (0.07)
Hospital LOS, days [3]	3 (0–99)	3 (0–91)	24 (5–99)
Mortality, n (%)	2 (4.0)	2 (4.5)	0

[1] Data is presented as mean (SD) unless otherwise indicated; [2] Two of the ICU patients were transferred from other hospitals and were excluded from CURB-65 calculations; [3] Data is presented as median and range. Key: AMAU, Acute Medical Assessment Unit; APACHE, Acute Physiology and Chronic Health Evaluation; COPD, chronic obstructive pulmonary disease; CURB, confusion urea respiratory rate blood pressure; ICU, intensive care unit; LOS, length of stay; SAPS, simplified acute physiology score; SOFA, sequential organ failure assessment.

The ICU cohort exhibited more severe hematological parameters, including a significantly higher mean C-reactive protein concentration ($p = 0.027$; Table 2). *Streptococcus pneumonia* was the most common pathogen identified in the AMAU patients (11%), followed by *Legionella* (9%) and *Haemophilus influenzae* (7%), and 11% of the patients had viral pathogens identified (*Adenovirus*, *Influenza A*, *Parainfluenza* and *Rhinovirus*). Although *Pseudomonas aeruginosa* was the most common pathogen identified in the ICU patients, the role in causing the initial pneumonia was unclear.

3.2. Vitamin C and Protein Carbonyls

The vitamin C status of community-acquired pneumonia patients admitted to hospital was 23 ± 14 µmol/L; this was significantly lower than healthy controls (56 ± 24 µmol/L; $p < 0.001$; Figure 1a). The patients admitted to the ICU had significantly lower vitamin C status than those admitted to AMAU (11 ± 3 µmol/L vs. 24 ± 14 µmol/L; $p = 0.02$). Protein carbonyls, an established biomarker of oxidative stress, were significantly elevated in patients with pneumonia compared with healthy controls (468 ± 305 vs. 159 ± 39 pmol/mg protein, respectively; $p < 0.001$; Figure 1b).

Table 2. Participant hematological parameters.

Parameter	Total Cohort (n = 50)	AMAU (n = 44)	ICU (n = 6)
White cell count (×10^9/L) [1]	13 (6)	13 (5)	18 (13)
Neutrophils (×10^9/L)	11 (5)	11 (5)	15 (10)
Hemoglobin (g/L)	130 (17)	130 (17)	125 (26)
Platelets (×10^9/L)	241 (117)	244 (91)	218 (227)
Urea (mmol/L)	8.4 (6.5)	7.4 (4.1)	15 (13)
Creatinine (µmol/L)	107 (61)	98 (29)	168 (138)
Bilirubin (µmol/L)	19 (11)	18 (9)	25 (13)
C-reactive protein (mg/L)	165 (127)	152 (127)	261 (78) [2]
Alanine transaminase (U/L)	34 (21)	33 (21)	35 (23)
Alkaline phosphatase (U/L)		112 (53)	
Lactate (mmol/L)			1.5 (0.8)
PaO$_2$ (mmHg)			79 (19)
PaO$_2$/FiO$_2$			212 (59)

[1] Data is presented as mean (SD), [2] $p = 0.027$ relative to AMAU value. Key: AMAU, Acute Medical Assessment Unit; ICU, intensive care unit.

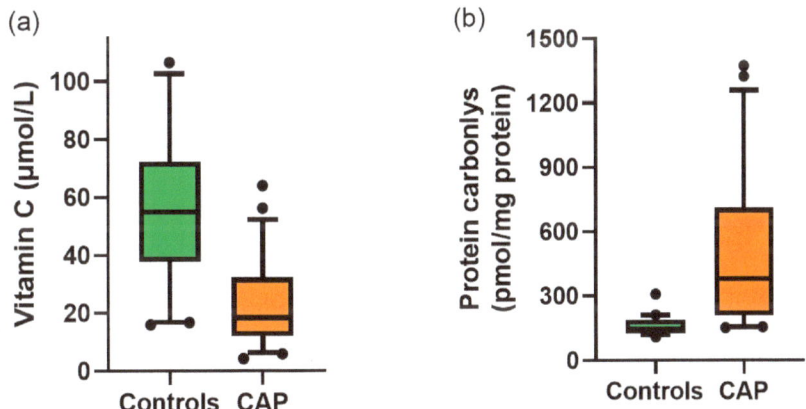

Figure 1. Vitamin C status and protein carbonyl concentrations in the community-acquired pneumonia (CAP) cohort and healthy controls. (a) Vitamin C was measured using HPLC with electrochemical detection, $p < 0.001$, $n = 50$ for both controls and CAP. (b) Protein carbonyls were measured using ELISA; $p < 0.001$, $n = 50$ for controls, $n = 46$ for CAP. Box plots show median with 25th and 75th percentiles as boundaries, and whiskers are the 5th and 95th percentiles, with symbols indicating outlying data points.

The pneumonia cohort comprised 96% patients with inadequate vitamin C status (i.e., <50 µmol/L), 62% with hypovitaminosis C (i.e., <23 µmol/L) and 22% with frank deficiency (i.e., <11 µmol/L; Figure 2). In contrast, the healthy controls comprised only 8% with hypovitaminosis C and no cases of deficiency.

Subsequent samples were collected from 14 (28%) of the participants (mean 2.7 ± 1.7 days, range 1–7 days); there were no statistically significant differences between baseline and subsequent samples for either vitamin C status or protein carbonyl concentrations (Table 3).

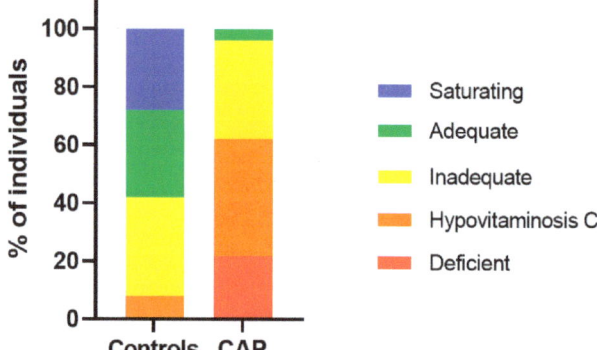

Figure 2. Percentage of individuals from the community-acquired pneumonia (CAP) cohort and healthy controls in different vitamin C categories. Vitamin C categories are presented as saturating (>70 µmol/L), adequate (between 70 and 50 µmol/L), inadequate (between 50 and 23 µmol/L), hypovitaminosis C (between 23 and 11 µmol/L), deficient (<11 µmol/L).

Table 3. Vitamin C status and protein carbonyl concentrations measured over time.

Biomarker	Baseline Sample [1]	Second Sample [2]	p Value
Vitamin C (µmol/L)	20 (7)	22 (7)	0.6
Protein carbonyls (pmol/mg protein)	541 (157)	625 (252)	0.6

[1] Data expressed as mean (95% CI); [2] Mean 2.7 ± 1.7 days (range 1–7 days).

3.3. Biomarker Correlations with Clinical and Physiological Parameters

There was no significant correlation between vitamin C status and CURB-65 scores ($p = 0.3$); however, there was a significant correlation with systolic blood pressure ($R = 0.33$, $p = 0.02$) and a trend towards significance with diastolic blood pressure ($R = 0.26$, $p = 0.07$). There was no significant correlation between vitamin C status and C-reactive protein concentrations ($R = 0.25$, $p = 0.09$). In contrast, there was a significant correlation between protein carbonyls and the CURB-65 score ($R = 0.4$, $p = 0.006$), as well as with urea and creatinine ($R = 0.50$–0.58, $p < 0.001$). There was no correlation between protein carbonyls and vitamin C status in the pneumonia cohort ($p = 0.3$); however, an inverse correlation between protein carbonyls and vitamin C status was observed in the healthy controls ($R = -0.38$, $p = 0.006$).

4. Discussion

Our study shows that patients with community-acquired pneumonia have significantly depleted vitamin C status (mean of 23 µmol/L) and a high prevalence of hypovitaminosis C and deficiency (62% and 22%, respectively). Lower vitamin C status was evident with increasing severity of the condition, as shown by the ICU patients having significantly lower vitamin C status than the rest of the hospitalized cohort. Our data is in agreement with two early observational studies investigating vitamin C status in patients with pneumonia [12,13]. Vitamin C concentrations of 31 µmol/L were reported in 11 patients with pneumonia, compared with concentrations of 66 µmol/L in 20 healthy controls [12]. In a very early study from the 1950s, ascorbate concentrations of 17 µmol/L in 7 acute patients who died, 24 µmol/L in 15 acute survivors, and 34 µmol/L in 13 convalescent cases were compared with 49 µmol/L in 28 healthy controls [13]. Thus, this study supports our finding of lower vitamin C status in more severe cases. These investigators also reported elevated concentrations of oxidized vitamin C (dehydroascorbic acid) in the patient samples, suggesting enhanced oxidative stress; however, the high levels reported in this study are likely an ex vivo artifact of the assay method used [21].

We were able to collect subsequent samples from a subgroup of the patients, which showed no change in vitamin C status in samples collected up to a week later. This is in agreement with an earlier intervention study by Hunt et al., who reported baseline vitamin C levels of 23 µmol/L in 57 elderly people with pneumonia or bronchitis, while two weeks later levels remained in the hypovitaminosis C range (i.e., 19 µmol/L) in the participants who did not receive vitamin C (n = 29) [14]. Another study also showed hypovitaminosis C in 70 patients with acute pneumonia at days 5 and 10 [15]. By week four, both of these studies reported that vitamin C status was still low and only approaching baseline levels [14,15]. This indicates that the vitamin C status of patients with pneumonia is likely to remain low for a significant duration following their illness.

In our study we measured protein carbonyls as a marker of oxidative stress. Protein carbonyls can be formed by a variety of reactive oxygen species and via a number of different reaction pathways including direct oxidation of specific amino acids, oxidative cleavage of the protein backbone or reaction of reactive sugar- and lipid-derived aldehydes with specific amino acids [22]. We found significantly elevated protein carbonyls in the patients with pneumonia compared with healthy controls. Elevated protein carbonyls have been observed previously in critically ill patients with sepsis [23]. The patients with the highest protein carbonyl values measured in our study had hypovitaminosis C. Elevated oxidative stress could be both a cause and a consequence of the low vitamin C status observed in the patients. Interestingly, a pre-clinical animal model indicated that administration of high-dose vitamin C to mice with sepsis decreased protein carbonyl levels in the most severely ill [24]. This has not yet been demonstrated in human studies; however, based on the potent antioxidant properties of vitamin C, it is possible that vitamin C administration to patients with pneumonia could decrease markers of excessive oxidative stress.

Vitamin C is known to have numerous immune supporting functions, including enhancing various leukocyte functions such as chemotaxis and microbial killing (reviewed in [10]). It may also be able to support resolution of the inflammatory process by enhancing neutrophil apoptosis and clearance from the lungs [25,26], as well as limiting generation of neutrophil extracellular traps (NETs), which are thought to enhance tissue damage and prolong lung inflammation [27,28]. Although we did not measure the vitamin C content of leukocytes, Hunt et al. have shown that the vitamin C content of leukocytes is low in patients with acute respiratory infections and these remain low at week 2, although some recovery is observed by week 4 [14]. It is possible that these depleted vitamin C levels may affect neutrophil function [10]. The vitamin C content of neutrophils has also been measured during upper respiratory tract infections such as the common cold [29,30]. Although vitamin C levels do decrease in leukocytes during the common cold, the levels recover more rapidly (i.e., within 4–5 days) than was observed for leukocytes from pneumonia patients. This indicates a prolonged burden on the immune cells of patients with pneumonia, which may affect their recovery.

Surprisingly few vitamin C intervention studies have been carried out in patients with pneumonia [31,32]. Administration of vitamin C at a dose of 200 mg/d to 28 elderly patients with pneumonia and bronchitis restored saturating vitamin C status within two weeks and also improved leukocyte vitamin C concentrations [14]. This study also showed a decreased respiratory symptom score in the most severely ill and a trend towards decreased mortality. Another intervention study showed a dose dependent decrease in duration of hospital stay from 24 days in the control group to 19 days in the lower vitamin C group (250–800 mg/d) and 15 days in the higher vitamin C group (500–1600 mg/d) [15]. Thus, administration of vitamin C to depleted pneumonia patients may improve their clinical outcomes. More well-controlled trials are required to test this [32].

Sepsis is a common complication of severe pneumonia, often requiring admission to the ICU. We have previously shown that critically ill patients with sepsis have depleted vitamin C status despite receiving recommended enteral and parenteral intakes of vitamin C (up to a mean of 200 mg/d) [33]. Other clinical research has indicated that critically ill patients likely need at least 10-fold more vitamin C (i.e., 2–3 g/d) to compensate for the enhanced requirements for the vitamin during the inflammatory process [34,35]. Therefore, it is likely that pneumonia patients who have progressed to sepsis and have been admitted to the ICU will require gram intravenous (IV) doses of vitamin C to restore adequate vitamin C status. One trial has shown improved radiologic score and decreased mortality in severe pneumonia cases in the ICU who were administered a combination containing IV vitamin C at a dose of 6 g/d [36]. A number of other clinical trials of patients with sepsis and septic shock have also indicated improved patient outcomes with administration of gram doses of IV vitamin C [11]. The decreased requirement for vasopressor drugs observed in some trials may reflect the ability of vitamin C to aid in endogenous vasopressor synthesis via its enzyme cofactor functions [37]. In support of this premise, we observed a positive correlation between vitamin C status and blood pressure in the patients with pneumonia.

Although the samples in our study were collected prior to the SARS-CoV-2 outbreak, it is likely that people with COVID-19-associated pneumonia and sepsis would have similarly low vitamin C status and high oxidative stress. Early case reports from the 1940s indicated that IV administration of gram doses of vitamin C to cases of viral pneumonia rapidly improved common symptoms [38]. There are currently a number of intervention trials up and running around the world that will specifically test IV vitamin C for COVID-19-related pneumonia and sepsis. Furthermore, it is likely that patients with other severe infectious conditions may also have low vitamin C status. This has been previously demonstrated in patients with tuberculosis, bacterial meningitis, tetanus and typhoid fever [12,13]. These patients would also likely benefit from additional vitamin C supplementation.

A limitation of our study was the use of non-fasting plasma samples for analysis of vitamin C. However, as these were severely ill hospitalized patients it was felt that fasting was not appropriate. Therefore, we collected non-fasting samples from the healthy controls for an equivalent comparison. The number of participants was relatively low, particularly for the ICU subgroup comparisons; however, the differences in biomarker values between the patients and healthy controls were still highly significant.

5. Conclusions

Patients with pneumonia exhibit low vitamin C status and an elevated prevalence of hypovitaminosis C and deficiency compared with healthy controls. This indicates an enhanced requirement for the vitamin during their illness. Due to the important roles that vitamin C plays in the immune system, low vitamin C status is possibly both a cause and a consequence of the disease. The patients also exhibited elevated oxidative stress as evidenced by significantly higher protein carbonyl concentrations than healthy controls. Elevated oxidative stress could be both a cause and a consequence of the low vitamin C status observed in the patients. Therefore, these patients would likely benefit from additional vitamin C supplementation to restore their blood and tissue levels to optimal. This may decrease excessive oxidative stress and aid in their recovery.

Author Contributions: Conceptualization, A.C.C., S.T.C.; methodology, S.T.C., A.C.C., L.D., E.S.; investigation, L.D., E.S.; data curation, L.D., A.C.C.; formal analysis, A.C.C.; writing—original draft preparation, A.C.C.; writing—review and editing, S.T.C., E.S., L.D.; supervision, A.C.C., S.T.C.; project administration, A.C.C.; funding acquisition, A.C.C. All authors have read and agreed to the published version of the manuscript.

Funding: This research was funded by the Health Research Council of New Zealand (grant number 16/037) and the Canterbury Medical Research Foundation (grant number 15/06).

Acknowledgments: A.C. is a recipient of a Sir Charles Hercus Health Research Fellowship from the Health Research Council of New Zealand. Thank you to Bruce Dobbs for setting up the patient database, Marguerite DeAbaffy for helping to recruit patients and collect blood samples, and Kate Vick for processing the patient samples.

Conflicts of Interest: The authors declare no conflict of interest.

References

1. Musher, D.M.; Thorner, A.R. Community-acquired pneumonia. *N. Engl. J. Med.* **2014**, *371*, 1619–1628. [CrossRef] [PubMed]
2. Lai, C.C.; Liu, Y.H.; Wang, C.Y.; Wang, Y.H.; Hsueh, S.C.; Yen, M.Y.; Ko, W.C.; Hsueh, P.R. Asymptomatic carrier state, acute respiratory disease, and pneumonia due to severe acute respiratory syndrome coronavirus 2 (SARS-CoV-2): Facts and myths. *J. Microbiol. Immunol. Infect* **2020**. [CrossRef] [PubMed]
3. World Health Organization. *Global Health Estimates 2016: Deaths by Cause, Age, Sex, by Country and by Region, 2000–2016*; World Health Organization: Geneva, Switzerland, 2018.
4. GBD 2016 Causes of Death Collaborators. Global, regional, and national age-sex specific mortality for 264 causes of death, 1980–2016: A systematic analysis for the Global Burden of Disease Study 2016. *Lancet* **2017**, *390*, 1151–1210. [CrossRef]
5. GBD 2016 Lower Respiratory Infections Collaborators. Estimates of the global, regional, and national morbidity, mortality, and aetiologies of lower respiratory infections in 195 countries, 1990–2016: A systematic analysis for the Global Burden of Disease Study 2016. *Lancet Infect Dis.* **2018**, *18*, 1191–1210. [CrossRef]
6. Burton, D.C.; Flannery, B.; Bennett, N.M.; Farley, M.M.; Gershman, K.; Harrison, L.H.; Lynfield, R.; Petit, S.; Reingold, A.L.; Schaffner, W.; et al. Socioeconomic and racial/ethnic disparities in the incidence of bacteremic pneumonia among US adults. *Am. J. Public Health* **2010**, *100*, 1904–1911. [CrossRef]
7. Chambers, S.; Laing, R.; Murdoch, D.; Frampton, C.; Jennings, L.; Karalus, N.; Mills, G.; Town, I. Maori have a much higher incidence of community-acquired pneumonia and pneumococcal pneumonia than non-Maori. *N. Z. Med. J.* **2006**, *119*, U1978.
8. Hemilä, H. Vitamin C and infections. *Nutrients* **2017**, *9*, 339. [CrossRef]
9. Myint, P.K.; Wilson, A.M.; Clark, A.B.; Luben, R.N.; Wareham, N.J.; Khaw, K.T. Plasma vitamin C concentrations and risk of incident respiratory diseases and mortality in the European Prospective Investigation into Cancer-Norfolk population-based cohort study. *Eur. J. Clin. Nutr.* **2019**, *73*, 1492–1500. [CrossRef]
10. Carr, A.C.; Maggini, S. Vitamin C and immune function. *Nutrients* **2017**, *9*, 1211. [CrossRef]
11. Carr, A.C. Vitamin C in pneumonia and sepsis. In *Vitamin C: New Biochemical and Functional Insights. Oxidative Stress and Disease*; Chen, Q., Vissers, M., Eds.; CRC Press/Taylor & Francis: Boca Raton, FL, USA, 2020; pp. 115–135.
12. Bakaev, V.V.; Duntau, A.P. Ascorbic acid in blood serum of patients with pulmonary tuberculosis and pneumonia. *Int. J. Tuberc. Lung Dis.* **2004**, *8*, 263–266.
13. Chakrabarti, B.; Banerjee, S. Dehydroascorbic acid level in blood of patients suffering from various infectious diseases. *Proc. Soc. Exp. Biol. Med.* **1955**, *88*, 581–583. [CrossRef] [PubMed]
14. Hunt, C.; Chakravorty, N.K.; Annan, G.; Habibzadeh, N.; Schorah, C.J. The clinical effects of vitamin C supplementation in elderly hospitalised patients with acute respiratory infections. *Int. J. Vitam. Nutr. Res.* **1994**, *64*, 212–219. [PubMed]
15. Mochalkin, N.I. Ascorbic acid in the complex therapy of acute pneumonia. *Voenno-Meditsinskii Zhurnal* **1970**, *9*, 17–21, (English translation: http://www.mv.helsinki.fi/home/hemila/T5.pdf). [PubMed]
16. Halm, E.A.; Fine, M.J.; Marrie, T.J.; Coley, C.M.; Kapoor, W.N.; Obrosky, D.S.; Singer, D.E. Time to clinical stability in patients hospitalized with community-acquired pneumonia: Implications for practice guidelines. *JAMA* **1998**, *279*, 1452–1457. [CrossRef] [PubMed]
17. Niederman, M.S.; Mandell, L.A.; Anzueto, A.; Bass, J.B.; Broughton, W.A.; Campbell, G.D.; Dean, N.; File, T.; Fine, M.J.; Gross, P.A.; et al. Guidelines for the management of adults with community-acquired pneumonia. Diagnosis, assessment of severity, antimicrobial therapy, and prevention. *Am. J. Respir. Crit. Care Med.* **2001**, *163*, 1730–1754. [CrossRef] [PubMed]
18. Lim, W.S.; van der Eerden, M.M.; Laing, R.; Boersma, W.G.; Karalus, N.; Town, G.I.; Lewis, S.A.; Macfarlane, J.T. Defining community acquired pneumonia severity on presentation to hospital: An international derivation and validation study. *Thorax* **2003**, *58*, 377–382. [CrossRef]
19. Carr, A.C.; Pullar, J.M.; Moran, S.; Vissers, M.C. Bioavailability of vitamin C from kiwifruit in non-smoking males: Determination of 'healthy' and 'optimal' intakes. *J. Nutr. Sci.* **2012**, *1*, e14. [CrossRef]
20. Buss, H.; Chan, T.P.; Sluis, K.B.; Domigan, N.M.; Winterbourn, C.C. Protein carbonyl measurement by a sensitive ELISA method. *Free Radic. Biol. Med.* **1997**, *23*, 361–366. [CrossRef]

21. Pullar, J.M.; Bayer, S.; Carr, A.C. Appropriate handling, processing and analysis of blood samples is essential to avoid oxidation of vitamin C to dehydroascorbic acid. *Antioxidants* **2018**, *7*, 29. [CrossRef]
22. Weber, D.; Davies, M.J.; Grune, T. Determination of protein carbonyls in plasma, cell extracts, tissue homogenates, isolated proteins: Focus on sample preparation and derivatization conditions. *Redox Biol.* **2015**, *5*, 367–380. [CrossRef]
23. Winterbourn, C.C.; Buss, I.H.; Chan, T.P.; Plank, L.D.; Clark, M.A.; Windsor, J.A. Protein carbonyl measurements show evidence of early oxidative stress in critically ill patients. *Crit. Care Med.* **2000**, *28*, 143–149. [CrossRef] [PubMed]
24. Kim, J.; Arnaout, L.; Remick, D. Hydrocortisone, ascorbic acid and thiamine (HAT) therapy decreases oxidative stress, improves cardiovascular function and improves survival in murine sepsis. *Shock* **2020**, *53*, 460–467. [CrossRef] [PubMed]
25. Vissers, M.C.; Wilkie, R.P. Ascorbate deficiency results in impaired neutrophil apoptosis and clearance and is associated with up-regulation of hypoxia-inducible factor 1alpha. *J. Leukoc. Biol.* **2007**, *81*, 1236–1244. [CrossRef] [PubMed]
26. Fisher, B.J.; Kraskauskas, D.; Martin, E.J.; Farkas, D.; Wegelin, J.A.; Brophy, D.; Ward, K.R.; Voelkel, N.F.; Fowler, A.A., 3rd; Natarajan, R. Mechanisms of attenuation of abdominal sepsis induced acute lung injury by ascorbic acid. *Am. J. Physiol. Lung Cell Mol. Physiol.* **2012**, *303*, L20–L32. [CrossRef] [PubMed]
27. Mohammed, B.M.; Fisher, B.J.; Kraskauskas, D.; Farkas, D.; Brophy, D.F.; Fowler, A.A.; Natarajan, R. Vitamin C: A novel regulator of neutrophil extracellular trap formation. *Nutrients* **2013**, *5*, 3131–3151. [CrossRef]
28. Bozonet, S.M.; Carr, A.C. The role of physiological vitamin C concentrations on key functions of neutrophils isolated from healthy individuals. *Nutrients* **2019**, *11*, 1363. [CrossRef]
29. Hume, R.; Weyers, E. Changes in leucocyte ascorbic acid during the common cold. *Scott Med. J.* **1973**, *18*, 3–7. [CrossRef]
30. Wilson, C.W. Ascorbic acid function and metabolism during colds. *Ann. N. Y. Acad. Sci.* **1975**, *258*, 529–539. [CrossRef]
31. Hemilä, H.; Louhiala, P. Vitamin C for preventing and treating pneumonia. *Cochrane Database Syst. Rev.* **2013**, *8*, Cd005532.
32. Padhani, Z.A.; Moazzam, Z.; Ashraf, A.; Bilal, H.; Salam, R.A.; Das, J.K.; Bhutta, Z.A. Vitamin C supplementation for prevention and treatment of pneumonia. *Cochrane Database Syst. Rev.* **2020**, *4*, 1–39.
33. Carr, A.C.; Rosengrave, P.C.; Bayer, S.; Chambers, S.; Mehrtens, J.; Shaw, G.M. Hypovitaminosis C and vitamin C deficiency in critically ill patients despite recommended enteral and parenteral intakes. *Crit. Care* **2017**, *21*, 300. [CrossRef] [PubMed]
34. Long, C.L.; Maull, K.I.; Krishnan, R.S.; Laws, H.L.; Geiger, J.W.; Borghesi, L.; Franks, W.; Lawson, T.C.; Sauberlich, H.E. Ascorbic acid dynamics in the seriously ill and injured. *J. Surg. Res.* **2003**, *109*, 144–148. [CrossRef]
35. de Grooth, H.J.; Manubulu-Choo, W.P.; Zandvliet, A.S.; Spoelstra-de Man, A.M.E.; Girbes, A.R.; Swart, E.L.; Oudemans-van Straaten, H.M. Vitamin-C pharmacokinetics in critically ill patients: A randomized trial of four intravenous regimens. *Chest* **2018**, *153*, 1368–1377. [CrossRef] [PubMed]
36. Kim, W.Y.; Jo, E.J.; Eom, J.S.; Mok, J.; Kim, M.H.; Kim, K.U.; Park, H.K.; Lee, M.K.; Lee, K. Combined vitamin C, hydrocortisone, and thiamine therapy for patients with severe pneumonia who were admitted to the intensive care unit: Propensity score-based analysis of a before-after cohort study. *J. Crit. Care* **2018**, *47*, 211–218. [CrossRef] [PubMed]
37. Carr, A.C.; Shaw, G.M.; Fowler, A.A.; Natarajan, R. Ascorbate-dependent vasopressor synthesis: A rationale for vitamin C administration in severe sepsis and septic shock? *Crit. Care* **2015**, *19*, e418. [CrossRef]
38. Klenner, F.R. Virus pneumonia and its treatment with vitamin C. *South Med. Surg.* **1948**, *110*, 36–38.

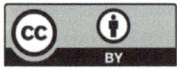

© 2020 by the authors. Licensee MDPI, Basel, Switzerland. This article is an open access article distributed under the terms and conditions of the Creative Commons Attribution (CC BY) license (http://creativecommons.org/licenses/by/4.0/).

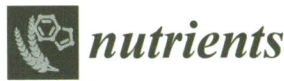

Article

A Cecal Slurry Mouse Model of Sepsis Leads to Acute Consumption of Vitamin C in the Brain

David C. Consoli [1], Jordan J. Jesse [2], Kelly R. Klimo [3], Adriana A. Tienda [1], Nathan D. Putz [2], Julie A. Bastarache [2] and Fiona E. Harrison [1,*]

1. Division of Diabetes, Endocrinology, and Metabolism; Vanderbilt University Medical Center, Nashville, TN 37232, USA; david.c.consoli@vanderbilt.edu (D.C.C.); adriana.a.tienda@vumc.org (A.A.T.)
2. Division of Allergy, Pulmonary, and Critical Care Medicine; Vanderbilt University Medical Center, Nashville, TN 37232, USA; jordan.jesse@vumc.org (J.J.J.); nathan.putz@vumc.org (N.D.P.); julie.bastarache@vumc.org (J.A.B.)
3. Undergraduate Program in Neuroscience, Vanderbilt University, Nashville, TN 37232, USA; Kelly.klimo@vanderbilt.edu
* Correspondence: fiona.harrison@vumc.org; Tel.: +1-615-875-5547

Received: 2 March 2020; Accepted: 23 March 2020; Published: 26 March 2020

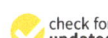

Abstract: Vitamin C (ascorbate, ASC) is a critical antioxidant in the body with specific roles in the brain. Despite a recent interest in vitamin C therapies for critical care medicine, little is known about vitamin C regulation during acute inflammation and critical illnesses such as sepsis. Using a cecal slurry (CS) model of sepsis in mice, we determined ASC and inflammatory changes in the brain following the initial treatment. ASC levels in the brain were acutely decreased by approximately 10% at 4 and 24 h post CS treatment. Changes were accompanied by a robust increase in liver ASC levels of up to 50%, indicating upregulation of synthesis beginning at 4 h and persisting up to 7 days post CS treatment. Several key cytokines interleukin 6 (IL-6), interleukin 1β (IL-1β), tumor necrosis factor alpha (TNFα), and chemokine (C-X-C motif) ligand 1 (CXCL1, KC/Gro) were also significantly elevated in the cortex at 4 h post CS treatment, although these levels returned to normal by 48 h. These data strongly suggest that ASC reserves are directly challenged throughout illness and recovery from sepsis. Given the timescale of this response, decreases in cortical ASC are likely driven by hyper-acute neuroinflammatory processes. However, future studies are required to confirm this relationship and to investigate how this deficiency may subsequently impact neuroinflammation.

Keywords: vitamin C; ascorbate; sepsis; brain; cecal slurry; inflammation; cytokines; mouse

1. Introduction

Sepsis is estimated to affect more than 30 million people and account for more than 5 million deaths annually [1]. During this critical illness, the robust inflammatory response of the immune system includes release of multiple cytokines and other signaling molecules that can ultimately lead to severe tissue injury and multiple organ failure [2–4]. This damage extends to the brain as evidenced by delirium in the majority of patients [5]. Despite the advances in clinical understanding of delirium during sepsis, little is known about the cellular and molecular underpinnings of acute brain dysfunction in critically ill patients. Sepsis patients often exhibit low plasma levels of vitamin C (ascorbate, ASC) [6–9]. In one study, as many as 88% of sepsis patients had subnormal plasma levels of ASC (<23 μM) and up to 38% had severe ASC deficiency (<11 μM) [10], suggesting high demand for ASC during septic insult. Lower plasma levels of ASC are also associated with increased incidence of multiple organ failure and decreased survival [11]. The brain is particularly susceptible to this dysregulated inflammatory response and to suboptimal ASC levels, because higher oxidative stress levels in the brain are especially damaging to its enriched lipid composition and nutrient-demanding metabolic rate [12,13]. Up to 30% of patients are reported to experience cognitive deficits following recovery from sepsis [14–16], and several studies using rodent sepsis models have shown that acute illness damages cognition in surviving animals [17–19].

ASC is a critical antioxidant for cellular function and has an emerging role in immune function [20]. Preclinical studies have shown a variety of beneficial effects on the pathophysiological changes in sepsis, including protection against microvascular dysfunction and deficits in vasoconstriction [21–23] by preserving tight endothelial barrier function and capillary blood flow [24–26]. ASC administration during sepsis also attenuates acute lung injury [27] and improves multiple organ dysfunction syndrome in animal models of sepsis [28,29]. The role of intravenous ASC in clinical practice to improve short term patient recovery is still under clinical investigation [30,31]. ASC accumulates to high levels in the brain via the sodium-dependent vitamin C transporter 2 (SVCT2) in a two-step, energy-dependent process from blood into the choroid plexus cerebral spinal fluid and then into neurons [32]. In the brain, ASC serves two primary roles as a neuroprotector and neuromodulator [32–34]. ASC maintains blood–brain barrier integrity by preserving tight endothelial barriers [35,36] and maintaining capillary blood flow [37]. ASC is a critical enzymatic co-factor in neurotransmitter synthesis and DNA methylation [32,38], and is intimately involved in preserving glutamatergic neurotransmission through the glutamate-uptake ASC-release exchange [39–41]. Despite the interest in ASC as a treatment for preventing organ failure in sepsis, the roles of ASC in the brain, and the number of patients experiencing cognitive deficits following recovery from the acute trauma, the effects of sepsis on the brain are understudied. Furthermore, the specific role of ascorbate in sepsis-induced brain dysfunction has not been studied. Here, we utilized a cecal slurry (CS) model of sepsis in mice to observe changes in ASC and inflammatory response in the brain during and following sepsis. We hypothesized that ASC is depleted in sepsis, and sought to define a timeline for changes in ASC level and cytokine release, particularly in the brain.

2. Materials and Methods

2.1. Mouse CS or LPS Treatment

All experiments conducted with live mice were reviewed and approved by the Vanderbilt Institutional Animal Care and Use Committee. Cecal slurry (CS) was used to induce acute peritonitis in mice as a model of sepsis as previously described [42–44]. C57/Bl6J donor mice at six weeks of age were obtained from Jackson Laboratory (#000664) and euthanized within 7 days of arrival. Cecal contents were collected and resuspended in 5% dextrose at 80 mg/mL, then filtered through a 100 μm filter. Aliquots were stored at -80 °C until ready for use.

All mice for treatment groups were bred in house from C57/Bl6J mice originally obtained from Jackson Laboratory. Mice at 10–12 weeks of age were treated with CS (1.5 mg/g; i.p.) or the vehicle 5% dextrose for control groups. Another widely used model of peripheral inflammatory response utilizes lipopolysaccharide (LPS) administration. For LPS studies, mice at 6–8 weeks of age received LPS (3.75 μg/g; i.p.) or saline. Control and treated mice were distributed across cages and provided with supplemental nutrition on the floor of the cage (DietGel 76A, Clear H_2O) to promote survival.

2.2. Evaluation of Sickness Score

An observer blinded to treatment groups scored the mice on the severity of sepsis using a 12-point scale of sickness severity, where 12 is healthy with normal activity and 0 is moribund [45,46]. In brief, the score is determined by response to finger poke (4 for normal, 3 for decreased, 2 for severely decreased, or 1 for minimal response), signs of encephalopathy (4 for normal, 3 for tremors or staggering, 2 for twisting movements, or 1 for turning), and general appearance (score is decreased by 1 for each display of piloerection, periorbital exudates, respiratory distress, or diarrhea). All mice were monitored closely for 48 h or until mice recovered to a normal score of 12. CS-treated mice that never received a score below 10 or died prior to the assigned timepoint were excluded from analysis.

2.3. Tissue Collection

Mice were anesthetized with isoflurane then euthanized by decapitation at 4, 24, 48 h or 7 days post-injection. Control mice were euthanized at each timepoint and data collapsed into one group. Tissue samples were collected, flash-frozen on dry ice, and stored at −80 °C for further analysis.

2.4. Ascorbic Acid HPLC

Sample extracts were prepared by adding 10 μl extraction buffer (7:2 25% *w/v* metaphosphoric acid: 100 mM sodium phosphate, 0.05 mM EDTA pH 8.0) per mg of wet tissue to normalize by weight. Samples were homogenized with 0.5 mm ceria-stabilized zirconium oxide beads (Next Advance, Inc.) in a bullet homogenizer, centrifuged at 10,000 rpm, and the clear supernatant transferred into a fresh tube. Concentrations of ASC were measured at 1:100 dilution in triplicate with ion pair HPLC, using tetrapentyl ammonium bromide as the ion pair reagent and electrochemical detection as previously described [47,48].

2.5. Determination of Gene Expression

RNA was extracted using an RNeasy Mini Kit (Qiagen). qPCR was performed using a PrimePCR Probe Assay consisting of iScript cDNA synthesis, PrimePCR Probes (PrimePCR™ Probe Assay: Slc23a1, Mouse), and Sso Advanced Universal Supermix (Bio Rad).

2.6. Measurement of Oxidative Stress Markers

Malondialdehyde, a lipid peroxidation end product, was measured by fluorescent spectrophotometric assay of thiobarbituric acid reactive substances (TBARS) as previously described [49]. Sulfhydryls were measured by reduction of 5,5′-dithiobis (2-nitrobenzoic acid) (DTNB) to 2-nitro-5-thiobenzoate (TNB) anion by thiol groups and spectrophotometric analysis [50,51].

2.7. Measurement of Cytokine Expression

Frozen mouse tissues were homogenized in volumes of RIPA buffer (Thermo Fisher Scientific) normalized by tissue weight. Tissue levels of IFN-γ, IL-1b, IL-6, KC/GRO, IL-10, and TNF-alpha were assayed in duplicate using a V-PLEX Custom Mouse Cytokine Kit, (Meso Scale Diagnostics, LLC) according to the manufacturer's instructions [52].

2.8. Statistical Analyses

Statistical analyses were performed using Graphpad Prism software (version 8.3.0). Data were first checked for equality of group variances using the Brown–Forsyth test and analyzed using parametric statistics. We did not expect any differences in response to CS according to sex, and all data were first analyzed using a multivariate ANOVA analysis, including sex as an additional variable. There were no main effects of sex on any of the key outcomes (sickness score, weight loss, ASC levels) so data were combined for all subsequent analysis. For outcomes following CS treatment, data were analyzed with univariate ANOVA with group (encompassing treatments and time post treatment) as the main independent variable. Significant omnibus ANOVA were followed with Dunnett's post hoc analyses to test difference from the control group. Independent t-tests were used to test effects of LPS versus treatment with the vehicle. Numerical outliers that likely reflected experimental error were identified and removed using ROUT (Q = 5%). Error bars are shown as SEM or SD as indicated in figure legends.

3. Results

3.1. Cecal Slurry Treatment Induces Acute Peritonitis and Weight Loss

Mice that received cecal slurry (CS) treatment became severely lethargic and exhibited decreased responses to stimuli, signs of encephalopathy, and worsened appearance by 12 h (Figure 1A). Sickness scores decreased as early as 4 h, began to recover by 24 h, and returned to normal appearance and activity by 48 h (Figure 1B; CS Treatment $F_{(1, 63)} = 113.8$, $p < 0.001$; Time $F_{(5, 59)} = 15.61$, $p < 0.001$). CS treatment also caused significant weight loss that persisted to 48 h, although mice regained weight by 7 days post CS treatment (Figure 1C; CS Treatment $F_{(1, 63)} = 121.3$, $p < 0.001$; Time $F_{(5, 59)} = 24.06$, $p < 0.001$). Out of 55 CS treated mice, only two mice died before their scheduled timepoint. This mild 1.5 mg/g dose was chosen to optimize survival to 7 days post CS treatment. The 4% mortality rate at this dose is low compared to other studies utilizing this CS model (2.0 mg/g, up to 67% by 48 h) [42,44].

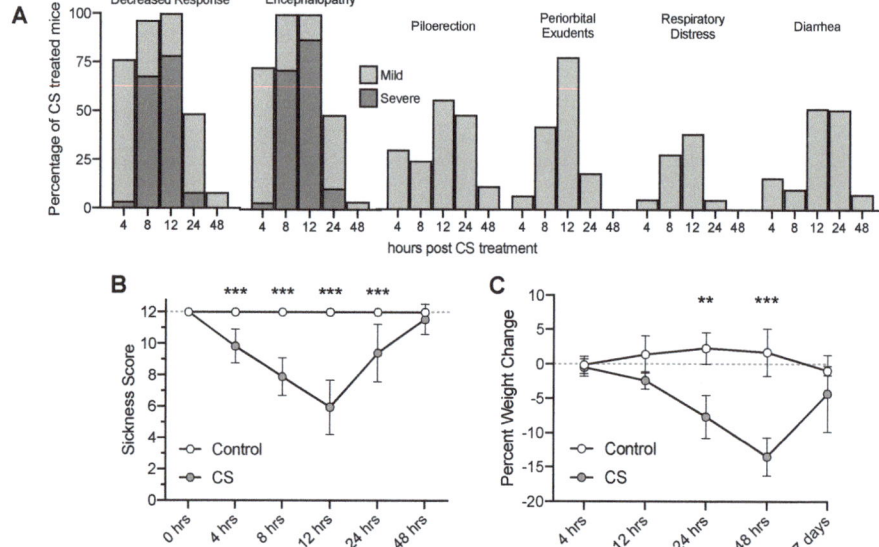

Figure 1. Observed sickness scores of mice and percent weight change over time following Cecal Slurry (CS) treatment. (**A**) Percentage of mice showing sickness behaviors and appearances. (**B**) Clinical Sickness Scores. (**C**) Weight loss. ** $p < 0.01$*** $p < 0.001$. Error bars plotted as mean ± SD.

3.2. Tissue ASC Concentrations Following CS Treatment

There was a small (~10% at 4 h) but significant decrease in cortical ASC at 4 and 24 h following CS treatment compared to controls (Figure 2A, $F_{(4, 54)} = 3.216$, $p = 0.0193$,), indicating consumption of brain ASC reserves. Liver ASC levels were significantly increased following CS treatment (~50% at 24 h) indicating robust upregulation of ASC synthesis (Figure 2B, $F_{(4, 54)} = 5.090$, $p = 0.0015$) that persisted to 7 days post CS treatment. No significant differences in ASC levels were observed in peripheral organs of CS-treated mice compared to controls, although levels varied post CS treatment (kidney: Figure 2C, $F_{(4, 54)} = 2.153$, $p = 0.0867$; lung: Figure 2D, $F_{(4, 55)} = 3.188$, $p = 0.020$). We hypothesized that a decrease in ASC levels in the brain would result in upregulation of SVCT2 expression, though no significant changes were observed in hippocampal SVCT2 expression in response to CS treatment (Figure 2E, $F_{(4, 38)} = 2.235$, $p = 0.0833$).

No decrease in brain ASC level was observed at 4 h following LPS treatment (Figure 2F, $t(10) = 0.842$, $p = 0.4197$). However, LPS treatment also induced upregulation of ASC synthesis in liver (Figure 2G, t(10) = 4.913, $p < 0.001$). No changes were observed in lung (Figure 2H, t(9) = 0.246, $p = 0.8111$), or kidney (Figure 2I, t(10) = 2.066, $p = 0.0658$).

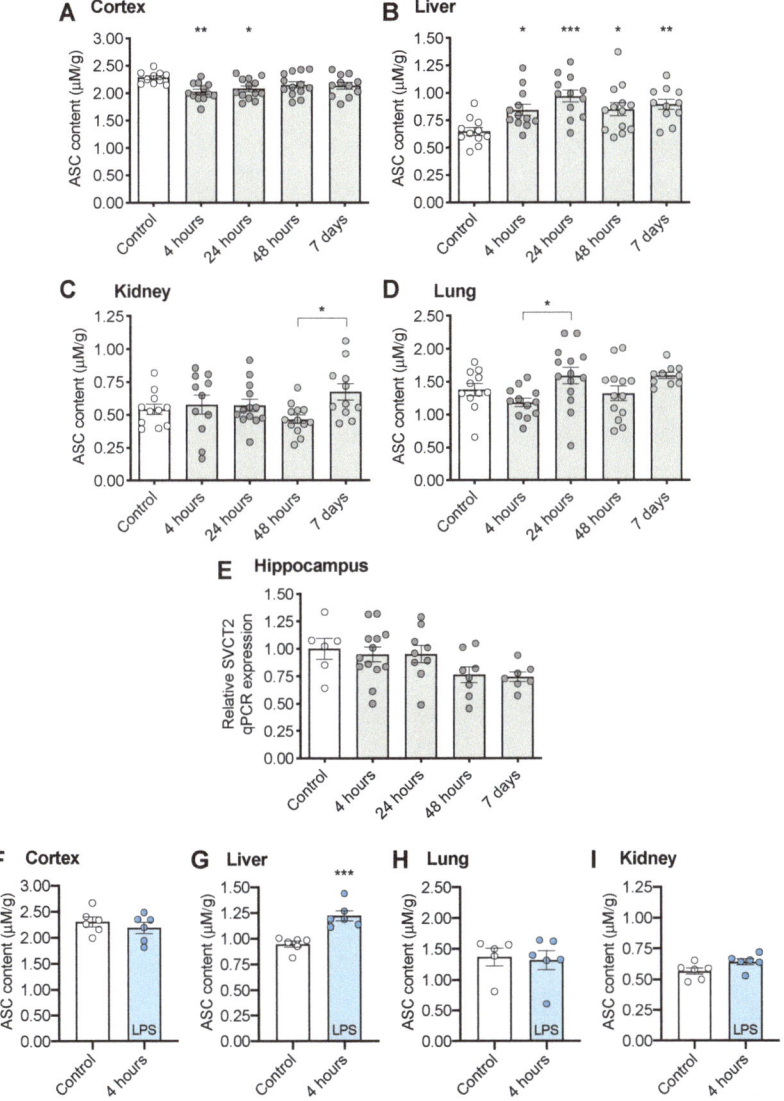

Figure 2. Tissue ASC (ascorbate) concentrations following CS treatment in (**A**) cortex, (**B**) liver, (**C**) kidney, (**D**) lung. (**E**) Sodium-dependent vitamin C transporter 2, SVCT2 gene expression in brain following CS treatment. Tissue ASC concentrations following LPS treatment (**F**) brain, (**G**) liver, (**H**) lung, and (**I**) kidney. * $p < 0.05$ ** $p < 0.01$ *** $p < 0.001$ from control following significant ANOVA results unless otherwise indicated. Error bars plotted as mean ± SEM.

3.3. CS Treatment Does Not Induce Changes in Oxidative Stress Measurements

CS treatment did not increase either of the oxidative stress markers malondialdehyde (cortex: Figure 3A, $F_{(4, 33)} = 2.092$, $p = 0.1042$; Liver: Figure 3B, $F_{(4, 33)} = 1.833$, $p = 0.1459$) or sulfhydryls (cortex: Figure 3C, $F_{(4, 30)} = 0.6471$, $p = 0.6333$; Liver: Figure 3D, $F_{(4, 35)} = 2.210$, $p = 0.0880$) in the brain.

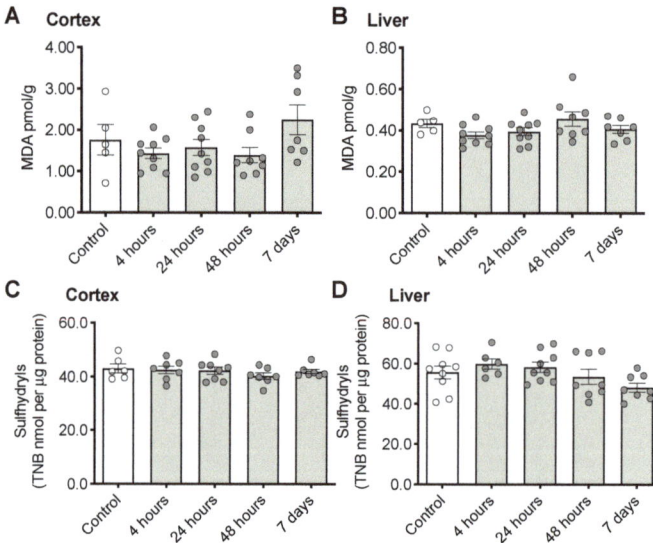

Figure 3. Indicators of oxidative stress following CS treatment. Malondialdehyde (MDA) in cortex (**A**) and liver (**B**) or sulfhydryls in cortex (**C**) and liver (**D**). Error bars plotted as mean ± SEM.

3.4. CS Treatment Initiates an Inflammatory Response in the Brain

In cortex, expression of several proinflammatory cytokines was elevated at 4 h post CS treatment including interleukin 6 (IL-6: $F_{(4, 31)} = 8.356$, $p < 0.001$), interleukin 1β (IL-1β: $F_{(4, 31)} = 9.742$, $p < 0.001$), tumor necrosis factor alpha (TNFα: $F_{(4, 33)} = 4.261$, $p = 0.0069$), and chemokine (C-X-C motif) ligand 1 (CXCL1, KC/Gro: $F_{(4, 30)} = 7.091$, $p < 0.001$) (Figure 4A–D). Cytokine expression levels returned to normal by 48 h post CS treatment. More modest increases in interferon gamma (INFγ: $F_{(4, 33)} = 0.9214$, $p = 0.4632$) and interleukin 10 (IL-10: $F_{(4, 32)} = 1.442$, $p = 0.2430$) were not statistically significant (Figure 2E,F).

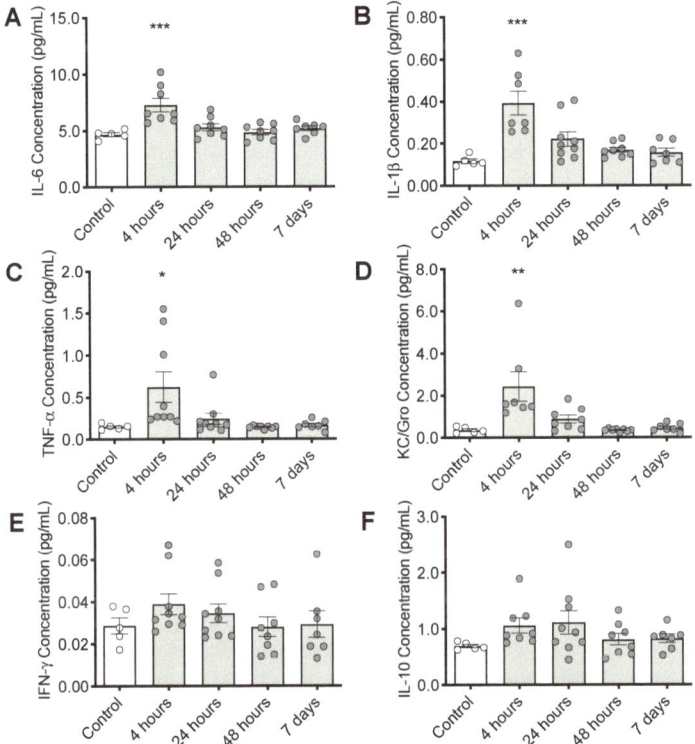

Figure 4. Timeline of inflammatory changes in the brain following CS treatment. Cortical cytokine levels of (**A**) interleukin 6 (IL-6), (**B**) interleukin 1β (IL-1β), (**C**) tumor necrosis factor alpha (TNFα), and (**D**) chemokine (C-X-C motif) ligand 1 (CXCL1, KC/Gro), (**E**) Interferon gamma (INFγ) and (**F**) interleukin 10 (IL-10) * $p < 0.05$, ** $p < 0.01$, *** $p < 0.001$. Error bars plotted as mean ± SEM.

4. Discussion

Despite significant clinical interest in ASC as a potential therapeutic adjuvant, the role of ASC in sepsis, particularly in the brain, has not been well studied. The present study highlights the potential rapid, although modest, consumption of ASC stores during and following sepsis co-occurring with the associated inflammatory changes that occur in the brain.

Mice and most other rodent species possess the gene encoding gulonolactone oxidase, an enzyme responsible for catalyzing the final step in ASC synthesis in the liver [53–56]. Synthesis can be upregulated to provide higher tissue levels in the liver under periods of increased physiological need, such as pregnancy [57]. ASC depletion in the brain is rare in non-genetically modified mice, however, increased liver levels indicate upregulation of ASC synthesis to prevent depletion. In the brain, high concentrations are critical for maintaining optimal brain function and preventing oxidative damage [32,33,58]. CS treatment resulted in an approximately 10% decrease in ASC in cortex (Figure 2A) even in this relatively mild sepsis model, and despite upregulation of synthesis in the liver. The two-step transport system of ASC into the brain by SVCT2 from blood into the choroid plexus cerebral spinal fluid and then into neurons allows for preservation of ASC at the expense of other tissues [32]. It is possible that other brain regions, such as the hippocampus, may have different levels of susceptibility to ASC depletion due to varying proximity to the ventricles and choroid plexus, and future studies should address different brain areas, including hippocampus, in analysis.

Over this short time interval, we did not observe decreased ASC levels in most peripheral organs including lung and kidney (Figure 2C,D) and heart, muscle, spleen, and adrenal gland (data not shown). We observed a significant increase in liver ASC by 4 h in both CS- and LPS-treated mice (Figure 2B,G). Our data confirm results of prior work in which an LPS-induced increase in liver ASC was observed from 3 h post LPS treatment [59]. LPS treatment did not fully recapitulate the ASC changes we observed with CS treatment, possibly due to the dose initiating a lower neuroinflammatory effect or different pathways, although this was not directly tested. While no changes were observed in brain in that study [59], the lack of cortical ASC deficiency in the LPS model may be a limitation of intraperitoneal LPS as a model of sepsis. We hypothesize that increased synthesis in the liver provided sufficient circulating levels to replenish (brain) or protect (lung, kidneys) peripheral tissues during the time period and for the dose studied. It took more than 24 h to replenish brain ASC, possibly due to slower brain uptake, since ASC must first accumulate in the cerebral spinal fluid. Future experiments should be performed in genetically modified mice that are, like humans, incapable of synthesizing ASC (e.g., gulonolactone oxidase knockout mice) [47,60], and are therefore unable to upregulate hepatic synthesis to meet increased need. Such models could also be used to establish a timeline of circulating ASC levels in plasma as well as testing whether a clinically relevant ASC pretreatment [61] is capable of protecting against decreased brain ASC, neuroinflammatory changes, or severity of observed sickness. If peripheral ASC administration is unable to change cortical ASC levels, this would suggest blood–brain barrier transport of ASC is limiting early in sepsis or that there is high uptake by other organs. However, if neuroinflammation is improved by pretreatment with ASC, this would suggest that ASC deficiency may be directly associated with sepsis-associated neuroinflammation.

The CS dosing regimen used (1.5 mg/g) causes a mild sickness response, chosen to optimize recovery and survival to 7 days post treatment. Nevertheless, this modest insult was still sufficient to deplete ASC and increase cytokine production in the brain at 4 h after injection (Figure 4), when the mice are just starting to become systemically ill. This finding suggests that the brain is adversely affected by systemic inflammation in the earliest stages of illness. The release of cytokines in the brain at this time indicates activation of brain macrophages and resident microglia, which generate reactive oxygen species. The observed ASC depletion likely indicates ASC plays a primary role in electron donation to neutralize these free radicals, and that the oxidative stress was sufficient to overwhelm ASC recycling capacity. While future studies will need to clarify the relationship between ASC deficiency and neuroinflammation, it is most likely that ASC deficiency is driven by the acute neuroinflammatory response and associated generation of radical species. Oxidative stress is a key component of clinical sepsis [62], and although the global oxidative measurements did not show elevations in brain or liver oxidative stress under these conditions, any reduction in brain ASC and especially upregulation of liver ASC synthesis indicates elevated oxidative challenge. The measures of global tissue MDA may not have been sensitive enough to detect localized increases in oxidative stress in specific cells (endothelium, for example) or tissue compartments. Despite the activated immune response and challenge of brain ASC stores, we did not observe upregulation of the sodium-dependent vitamin C transporter SVCT2 in brain tissue. To confirm the association between ASC consumption and acute inflammatory challenge in a second model, we used LPS to induce endotoxemia and systemic inflammation. LPS treatment was also sufficient to upregulate liver ASC synthesis by 4 h. Whether higher doses of CS or LPS would cause further or prolonged depletion of brain ASC in a more severe illness model should be studied in future experiments.

ASC deficiency is well defined in critical care patient populations [6–10]. Many preclinical studies have shown that early ASC supplementation or IV treatment can protect against vascular and organ dysfunctions associated with sepsis [22,23,26]. One possible explanation for the potential beneficial effects of ASC is that hospitalized patients who develop sepsis are more likely to have underlying ASC deficiency, either as a result of chronic illness, co-morbidities, or poor diet. However, our results and many others suggest that ASC depletion is directly caused by the illness itself, likely due to massive inflammatory challenge, endothelial breakdown, and elevated oxidative stress [35,37]. Although some clinical studies have associated lower plasma levels of ASC with increased incidence of multiple organ failure and decreased survival [11], several phase I clinical studies have shown that IV administration of ASC during sepsis does not improve or worsen short term survival outcomes [8,31,63]. Overall survivability during sepsis is dependent on a variety of factors including antibiotics administration, prior health status, prior injury or illness, and age [64]. While maintenance of ASC levels during sepsis may not directly impact acute survival, it may be critical to protection against inflammatory damage following sepsis, especially in the brain [14]. Future studies will seek to understand how ASC is involved in the acute inflammatory response and the implications for long term cognitive dysfunction following recovery.

Author Contributions: Conceptualization, F.E.H., J.A.B. and D.C.C.; statistical analyses, F.E.H. and D.C.C.; experimental investigation, D.C.C., J.J.J., N.D.P., K.R.K., and A.A.T.; writing—original draft preparation, D.C.C.; writing—review and editing, F.E.H. and J.A.B.; funding acquisition, F.E.H. and J.A.B. All authors have read and agreed to the published version of the manuscript.

Funding: This research was funded by R01 HL135849-03 and HL135849-02S1 to Lorraine Ware and Julie Bastarache, and VA Merit I01 CX001610 to James M May.

Acknowledgments: The authors would like to thank Jordyn M Wilcox, Shilpy Dixit, Krista C Paffenroth, and John E Dugan for technical assistance in generating data for this manuscript, and James M May for providing valuable feedback on early versions of the manuscript.

Conflicts of Interest: The authors declare no conflict of interest. The funders had no role in the design of the study; in the collection, analyses, or interpretation of data; in the writing of the manuscript, or in the decision to publish the results.

References

1. Fleischmann, C.; Scherag, A.; Adhikari, N.K.J.; Hartog, C.S.; Tsaganos, T.; Schlattmann, P.; Angus, D.C.; Reinhart, K. Assessment of global incidence and mortality of hospital-treated sepsis current estimates and limitations. *Am. J. Respir. Crit. Care Med.* **2016**, *193*, 259–272. [CrossRef] [PubMed]
2. Kuhn, S.O.; Meissner, K.; Mayes, L.M.; Bartels, K. Vitamin C in sepsis. *Curr. Opin. Anaesthesiol.* **2018**, *31*, 55–60. [CrossRef] [PubMed]
3. Ince, C.; Mayeux, P.R.; Nguyen, T.; Gomez, H.; Kellum, J.A.; Ospina-Tascón, G.A.; Hernandez, G.; Murray, P.; De Backer, D. The endothelium in sepsis. *Shock* **2016**, *45*, 259–270. [CrossRef] [PubMed]
4. Biesalski, H.K.; McGregor, G.P. Antioxidant therapy in critical care–Is the microcirculation the primary target? *Proc. Crit. Care Med.* **2007**, *35*, S577–S583. [CrossRef] [PubMed]
5. Zampieri, F.G.; Park, M.; Machado, F.S.; Azevedo, L.C.P. Sepsis-associated encephalopathy: Not just delirium. *Clinics* **2011**, *66*, 1825–1831. [CrossRef]
6. Borrelli, E.; Roux-Lombard, P.; Grau, G.E.; Girardin, E.; Ricou, B.; Dayer, J.M.; Suter, P.M. Plasma concentrations of cytokines, their soluble receptors, and antioxidant vitamins can predict the development of multiple organ failure in patients at risk. *Crit. Care Med.* **1996**, *24*, 392–397. [CrossRef]
7. Galley, H.F.; Davies, M.J.; Webster, N.R. Ascorbyl radical formation in patients with sepsis: Effect of ascorbate loading. *Free Radic. Biol. Med.* **1996**, *20*, 139–143. [CrossRef]
8. Fujii, T.; Udy, A.A.; Deane, A.M.; Luethi, N.; Bailey, M.; Eastwood, G.M.; Frei, D.; French, C.; Orford, N.; Shehabi, Y.; et al. Vitamin C, Hydrocortisone and Thiamine in Patients with Septic Shock (VITAMINS) trial: Study protocol and statistical analysis plan. *Crit. Care Resusc.* **2019**, *21*, 119–125.
9. Hudson, E.P.; Collie, J.T.; Fujii, T.; Luethi, N.; Udy, A.A.; Doherty, S.; Eastwood, G.; Yanase, F.; Naorungroj, T.; Bitker, L.; et al. Pharmacokinetic data support 6-hourly dosing of intravenous vitamin C to critically ill patients with septic shock. *Crit. Care Resusc.* **2019**, *21*, 236–242.
10. Carr, A.C.; Rosengrave, P.C.; Bayer, S.; Chambers, S.; Mehrtens, J.; Shaw, G.M. Hypovitaminosis C and vitamin C deficiency in critically ill patients despite recommended enteral and parenteral intakes. *Crit. Care* **2017**, *21*, 300. [CrossRef] [PubMed]
11. Fowler, A.A.; Syed, A.A.; Knowlson, S.; Sculthorpe, R.; Farthing, D.; DeWilde, C.; Farthing, C.A.; Larus, T.L.; Martin, E.; Brophy, D.F.; et al. Phase I safety trial of intravenous ascorbic acid in patients with severe sepsis. *J. Transl. Med.* **2014**, *12*, 32. [CrossRef] [PubMed]

12. Magistretti, P.J.; Allaman, I. A Cellular Perspective on Brain Energy Metabolism and Functional Imaging. *Neuron* **2015**, *86*, 883–901. [CrossRef] [PubMed]
13. Cobley, J.N.; Fiorello, M.L.; Bailey, D.M. 13 reasons why the brain is susceptible to oxidative stress. *Redox Biol.* **2018**, *15*, 490–503. [CrossRef] [PubMed]
14. Calsavara, A.J.C.; Costa, P.A.; Nobre, V.; Teixeira, A.L. Factors Associated with Short and Long Term Cognitive Changes in Patients with Sepsis. *Sci. Rep.* **2018**, *8*, 4509. [CrossRef]
15. Iwashyna, T.J.; Ely, E.W.; Smith, D.M.; Langa, K.M. Long-term cognitive impairment and functional disability among survivors of severe sepsis. *JAMA—J. Am. Med. Assoc.* **2010**, *304*, 1787–1794. [CrossRef]
16. Annane, D.; Sharshar, T. Cognitive decline after sepsis. *Lancet Respir. Med.* **2015**, *3*, 61–69. [CrossRef]
17. Anderson, S.T.; Commins, S.; Moynagh, P.N.; Coogan, A.N. Lipopolysaccharide-induced sepsis induces long-lasting affective changes in the mouse. *Brain. Behav. Immun.* **2015**, *43*, 98–109. [CrossRef]
18. Zaghloul, N.; Addorisio, M.E.; Silverman, H.A.; Patel, H.L.; Valdés-Ferrer, S.I.; Ayasolla, K.R.; Lehner, K.R.; Olofsson, P.S.; Nasim, M.; Metz, C.N.; et al. Forebrain Cholinergic Dysfunction and Systemic and Brain Inflammation in Murine Sepsis Survivors. *Front. Immunol.* **2017**, *8*, 1673. [CrossRef]
19. Hippensteel, J.A.; Anderson, B.J.; Orfila, J.E.; McMurtry, S.A.; Dietz, R.M.; Su, G.; Ford, J.A.; Oshima, K.; Yang, Y.; Zhang, F.; et al. Circulating heparan sulfate fragments mediate septic cognitive dysfunction. *J. Clin. Investig.* **2019**, *129*, 1779–1784. [CrossRef]
20. Carr, A.C.; Maggini, S. Vitamin C and immune function. *Nutrients* **2017**, *9*, 1211. [CrossRef]
21. Armour, J.; Tyml, K.; Lidington, D.; Wilson, J.X. Ascorbate prevents microvascular dysfunction in the skeletal muscle of the septic rat. *J. Appl. Physiol.* **2001**, *90*, 795–803. [CrossRef] [PubMed]
22. Wu, F.; Wilson, J.X.; Tyml, K. Ascorbate protects against impaired arteriolar constriction in sepsis by inhibiting inducible nitric oxide synthase expression. *Free Radic. Biol. Med.* **2004**, *37*, 1282–1289. [CrossRef] [PubMed]
23. Mckinnon, R.L.; Lidington, D.; Tyml, K. Ascorbate inhibits reduced arteriolar conducted vasoconstriction in septic mouse cremaster muscle. *Microcirculation* **2007**, *14*, 697–707. [CrossRef] [PubMed]
24. Han, M.; Pendem, S.; Teh, S.L.; Sukumaran, D.K.; Wu, F.; Wilson, J.X. Ascorbate protects endothelial barrier function during septic insult: Role of protein phosphatase type 2A. *Free Radic. Biol. Med.* **2010**, *48*, 128–135. [CrossRef]
25. Tyml, K.; Li, F.; Wilson, J.X. Septic impairment of capillary blood flow requires nicotinamide adenine dinucleotide phosphate oxidase but not nitric oxide synthase and is rapidly reversed by ascorbate through an endothelial nitric oxide synthase-dependent mechanism. *Crit. Care Med.* **2008**, *36*, 2355–2362. [CrossRef]
26. Zhou, G.; Kamenos, G.; Pendem, S.; Wilson, J.X.; Wu, F. Ascorbate protects against vascular leakage in cecal ligation and puncture-induced septic peritonitis. *Am. J. Physiol.—Regul. Integr. Comp. Physiol.* **2012**, *302*, R409–R416. [CrossRef]
27. Fisher, B.J.; Seropian, I.M.; Kraskauskas, D.; Thakkar, J.N.; Voelkel, N.F.; Fowler, A.A.; Natarajan, R. Ascorbic acid attenuates lipopolysaccharide-induced acute lung injury. *Crit. Care Med.* **2011**, *39*, 1454–1460. [CrossRef]
28. Fisher, B.J.; Kraskauskas, D.; Martin, E.J.; Farkas, D.; Puri, P.; Massey, H.D.; Idowu, M.O.; Brophy, D.F.; Voelkel, N.F.; Fowler, A.A.; et al. Attenuation of sepsis-induced organ injury in mice by vitamin C. *J. Parenter. Enter. Nutr.* **2014**, *38*, 825–839. [CrossRef]
29. Gao, Y.-L.; Lu, B.; Zhai, J.-H.; Liu, Y.-C.; Qi, H.-X.; Yao, Y.; Chai, Y.-F.; Shou, S.-T. The Parenteral Vitamin C Improves Sepsis and Sepsis-Induced Multiple Organ Dysfunction Syndrome via Preventing Cellular Immunosuppression. *Mediat. Inflamm.* **2017**, *2017*, 4024672. [CrossRef]
30. Fujii, T.; Luethi, N.; Young, P.J.; Frei, D.R.; Eastwood, G.M.; French, C.J.; Deane, A.M.; Shehabi, Y.; Hajjar, L.A.; Oliveira, G.; et al. Effect of Vitamin C, Hydrocortisone, and Thiamine vs Hydrocortisone Alone on Time Alive and Free of Vasopressor Support among Patients with Septic Shock: The VITAMINS Randomized Clinical Trial. *JAMA—J. Am. Med. Assoc.* **2020**, *323*, 423–431. [CrossRef]
31. Fowler, A.A.; Truwit, J.D.; Hite, R.D.; Morris, P.E.; Dewilde, C.; Priday, A.; Fisher, B.; Thacker, L.R.; Natarajan, R.; Brophy, D.F.; et al. Effect of Vitamin C Infusion on Organ Failure and Biomarkers of Inflammation and Vascular Injury in Patients with Sepsis and Severe Acute Respiratory Failure: The CITRIS-ALI Randomized Clinical Trial. *JAMA—J. Am. Med. Assoc.* **2019**, *322*, 1261–1270. [CrossRef] [PubMed]
32. Harrison, F.E.; May, J.M. Vitamin C function in the brain: Vital role of the ascorbate transporter SVCT2. *Free Radic. Biol. Med.* **2009**, *46*, 719–730. [CrossRef]

33. Harrison, F.E.; Bowman, G.L.; Polidori, M.C. Ascorbic acid and the brain: Rationale for the use against cognitive decline. *Nutrients* **2014**, *6*, 1752. [CrossRef] [PubMed]
34. Ballaz, S.J.; Rebec, G.V. Neurobiology of vitamin C: Expanding the focus from antioxidant to endogenous neuromodulator. *Pharm. Res.* **2019**, *146*, 104321. [CrossRef] [PubMed]
35. Kuck, J.L.; Bastarache, J.A.; Shaver, C.M.; Fessel, J.P.; Dikalov, S.I.; May, J.M.; Ware, L.B. Ascorbic acid attenuates endothelial permeability triggered by cell-free hemoglobin. *Biochem. Biophys. Res. Commun.* **2018**, *495*, 433–437. [CrossRef]
36. Lin, J.L.; Huang, Y.H.; Shen, Y.C.; Huang, H.C.; Liu, P.H. Ascorbic acid prevents blood-brain barrier disruption and sensory deficit caused by sustained compression of primary somatosensory cortex. *J. Cereb. Blood Flow Metab.* **2010**, *30*, 1121–1136. [CrossRef]
37. Wilson, J.X.; Wu, F. Vitamin C in sepsis. *Subcell. Biochem.* **2012**, *56*, 67–83.
38. Young, J.I.; Züchner, S.; Wang, G. Regulation of the Epigenome by Vitamin C. *Annu. Rev. Nutr.* **2015**, *35*, 545–564. [CrossRef]
39. Wilson, J.X.; Peters, C.E.; Sitar, S.M.; Daoust, P.; Gelb, A.W. Glutamate stimulates ascorbate transport by astrocytes. *Brain Res.* **2000**, *858*, 61–66. [CrossRef]
40. May, J.M. Vitamin C transport and its role in the central nervous system. *Subcell. Biochem.* **2012**, *56*, 85–103.
41. Mi, D.J.; Dixit, S.; Warner, T.A.; Kennard, J.A.; Scharf, D.A.; Kessler, E.S.; Moore, L.M.; Consoli, D.C.; Bown, C.W.; Eugene, A.J.; et al. Altered glutamate clearance in ascorbate deficient mice increases seizure susceptibility and contributes to cognitive impairment in APP/PSEN1 mice. *Neurobiol. Aging* **2018**, *71*, 241–254. [CrossRef]
42. Shaver, C.M.; Paul, M.G.; Putz, N.D.; Landstreet, S.R.; Kuck, J.L.; Scarfe, L.; Skrypnyk, N.; Yang, H.; Harrison, F.E.; de Caestecker, M.P.; et al. Cell-free hemoglobin augments acute kidney injury during experimental sepsis. *Am. J. Physiol. Physiol.* **2019**, *317*, F922–F929. [CrossRef]
43. Meegan, J.E.; Shaver, C.M.; Putz, N.D.; Jesse, J.J.; Landstreet, S.R.; Lee, H.N.R.; Sidorova, T.N.; Brennan McNeil, J.; Wynn, J.L.; Cheung-Flynn, J.; et al. Cell-free hemoglobin increases inflammation, lung apoptosis, and microvascular permeability in murine polymicrobial sepsis. *PLoS ONE* **2020**, *15*, e0228727. [CrossRef]
44. Eric Kerchberger, V.; Bastarache, J.A.; Shaver, C.M.; Nagata, H.; Brennan McNeil, J.; Landstreet, S.R.; Putz, N.D.; Kuang Yu, W.; Jesse, J.; Wickersham, N.E.; et al. Haptoglobin-2 variant increases susceptibility to acute respiratory distress syndrome during sepsis. *JCI Insight* **2019**, *4*, 21. [CrossRef]
45. Su, G.; Atakilit, A.; Li, J.T.; Wu, N.; Luong, J.; Chen, R.; Bhattacharya, M.; Sheppard, D. Effective treatment of mouse sepsis with an inhibitory antibody targeting integrin αvβ5. *Crit. Care Med.* **2013**, *41*, 546–553. [CrossRef]
46. Manley, M.O.; O'Riordan, M.A.; Levine, A.D.; Latifi, S.Q. Interleukin 10 extends the effectiveness of standard therapy during late sepsis with serum interleukin 6 levels predicting outcome. *Shock* **2005**, *23*, 521–526.
47. Harrison, F.E.; Yu, S.S.; Van Den Bossche, K.L.; Li, L.; May, J.M.; McDonald, M.P. Elevated oxidative stress and sensorimotor deficits but normal cognition in mice that cannot synthesize ascorbic acid. *J. Neurochem.* **2008**, *106*, 1198–1208. [CrossRef]
48. May, J.M.; Qu, Z.C.; Mendiratta, S. Protection and recycling of α-tocopherol in human erythrocytes by intracellular ascorbic acid. *Arch. Biochem. Biophys.* **1998**, *349*, 281–289. [CrossRef]
49. Harrison, F.E.; Hosseini, A.H.; McDonald, M.P.; May, J.M. Vitamin C reduces spatial learning deficits in middle-aged and very old APP/PSEN1 transgenic and wild-type mice. *Pharm. Biochem. Behav.* **2009**, *93*, 443–450. [CrossRef]
50. Sgaravatti, Â.M.; Magnusson, A.S.; Oliveira, A.S.; Mescka, C.P.; Zanin, F.; Sgarbi, M.B.; Pederzolli, C.D.; Wyse, A.T.S.; Wannmacher, C.M.D.; Wajner, M.; et al. Effects of 1,4-butanediol administration on oxidative stress in rat brain: Study of the neurotoxicity of γ-hydroxybutyric acid in vivo. *Metab. Brain Dis.* **2009**, *24*, 271–282. [CrossRef]
51. Aksenov, M.Y.; Markesbery, W.R. Changes in thiol content and expression of glutathione redox system genes in the hippocampus and cerebellum in Alzheimer's disease. *Neurosci. Lett.* **2001**, *302*, 141–145. [CrossRef]
52. Bastarache, J.A.; Koyama, T.; Wickersham, N.E.; Ware, L.B. Validation of a multiplex electrochemiluminescent immunoassay platform in human and mouse samples. *J. Immunol. Methods* **2014**, *408*, 13–23. [CrossRef] [PubMed]
53. Gabbay, K.H.; Bohren, K.M.; Morello, R.; Bertin, T.; Liu, J.; Vogel, P. Ascorbate synthesis pathway: Dual role of ascorbate in bone homeostasis. *J. Biol. Chem.* **2010**, *285*, 19510–19520. [CrossRef]

54. Levine, M.; Downing, D. New Concepts in the Biology and Biochemistry of Ascorbic Acid. *J. Nutr. Med.* **1992**, *3*, 361–362. [CrossRef]
55. Ching, S.; Mahan, D.C.; Dabrowski, K. Liver L-Gulonolactone Oxidase Activity and Tissue Ascorbic Acid Concentrations in Nursing Pigs and the Effect of Various Weaning Ages. *J. Nutr.* **2001**, *131*, 2002–2006. [CrossRef]
56. Ching, S.; Mahan, D.C.; Ottobre, J.S.; Dabrowski, K. Ascorbic Acid Synthesis in Fetal and Neonatal Pigs and in Pregnant and Postpartum Sows. *J. Nutr.* **2001**, *131*, 1997–2001. [CrossRef]
57. Harrison, F.E.; Dawes, S.M.; Meredith, M.E.; Babaev, V.R.; Li, L.; May, J.M. Low vitamin C and increased oxidative stress and cell death in mice that lack the sodium-dependent vitamin C transporter SVCT2. *Free Radic. Biol. Med.* **2010**, *49*, 821–829. [CrossRef]
58. Jackson, T.S.; Xu, A.; Vita, J.A.; Keaney, J.F. Ascorbate prevents the interaction of superoxide and nitric oxide only at very high physiological concentrations. *Circ. Res.* **1998**, *83*, 916–922. [CrossRef]
59. Kuo, S.-M.; Tan, C.-H.; Dragan, M.; Wilson, J.X. Endotoxin Increases Ascorbate Recycling and Concentration in Mouse Liver. *J. Nutr.* **2005**, *135*, 2411–2416. [CrossRef]
60. Maeda, N.; Hagihara, H.; Nakata, Y.; Hiller, S.; Wilder, J.; Reddick, R. Aortic wall damage in mice unable to synthesize ascorbic acid. *Proc. Natl. Acad. Sci. USA* **2000**, *97*, 841–846. [CrossRef]
61. Wilson, J.X. Evaluation of Vitamin C for Adjuvant Sepsis Therapy. *Antioxid. Redox Signal* **2013**, *19*, 2129–2140. [CrossRef] [PubMed]
62. Prauchner, C.A. Oxidative stress in sepsis: Pathophysiological implications justifying antioxidant co-therapy. *Burns* **2017**, *43*, 471–485. [CrossRef]
63. Ahn, J.H.; Oh, D.K.; Huh, J.W.; Lim, C.M.; Koh, Y.; Hong, S.B. Vitamin C alone does not improve treatment outcomes in mechanically ventilated patients with severe sepsis or septic shock: A retrospective cohort study. *J. Thorac. Dis.* **2019**, *11*, 1562–1570. [CrossRef] [PubMed]
64. Rhodes, A.; Evans, L.E.; Alhazzani, W.; Levy, M.M.; Antonelli, M.; Ferrer, R.; Kumar, A.; Sevransky, J.E.; Sprung, C.L.; Nunnally, M.E.; et al. Surviving Sepsis Campaign: International Guidelines for Management of Sepsis and Septic Shock: 2016. *Crit. Care Med.* **2017**, *45*, 486–552. [CrossRef] [PubMed]

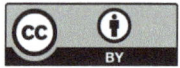 © 2020 by the authors. Licensee MDPI, Basel, Switzerland. This article is an open access article distributed under the terms and conditions of the Creative Commons Attribution (CC BY) license (http://creativecommons.org/licenses/by/4.0/).

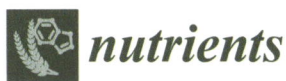

Article

Subphenotypes in Patients with Septic Shock Receiving Vitamin C, Hydrocortisone, and Thiamine: A Retrospective Cohort Analysis

Won-Young Kim *, Jae-Woo Jung, Jae Chol Choi, Jong Wook Shin and Jae Yeol Kim

Department of Internal Medicine, Chung-Ang University Hospital, Chung-Ang University College of Medicine, Seoul 06973, Korea; jwjung@cau.ac.kr (J.-W.J.); medics27@cau.ac.kr (J.C.C.); basthma@cau.ac.kr (J.W.S.); jykimmd@cau.ac.kr (J.Y.K.)
* Correspondence: wykim81@cau.ac.kr; Tel.: +82-2-6299-1439

Received: 13 November 2019; Accepted: 4 December 2019; Published: 5 December 2019

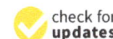

Abstract: This study aimed to identify septic phenotypes in patients receiving vitamin C, hydrocortisone, and thiamine using temperature and white blood cell count. Data were obtained from septic shock patients who were also treated using a vitamin C protocol in a medical intensive care unit. Patients were divided into groups according to the temperature measurements as well as white blood cell counts within 24 h before starting the vitamin C protocol. In the study, 127 patients included who met the inclusion criteria. In the cohort, four groups were identified: "Temperature $\geq$37.1 °C, white blood cell count $\geq$15.0 1000/mm^3" (group A; n = 27), "$\geq$37.1 °C, <15.0 1000/mm^3" (group B; n = 30), "<37.1 °C, $\geq$15.0 1000/mm^3" (group C; n = 35) and "<37.1 °C, <15.0 1000/mm^3" (group D; n = 35). The intensive care unit mortality rates were 15% for group A, 33% for group B, 34% for group C, and 49% for group D (p = 0.051). The temporal improvement in organ dysfunction and vasopressor dose seemed more apparent in group A patients. Our results suggest that different subphenotypes exist among sepsis patients treated using a vitamin C protocol, and clinical outcomes might be better for patients with the hyperinflammatory subphenotype.

Keywords: ascorbic acid; hydrocortisone; leukocytes; septic shock; temperature; thiamine

1. Introduction

Sepsis involves life-threatening organ dysfunction caused by a dysregulated host response to infection [1]. The global burden of sepsis is substantial, with an estimated 32 million cases and 5.3 million deaths per year [2]. In addition to the risk of short-term mortality, patients with sepsis experience various long-term complications and reduced quality of life. Thus, the cornerstones of sepsis treatment involve early identification, prompt antibiotic therapy, source control, and hemodynamic stability [3]. However, sepsis patients can still die of multiorgan dysfunction even if shock is prevented using these strategies.

Low-dose corticosteroids have been used as an adjuvant therapy for septic shock, as it downregulates the dysfunctional proinflammatory response and limits the anti-inflammatory response [4,5], increases adrenergic responsiveness [6], and preserves the endothelial glycocalyx [7]. Meanwhile, doses of corticosteroid in current guidelines do not consider the increased half-life of cortisol in the critically ill and may further increase central adrenocortical inhibition [8]. Two large randomized controlled trials have recently examined the effects of low-dose corticosteroids on mortality after septic shock [9,10], albeit with conflicting results. The APROCCHSS trial [10] reported that this treatment improved survival, whereas the ADRENAL trial [9] failed to detect a significant survival difference. The two trials had different inclusion–exclusion criteria, sources of sepsis, baseline therapies, and modes of hydrocortisone administration [11,12]. Another explanation may be that the current definition of sepsis captures a heterogeneous patient population. For example, Antcliffe et al. recently found a significant interaction between the previously identified sepsis response signatures (SRS) endotype and hydrocortisone therapy, demonstrating higher mortality in SRS2 patients treated using corticosteroids than in those treated using a placebo [13]. Nevertheless, most sepsis trials have focused on a one-size-fits-all approach, which may partially explain the inconsistent results from the aforementioned studies [9,10]. Therefore, novel methods of identifying subphenotypes among sepsis patients might help improve their management.

Vitamin C also limits the expression of proinflammatory cytokines, directly scavenges reactive oxygen species, and maintains endothelial barrier function [14,15]. Furthermore, there is evidence that vitamin C may act synergistically with corticosteroids [16,17] and that thiamine and vitamin C act to limit oxidative injury [18]. In septic shock patients, thiamine was associated with improved lactate clearance and a reduction in mortality [19]. These findings have led to recent observational studies, which demonstrated that sepsis patients experienced a substantial survival benefit after receiving vitamin C, hydrocortisone, and thiamine (which we will refer to as a "vitamin C protocol") [20,21]. Several randomized controlled trials are currently underway to evaluate the effects of a vitamin C protocol on clinically important outcomes in sepsis. In the most recent CITRIS-ALI trial of patients with sepsis and acute respiratory distress syndrome (ARDS), a 96 h infusion of vitamin C compared with placebo did not significantly improve organ dysfunction scores or alter markers of inflammation and vascular injury [22]. However, the number of secondary outcomes including 28-day mortality, significantly favored vitamin C treatment. Moreover, differences in baseline characteristics of heterogeneous sepsis population may have influenced outcomes.

We hypothesize that subgroups exist within the septic phenotype receiving a vitamin C protocol, which will have variable physiological characteristics and clinical outcomes. In this study, body temperature and white blood cell count were used to classify these patients into novel subphenotypes.

2. Materials and Methods

2.1. Study Subjects, Study Design, and Treatment Protocol

This retrospective cohort study evaluated consecutive critically ill adults with sepsis or septic shock who were admitted to the medical intensive care unit (ICU) of an 835-bed university-affiliated tertiary hospital (Seoul, Korea) between September 2018 and August 2019. In September 2018, our institution adopted a vitamin C protocol as routine adjuvant therapy for septic shock due to experimental and emerging clinical data. The present study included consecutive patients who were treated with the vitamin C protocol, although patients were excluded if they were <19 years old, were not diagnosed with septic shock, and/or had a do-not-resuscitate order. Although this study did not evaluate the efficacy of the vitamin C protocol in septic shock, patients who were moribund and died within 24 h of receiving the protocol were also excluded.

Baseline demographics and physiological characteristics (i.e., vital signs, laboratory results) were compared between ICU survivors and non-survivors. In addition, the highest tympanic temperature measurements, as well as white blood cell counts from within 24 h before starting the vitamin C protocol, were compared between survivors and non-survivors. According to the temperature and white blood cell count, patients were divided into four groups. The primary study outcome was ICU mortality. The secondary outcomes included net fluid retention, vasopressor weaning, vasopressor-free days at day 28, ventilator weaning, ventilator-free days at day 28, hospital mortality, changes in the sequential organ failure assessment (SOFA) score [23] at day 4 relative to the start of the protocol, and changes in the norepinephrine equivalent dose and vasoactive-inotropic score at 24 h relative to the start of the protocol. Potential adverse effects of the vitamin C protocol were also analyzed. The study protocol was approved by the Institutional Review Board of Chung-Ang University Hospital (No.

1905-005-16264), and the requirement for written informed consent was waived due to the retrospective observational nature of the study.

The vitamin C protocol consisted of a combination of intravenous vitamin C (1.5 g every 6 h for 4 days), hydrocortisone (50 mg every 6 h for 7 days), and thiamine (200 mg every 12 h for 4 days) [20,21]. All patients were managed by adherence to therapeutic recommendations based on the surviving sepsis campaign guidelines and the lung-protective ventilation strategy [24,25].

2.2. Data Collection and Definitions

Baseline data were collected regarding age, sex, body mass index, comorbidities, cause of sepsis, presence of nosocomial infection, concurrent bacteremia, ARDS and/or septic cardiomyopathy, and the patients' status within 24 h after ICU admission (mechanical ventilation, neuromuscular blockers, and/or renal replacement therapy). In addition, illness severity at the time of ICU admission was assessed by using the acute physiology and chronic health evaluation (APACHE) II score [26] and the SOFA score. Moreover, the time of septic shock onset, the time of starting the vitamin C protocol, and the vital signs and laboratory data from within 24 h before starting the vitamin C protocol were extracted. Intake and output of all fluids (urine volume, dialysis volume, drainage volume, and stool weight) were determined hourly for the first 4 days. The severity of organ dysfunction was assessed by calculating the SOFA score for the first 4 days. The hourly dosage of vasopressors was recorded as the norepinephrine equivalent dose [27] and the vasoactive-inotropic score [28]. We used the vasoactive-inotropic score to include vasopressin, which is commonly used in current practice. Sepsis and septic shock were defined using the third international consensus definitions for sepsis and septic shock (Sepsis-3) [1]. Twenty-two of 127 (17%) patients had a serum lactate level <2 mmol/L, although they were included in the study due to persisting hypotension requiring high-dose vasopressors. An immunocompromised status was diagnosed if there was an underlying disease or condition that affected the immune system (human immunodeficiency virus infection, malignancy, or severe neutropenia) or if immunosuppressive therapy was being administered. Nosocomial infections were defined as those occurring within 48 h of hospital admission. The consensus definition was used to identify ARDS [29]. Echocardiographic findings of septic cardiomyopathy were defined as left ventricular, right ventricular, or biventricular dysfunction [30]. The success of vasopressor weaning was defined as the ability of the patient to maintain normal pressure for 48 h without any vasopressor support. Ventilator weaning was identified based on the patient's ability to breathe for 48 h without any form of ventilator support. Acute kidney injury was defined based on the KDIGO (Kidney Disease: Improving Global Outcomes) criteria [31]. Superinfection was diagnosed if a new microbiological infection occurred 48 h or more after admission.

2.3. Statistical Analysis

Continuous variables were presented as median (interquartile range [IQR]) or as mean ± standard deviation and were compared using the Mann-Whitney U test. Categorical variables were presented as number (percentage) and were compared using the chi-squared or Fisher's exact test, as appropriate. The Kruskal-Wallis test was used to compare continuous variables among more than two groups. The cutoff temperature and white blood cell count values were the median values of study patients. Kaplan-Meier survival estimates were built stratified by initial temperature and white blood cell count to analyze their discriminating power in terms of predicting ICU mortality. All tests of significance were two-tailed, and differences were considered statistically significant at p-values of <0.05. All analyses were performed using IBM SPSS software (version 25.0; IBM Corp., Armonk, NY, USA).

3. Results

Among the 233 sepsis or septic shock patients admitted to ICU, 127 eligible patients were identified, including 84 patients (66%) who survived their ICU admission and 43 patients (34%) who died in the

ICU. Seven patients with septic shock died within 24 h of receiving vitamin C protocol and were not included in the analysis (the baseline characteristics of these patients are detailed in Table S1).

3.1. Comparisons between Survivors and Non-Survivors

The patients' characteristics from before starting the vitamin C protocol are shown in Table 1 according to survival status. No significant differences were observed between the survivors and non-survivors in terms of age, sex, body mass index, or comorbidities. Regarding the distribution of sepsis causes, the survivors were more likely to have urosepsis, while the non-survivors were more likely to have pneumonia. As expected, the non-survivors required more mechanical ventilation, neuromuscular blockers, and renal replacement therapy within 24 h of ICU admission and had significantly higher vasopressor doses. Before vitamin C protocol initiation, the survivors had a significantly higher median temperature (37.2 °C (IQR: 36.8–38.0 °C) vs. 36.9 °C (IQR: 36.4–37.8 °C); $p = 0.01$). The survivors tended to have non-significantly higher median values for white blood cell count (15.5 (IQR: 9.3–21.9) 1000/mm^3 vs. 10.9 (IQR: 4.1–20.9) 1000/mm^3; $p = 0.08$). Among other vital signs and laboratory data, the survivors had significantly higher PaO_2/FiO_2, while the non-survivors had significantly higher respiratory rate and serum lactate. Echocardiographic findings were available for 68 patients (54%), with no significant differences in left ventricular systolic function or the proportion of patients with septic cardiomyopathy. There was also no difference in median time from onset of shock to vitamin C protocol administration (5 (IQR: 1–12) h vs. 7 (IQR: 3–12) h; $p = 0.27$).

Table 1. Pre-vitamin C protocol characteristics according to the ICU survival status after septic shock.

Variable	Total ($n = 127$)	Survivors ($n = 84$)	Non-Survivors ($n = 43$)	p
Age, years	77 (68–83)	77 (68–82)	79 (68–84)	0.61
Male sex	75 (59)	47 (56)	28 (65)	0.32
Body mass index, kg/m^2	21.3 (18.1–24.2)	21.3 (17.9–24.2)	21.1 (18.6–23.3)	0.98
Comorbidities				
Diabetes	44 (35)	28 (33)	16 (37)	0.66
Chronic heart failure	15 (12)	8 (10)	7 (16)	0.26
Chronic neurologic disease	38 (30)	26 (31)	12 (28)	0.72
Chronic lung disease	20 (16)	11 (13)	9 (21)	0.25
Liver cirrhosis	10 (8)	5 (6)	5 (12)	0.31
Chronic kidney disease	27 (21)	15 (18)	12 (28)	0.19
Malignancy	29 (23)	18 (21)	11 (26)	0.60
Immunocompromised	29 (23)	17 (20)	12 (28)	0.33
Nosocomial infection	49 (39)	29 (35)	20 (47)	0.19
Cause of sepsis				
Pneumonia	56 (44)	32 (38)	24 (56)	0.06
Urosepsis	35 (28)	30 (36)	5 (12)	0.004
Gastrointestinal/biliary	24 (19)	18 (21)	6 (14)	0.31
Skin/soft tissue	8 (6)	4 (5)	4 (9)	0.44
Concurrent bacteremia	36 (28)	25 (30)	11 (26)	0.62
ARDS at ICU admission	10 (8)	5 (6)	5 (12)	0.31
APACHE II score	28 (20–34)	25 (18–30)	31 (28–39)	<0.001
SOFA score	12 (10–14)	11 (10–12)	13 (12–15)	<0.001
Mechanical ventilation	87 (69)	48 (57)	39 (91)	<0.001
Neuromuscular blocker	35 (28)	15 (18)	20 (47)	0.001
Renal replacement therapy	41 (32)	11 (13)	30 (70)	<0.001

Table 1. Cont.

Variable	Total (n = 127)	Survivors (n = 84)	Non-Survivors (n = 43)	p
Vital signs and laboratory data				
Body temperature, °C	37.0 (36.7–38.0)	37.2 (36.8–38.0)	36.9 (36.4–37.8)	0.01
Mean arterial pressure, mmHg	60 (55–65)	60 (55–66)	58 (54–64)	0.20
Respiratory rate, breaths/min	28 (24–32)	27 (24–31)	30 (26–34)	0.03
PaO_2/FiO_2	214 (130–314)	240 (157–350)	147 (103–272)	0.007
Bicarbonate, mEq/L	19.2 (16.3–22.0)	19.4 (16.3–22.8)	19.0 (16.1–21.2)	0.59
Creatinine, mg/dL	1.4 (0.9–2.2)	1.3 (0.7–2.0)	1.7 (1.1–2.5)	0.11
White cell count, $1000/mm^3$	14.4 (8.0–21.8)	15.5 (9.3–21.9)	10.9 (4.1–20.9)	0.08
Total bilirubin, mg/dL	0.9 (0.5–1.6)	0.8 (0.5–1.6)	0.9 (0.5–1.9)	0.36
C-reactive protein, mg/L	135 (82–223)	137 (85–247)	133 (82–197)	0.74
Lactate, mmol/L	4.0 (2.5–7.0)	3.3 (2.3–6.4)	6.1 (3.9–8.5)	0.001
Norepi eq dose, ug/min	15.0 (9.4–21.3)	13.0 (5.6–18.7)	21.1 (12.9–32.4)	<0.001
Vasoactive-inotropic score	30.0 (18.6–48.7)	23.5 (14.1–44.1)	46.4 (26.7–74.7)	<0.001
Echocardiography (n = 47/21) [1]				
Ejection fraction, %	56 (42–63)	57 (44–63)	55 (42–61)	0.55
Septic cardiomyopathy	22 (32)	13 (28)	9 (43)	0.22
Time from shock onset to vitamin C protocol, h	6 (2–12)	5 (1–12)	7 (3–12)	0.27

The data are presented as median (interquartile range) or number (percentage). ICU: Intensive care unit; ARDS: Acute respiratory distress syndrome; APACHE: Acute Physiology and Chronic Health Evaluation; SOFA: Sequential Organ Failure Assessment; PaO_2: Arterial partial pressure of oxygen; FiO_2: Fraction of inspired oxygen; Norepi eq: Norepinephrine equivalent. [1] No. of patients was 47 for survivors and 21 for non-survivors.

3.2. Baseline Characteristics and Clinical Outcomes between Study Groups

The median temperature and white blood cell count of study patients were 37.0 °C (IQR: 36.7–38.0 °C) and 14.4 (IQR: 8.0–21.8) $1000/mm^3$, respectively. Analysis of the baseline temperature and white blood cell count in the cohort found four study groups. Group A (n = 27; 21%) was characterized by a high presenting temperature (≥37.1 °C) with a high white blood cell count (≥15.0 $1000/mm^3$). These patients could be referred to as the "hyperinflammatory" subphenotype. Similar to group A, group B (n = 30; 24%) also presented with a high temperature (≥37.1 °C) but with a low white blood cell count (<15.0 $1000/mm^3$). Group C (n = 35; 28%) presented with a low temperature (<37.1 °C) but with a high white blood cell count (≥15.0 $1000/mm^3$). Lastly, group D (n = 35; 28%) was characterized by low presenting temperature (<37.1 °C) with a low white blood cell count (<15.0 $1000/mm^3$). These patients could be referred to as the "hypoinflammatory" subphenotype. When we included the patients who died within 24 h of receiving protocol, the median temperature and white blood cell count were 37.0 °C (IQR: 36.7–38.0 °C) and 14.9 (IQR: 8.1–21.9) $1000/mm^3$, respectively.

Table 2 shows the pre-vitamin C protocol characteristics of the patients according to study groups. In the cohort, group D patients had a significantly lower body mass index. There were no significant differences between the four groups in terms of the cause of sepsis, severity of illness (APACHE II and SOFA scores), patient's status within 24 h after ICU admission, vital signs, and laboratory data except for temperature, white blood cell count, and PaO_2/FiO_2. In the cohort, group A and B patients had a significantly higher temperature than group C and D patients ($p < 0.001$). The group A and C patients had significantly higher white blood cell counts than group B and D patients ($p < 0.001$). The group B patients had significantly lower PaO_2/FiO_2 than the other groups. In group B patients, there was a significant delay in the median interval from shock onset to protocol administration ($p = 0.03$). Table 3 shows the clinical outcomes stratified according to study group. The group A patients (hyperinflammatory subphenotype) tended to have the lowest mortality rates and highest vasopressor and ventilator weaning rates. The Kaplan-Meier survival curves, stratified according to study group, are shown in Figure 1 ($p = 0.09$). When the 24 h non-survivors were included, the ICU mortality rates were 30% for group A, 43% for group B, 46% for group C, and 57% for group D ($p = 0.18$).

Table 2. Pre-vitamin C protocol patient characteristics according to the study group.

Variable	Group A (n = 27)	Group B (n = 30)	Group C (n = 35)	Group D (n = 35)	p
Age, years	77 (70–82)	77 (66–81)	78 (68–84)	79 (64–85)	0.88
Male sex	17 (63)	18 (60)	20 (57)	20 (57)	0.96
Body mass index, kg/m^2	21.3 (17.9–23.3)	22.8 (19.6–25.2)	21.6 (19.6–25.1)	19.7 (17.5–22.3)	0.04
Comorbidities					
Diabetes	9 (33)	12 (40)	11 (31)	12 (34)	0.91
Chronic heart failure	2 (7)	4 (13)	5 (14)	4 (11)	0.87
Chronic neurologic disease	9 (33)	8 (27)	10 (29)	11 (31)	0.95
Chronic lung disease	7 (26)	2 (7)	8 (23)	3 (9)	0.09
Liver cirrhosis	1 (4)	1 (3)	5 (14)	3 (9)	0.38
Chronic kidney disease	3 (11)	6 (20)	8 (23)	10 (29)	0.41
Malignancy	6 (22)	6 (20)	8 (23)	9 (26)	0.96
Immunocompromised	5 (19)	6 (20)	7 (20)	11 (31)	0.56
Nosocomial infection	12 (44)	14 (47)	11 (31)	12 (34)	0.52
Cause of sepsis					
Pneumonia	11 (41)	15 (50)	13 (37)	17 (49)	0.68
Urosepsis	7 (26)	8 (27)	13 (37)	7 (20)	0.45
Gastrointestinal/biliary	7 (26)	6 (20)	5 (14)	6 (17)	0.69
Skin/soft tissue	0	4 (13)	1 (3)	3 (9)	0.17
Concurrent Bacteremia	5 (19)	8 (27)	14 (40)	9 (26)	0.29
ARDS at ICU admission	2 (7)	3 (10)	3 (9)	2 (6)	0.97
APACHE II score	30 (26–35)	28 (21–34)	28 (19–33)	26 (19–32)	0.45
SOFA score	11 (10–13)	13 (11–14)	12 (11–13)	12 (10–14)	0.15
Mechanical ventilation	21 (78)	23 (77)	22 (63)	21 (60)	0.30
Neuromuscular blocker	8 (30)	11 (37)	10 (29)	6 (17)	0.36
Renal replacement therapy	7 (26)	8 (27)	14 (40)	12 (34)	0.58
Vital signs and laboratory data					
Body temperature, °C	37.8 (37.4–38.2)	38.2 (37.8–38.5)	36.8 (36.4–36.9)	36.7 (36.5–37.0)	<0.001
Mean arterial pressure, mmHg	59 (57–66)	60 (52–64)	62 (56–68)	58 (53–64)	0.35
Respiratory rate, breaths/min	28 (26–33)	29 (27–34)	27 (24–32)	26 (24–31)	0.14
PaO$_2$/FiO$_2$	232 (152–314)	158 (99–208)	260 (162–340)	250 (120–351)	0.048
Bicarbonate, mEq/L	19.5 (17.1–22.4)	19.2 (16.3–20.7)	19.0 (14.4–20.9)	19.5 (17.4–22.8)	0.75
Creatinine, mg/dL	1.5 (0.7–1.9)	1.4 (1.0–1.9)	1.4 (1.0–2.6)	1.3 (0.7–2.2)	0.84
White cell count, 1000/mm^3	21.9 (19.1–29.8)	8.1 (3.7–10.9)	21.9 (16.5–27.7)	8.1 (3.2–11.6)	<0.001
Total bilirubin, mg/dL	0.7 (0.4–1.3)	1.0 (0.6–1.9)	0.7 (0.5–2.6)	1.0 (0.6–1.5)	0.26
C-reactive protein, mg/L	135 (57–239)	150 (95–302)	140 (92–221)	115 (75–186)	0.20
Lactate, mmol/L	3.9 (2.6–7.0)	4.0 (3.1–6.1)	4.2 (2.3–6.9)	3.2 (2.1–7.2)	0.72
Norepi eq dose, ug/min	16.0 (10.2–19.1)	14.9 (10.4–21.1)	16.0 (9.6–28.3)	14.8 (6.5–20.7)	0.70
Vasoactive-inotropic score	32.0 (21.6–48.1)	25.9 (17.0–45.6)	38.0 (18.9–50.6)	27.0 (13.5–49.3)	0.71
Echocardiography (n = 17/15/21/15) [1]					
Ejection fraction, %	56 (36–64)	54 (37–63)	56 (42–60)	59 (54–64)	0.40
Septic cardiomyopathy	7 (41)	6 (60)	6 (29)	3 (20)	0.52
Time from shock onset to vitamin C protocol, h	7 (3–12)	11 (4–20)	4 (1–8)	4 (1–8)	0.03

The data are presented as median (interquartile range) or number (percentage). ARDS: Acute respiratory distress syndrome; ICU: Intensive care unit; APACHE: Acute Physiology and Chronic Health Evaluation; SOFA: Sequential Organ Failure Assessment; PaO$_2$: Arterial partial pressure of oxygen; FiO$_2$: Fraction of inspired oxygen; Norepi eq: Norepinephrine equivalent. [1] No. of patients was 17 for Group A, 15 for Group B, 21 for Group C, and 15 for Group D.

Table 3. Clinical outcomes according to study group.

Variable	Group A (n = 27)	Group B (n = 30)	Group C (n = 35)	Group D (n = 35)	p
Net fluid retention [1], mL					
Day 1	1363 (183–2145)	2355 (1584–3169)	2215 (296–2954)	1839 (977–3058)	0.12
Day 2	674 (−13–1281)	723 (−252–1624)	650 (−12–1434)	1335 (476–2030)	0.34
Day 3	610 (−279–932)	230 (−388–750)	390 (−94–947)	560 (−138–1713)	0.43
Day 4	234 (−238–696)	280 (−255–850)	392 (−379–1178)	453 (−210–1139)	0.79
Vasopressor weaning	24 (89)	20 (69)	23 (66)	22 (63)	0.12
Vasopressor-free days at day 28	21.4 ± 9.0	17.2 ± 12.1	16.7 ± 12.3	15.3 ± 12.5	0.30
Ventilator weaning (n = 21/22/22/21) [2,3]	15 (71)	14 (64)	8 (36)	6 (29)	0.01
Ventilator-free days at day 28	13.1 ± 11.1	13.4 ± 10.8	8.2 ± 11.2	5.6 ± 9.5	0.07
ICU mortality	4 (15)	10 (33)	12 (34)	17 (49)	0.051
Hospital mortality	6 (22)	13 (43)	15 (43)	19 (54)	0.09
Superinfection	4 (15)	6 (20)	3 (9)	6 (17)	0.62

The data are presented as median (interquartile range), mean ± standard deviation, or number (percentage). ICU: Intensive care unit. [1] The net fluid retention was determined as the difference between intake and output of all fluids (urine volume, dialysis volume, drainage volume, and stool weight). [2] Ventilator weaning was defined as the patient's ability to breathe for 48 h without any ventilator support. [3] No. of patients was 21 for Group A, 22 for Group B, 22 for Group C, and 21 for Group D.

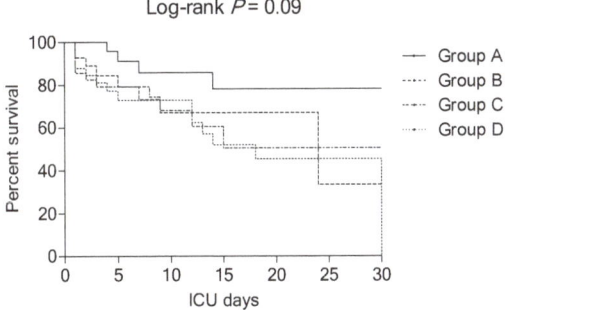

Figure 1. Kaplan-Meier curves for patients stratified according to the study group. ICU: Intensive care unit.

3.3. Physiological Characteristics between Study Groups

There was no significant difference among the study groups in terms of median change in the SOFA score on day 4 relative to day 1 ($p = 0.80$; Kruskal-Wallis test). However, Δ 4 d SOFA scores tended to be higher in group A patients (4 (range 1–5)) compared with that of the group D patients (1 [range 0–3]; $p = 0.06$) (Figure 2). Interestingly and also unexpectedly, there was a statistically significant difference in improvement in SOFA score in group C patients, compared to group D patients ($p = 0.047$).

Figure 3 shows the median change of the vasopressor dose (in norepinephrine equivalents or vasoactive-inotropic score) over the first 24 h, according to the study group. Before the vitamin C protocol, no significant inter-group differences were observed in the median norepinephrine equivalent dose or the median vasoactive-inotropic score (Table 2). The norepinephrine equivalent doses decreased over time for all study groups, although there was no significant difference among the groups ($p = 0.16$; Kruskal-Wallis test). However, a significant inter-group difference was detected between group A and D patients ($p = 0.008$; Figure 3A). There was a significant difference among patients in terms of change in the vasoactive-inotropic score ($p = 0.01$; Kruskal-Wallis test), with significant inter-group differences between group A and B and group A and D patients ($p = 0.01$ and $p = 0.005$, respectively; Figure 3B). Other study group characteristics in the cohort are detailed in Table S2.

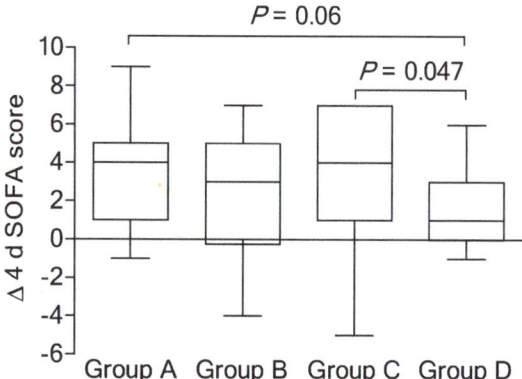

Figure 2. Median (interquartile range) changes in SOFA scores on day 4 relative to the scores on day 1, according to the study group. SOFA: Sequential Organ Failure Assessment.

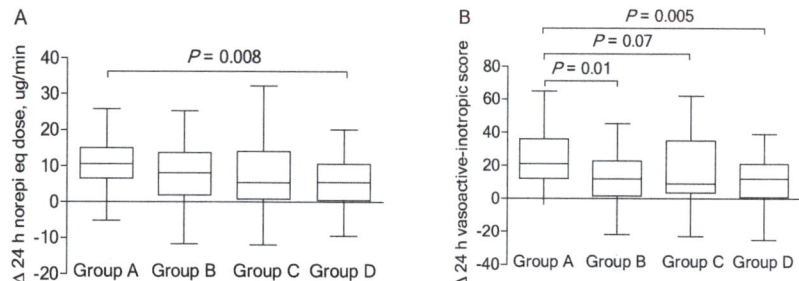

Figure 3. Median (interquartile range) change of the vasopressor dose (in norepinephrine equivalents (Norepi eq) or vasoactive-inotropic score) over the first 24 h according to the study group.

3.4. Septic Cardiomyopathy

Prior to vitamin C protocol administration, an echocardiography was performed in 68 of 127 (54%) patients. An echocardiographic finding of septic myocardial dysfunction was identified in 22 patients (Table S3). There was no significant difference in the proportion of patients with septic cardiomyopathy between the study groups (Table 2); however, the vasopressor weaning rate was highest (6/7; 86%), and the ICU mortality rate was lowest (1/7; 14%) in group A patients.

3.5. Adverse Events

Six of the 127 cohort patients (5%) developed acute kidney injury and needed renal replacement therapy throughout the study period. However, all of them were due to complications related to sepsis or underlying disease, and the relationship between toxicity and drug use was unclear. There was no significant difference between the study groups in terms of superinfection rates (15% vs. 20% vs. 9% vs. 17%; $p = 0.62$) (Table 3). Superinfection-related hospital mortality occurred in 5 (4%) patients (2 in group B and 3 in group D).

4. Discussion

The present study revealed subgroups in patients with septic shock who received the vitamin C protocol based on temperature and white blood cell count. We identified four subgroups of patients with considerable variations in their physiological differences. In addition, the groups exhibited different clinical outcomes to the vitamin C protocol, with the "hyperinflammatory" sepsis subphenotype potentially exhibiting a better clinical outcome. To the best of our knowledge, this is the first study to evaluate the subgroups in patients with septic shock receiving the vitamin C protocol.

Vitamin C exerts an anti-inflammatory effect by inhibiting the activation of nuclear factor kappa-B (NF-κB) [14,15], which modulates the transcription of several proinflammatory cytokines that promote antioxidant cellular injury [32] and endothelial dysfunction [33]. Vitamin C may also facilitate the production of catecholamines, vasopressin, and cortisol [34]. In this context, the primary anti-inflammatory action of corticosteroids involves suppressing the transcriptional activity of NF-κB and AP-1, which regulate the expression of cytokines, chemokines, inflammatory enzymes, cell adhesion molecules, coagulation factors, and receptors [35,36]. Furthermore, vitamin C may restore glucocorticoid receptor function [16], and corticosteroids increase cellular vitamin C uptake by increasing the expression of sodium-dependent vitamin C transporter-2 [17]. Moreover, thiamine exerts an anti-inflammatory effect by suppressing the oxidative stress-induced activation of NF-κB [37] and may act as a site-directed antioxidant [38]. Based on this information, our institution routinely started using the vitamin C protocol for septic shock in September 2018, as we believe that it is a combination of three safe, readily available, and inexpensive agents that target multiple pathways of the host's response to infection. In this setting, septic cardiomyopathy is a reversible phenomenon that is caused by myocardial depressant factors and inefficient metabolism [39]. Hao et al. also demonstrated that vitamin C significantly decreased myocardial oxidant injury, attenuated apoptosis, and maintained the functional integrity of mitochondria by limiting calcium overload and inhibiting the opening of the mitochondrial permeability transition pore [40]. In the present study, patients with the highest vasopressor dose were weaned-off and survived the ICU stay with apparent echocardiographic improvements (Table S3). There is no biologically plausible explanation for this observation, although we observed marked improvements in the course of septic cardiomyopathy among patients with the hyperinflammatory subphenotype. Despite the relatively small sample sizes of our study, these findings are of great interest, and further studies are needed to evaluate the role of vitamin C in septic cardiomyopathy.

Several studies have revealed that hypothermia during infection is associated with an increased risk of mortality, whereas patients with fever are associated with a lower risk compared to those with normothermia [41], which also supports the presence of different phenotypes among patients with sepsis. Temperature may also reflect a patient's underlying immunological state. Previous studies have investigated immunological differences between sepsis patients with and without fever based on their levels of pro- and anti-inflammatory cytokines [42,43], although the results failed to detect a significant difference in their cytokine profiles. There is a growing interest in immunomodulatory therapy, and accurate immunological phenotyping of sepsis patients is crucial [44]. Temperature itself may be useful for selecting immunosuppressive therapy in sepsis, even in the absence of specific cytokine abnormalities. In the present study, survivors had a significantly higher baseline temperature. However, there was heterogeneity in patients with an elevated baseline temperature (group A vs. group B). It is possible that the group A survivors tended to experience a gradual decrease in temperature (well-balanced inflammation); one can speculate, at least in part, why the group A patients exhibited better physiological characteristics and clinical outcomes than the group B patients. However, in the absence of a control group, it is not possible to draw associations between the vitamin C protocol's immunomodulatory effect and the better clinical outcomes in group A patients. Further studies are required to test this hypothesis.

Bhavani et al. reported that "hyperthermic, slow resolvers" had the highest levels of inflammatory markers, such as erythrocyte sedimentation rate and C-reactive protein, as well as the highest incidence of leukocytosis [45]. These "hyperthermic, slow resolvers" may represent the hyperinflammatory subphenotype. Sweeny et al. also identified an "inflammopathic" subtype from sepsis datasets, which included high disease severity, high bandemia, and high mortality [46]. In the present study, we identified a hyperinflammatory subphenotype (group A patients) that was accompanied by elevated baseline values for temperature and white blood cell count. It is difficult to directly compare the hyperinflammatory phenotypes observed with those seen in the study by Sweeny et al., which used a clustering analysis to pool data from 14 transcriptomic datasets ($n = 700$). Meanwhile, group A patients appeared to be related to better clinical outcomes and survival and temporal improvements in the SOFA score and short-term vasopressor dose. We speculate that the hyperinflammatory subphenotype would respond better than the hypoinflammatory subphenotype to immunomodulatory therapies, such as corticosteroids or vitamin C protocol. However, the lack of a comparator group does not allow one to make any inferences about the relationship between the subgroups and the treatment response. Of note, neither the demographics, the cause of sepsis, or the severity indices distinguished the septic phenotypes from each other, since the specified variables had similar values across the phenotypes (Table 2). Our data suggest that phenotype is not just an indicator of severity of illness as measured by classical prognostic factors. There were statistically significant differences in SOFA score improvement in group C patients. There is no possible explanation for these findings, although they did not lead to better clinical outcomes.

Patients with multiorgan dysfunction who survive the first 2 weeks of sepsis often develop persistent inflammation/immunosuppression and catabolism syndrome (PICS) [47]. In this context, vitamin C has immune-enhancing properties [48,49] and also improves chemotaxis, enhances lymphocyte function, and assists in phagocytosis and intracellular killing of bacteria [50]. Moreover, low-dose short-term corticosteroid treatment was not associated with an increased risk of secondary infections in recent randomized controlled trials [9,10,51], which suggests that a vitamin C protocol may prevent PICS. However, the long-term effects of vitamin C, which is temporarily supplemented for 4 days, are only speculative since the human body does not store it [52]. In addition, 35 of the 43 non-survivors (81%) in our study died within 14 days after starting the vitamin C protocol, which was related to refractory shock and multiorgan dysfunction, and we could not evaluate the efficacy of the protocol in PICS.

The present study has several limitations. First, the single-center retrospective design is associated with various risks of bias. The small sample size and low power may be the cause of various non-significant results. Second, we do not have inflammatory markers such as cytokines to explain the immunological basis for these subphenotypes. Third, the vitamin C levels were not measured. There is a possibility that there were differences between the groups regarding vitamin C levels. Fourth, the present analysis was based on a series of arbitrary classifiers (temperature and white blood cell count). We chose the median values of study patients for sufficiently large groups for statistical analysis, but categorization based on either high or low levels, including normal ranges in either category, may contribute to some overlap and inadequate separation of the study patients. For example, the group with a temperature of $\geq 37.1°C$ may include patients with relatively normal temperatures. However, the median temperatures of group A and B patients were significantly higher than those of group C and D patients. Thus, this limitation does not undermine the original conclusion of the study. Fifth, the ICU mortality rate was relatively high when compared with that seen in previous studies [20–22,53]. We suggest that this observation results from a higher level of illness severity in study patients (all of them were on vasopressors and their median APACHE II scores reached almost 30). Moreover, the overall mortality rate of sepsis and septic shock in our institution is about 20%. Lastly, a control group would be needed to assess the efficacy of the vitamin C protocol in septic shock, although that was not one of the objectives of this hypothesis-generating study, which aimed to identify potential subgroups of patients with septic shock. This information might help improve our understanding regarding the heterogeneity of sepsis patients and may provide the basis for designing future randomized controlled trials.

5. Conclusions

In conclusion, we identified septic subphenotypes in patients receiving vitamin C protocol with varying pathophysiologies and clinical outcomes. These findings may help guide future interventional studies targeting the immune response in septic shock patients. However, independent validation in a larger sample is needed to address the present study's findings.

Supplementary Materials: The following are available online at http://www.mdpi.com/2072-6643/11/12/2976/s1. Table S1: Pre-vitamin C protocol characteristics of the patients who died within 24 h of receiving protocol; Table S2: Change in physiological variables in the study groups; Table S3: Clinical characteristics including echocardiographic findings of 22 patients with septic cardiomyopathy.

Author Contributions: Conceptualization, W.-Y.K.; methodology, W.-Y.K.; formal analysis, W.-Y.K.; investigation, J.-W.J. and J.C.C.; resources, J.-W.J. and J.C.C.; data curation, W.-Y.K., J.-W.J., and J.C.C.; writing—original draft preparation, W.-Y.K.; writing—review and editing, J.W.S. and J.Y.K.; project administration, J.W.S. and J.Y.K.; funding acquisition, W.-Y.K.

Funding: This research was supported by the Chung-Ang University Research Grants in 2019.

Conflicts of Interest: The authors declare no conflict of interest. The funders had no role in the design of the study; in the collection, analyses, or interpretation of data; in the writing of the manuscript, or in the decision to publish the results.

References

1. Singer, M.; Deutschman, C.S.; Seymour, C.W.; Shankar-Hari, M.; Annane, D.; Bauer, M.; Bellomo, R.; Bernard, G.R.; Chiche, J.D.; Coopersmith, C.M.; et al. The third international consensus definitions for sepsis and septic shock (sepsis-3). *JAMA* **2016**, *315*, 801–810. [CrossRef] [PubMed]
2. Fleischmann, C.; Scherag, A.; Adhikari, N.K.; Hartog, C.S.; Tsaganos, T.; Schlattmann, P.; Angus, D.C.; Reinhart, K. International Forum of Acute Care Trialists. Assessment of global incidence and mortality of hospital-treated sepsis. Current estimates and limitations. *Am. J. Respir. Crit. Care Med.* **2016**, *193*, 259–272. [CrossRef] [PubMed]
3. Castellanos-Ortega, A.; Suberviola, B.; Garcia-Astudillo, L.A.; Holanda, M.S.; Ortiz, F.; Llorca, J.; Delgado-Rodríguez, M. Impact of the Surviving Sepsis Campaign protocols on hospital length of stay and mortality in septic shock patients: Results of a three-year follow-up quasi-experimental study. *Crit. Care Med.* **2010**, *38*, 1036–1043. [CrossRef] [PubMed]
4. Keh, D.; Boehnke, T.; Weber-Cartens, S.; Schulz, C.; Ahlers, O.; Bercker, S.; Volk, H.D.; Doecke, W.D.; Falke, K.J.; Gerlach, H. Immunologic and hemodynamic effects of "low-dose" hydrocortisone in septic shock: A double-blind, randomized, placebo-controlled, crossover study. *Am. J. Respir. Crit. Care Med.* **2003**, *167*, 512–520. [CrossRef]
5. Marik, P.E.; Pastores, S.M.; Annane, D.; Meduri, G.U.; Sprung, C.L.; Arlt, W.; Keh, D.; Briegel, J.; Beishuizen, A.; Dimopoulou, I.; et al. Recommendations for the diagnosis and management of corticosteroid insufficiency in critically ill adult patients: Consensus statements from an international task force by the American College of Critical Care Medicine. *Crit. Care Med.* **2008**, *36*, 1937–1949. [CrossRef]
6. Annane, D.; Bellissant, E.; Sebille, V.; Lesieur, O.; Mathieu, B.; Raphael, J.C.; Gajdos, P. Impaired pressor sensitivity to noradrenaline in septic shock patients with and without impaired adrenal function reserve. *Br. J. Clin. Pharmacol.* **1998**, *46*, 589–597. [CrossRef]
7. Chappell, D.; Jacob, M.; Hofmann-Kiefer, K.; Bruegger, D.; Rehm, M.; Conzen, P.; Welsch, U.; Becker, B.F. Hydrocortisone preserves the vascular barrier by protecting the endothelial glycocalyx. *Anesthesiology* **2007**, *107*, 776–784. [CrossRef]
8. Téblick, A.; Peeters, B.; Langouche, L.; Van den Berghe, G. Adrenal function and dysfunction in critically ill patients. *Nat. Rev. Endocrinol.* **2019**, *15*, 417–427. [CrossRef]
9. Venkatesh, B.; Finfer, S.; Cohen, J.; Rajbhandari, D.; Arabi, Y.; Bellomo, R.; Billot, L.; Correa, M.; Glass, P.; Harward, M.; et al. Adjunctive glucocorticoid therapy in patients with septic shock. *N. Engl. J. Med.* **2018**, *378*, 797–808. [CrossRef]
10. Annane, D.; Renault, A.; Brun-Buisson, C.; Megarbane, B.; Quenot, J.P.; Siami, S.; Cariou, A.; Forceville, X.; Schwebel, C.; Martin, C.; et al. Hydrocortisone plus fludrocortisone for adults with septic shock. *N. Engl. J. Med.* **2018**, *378*, 809–818. [CrossRef]
11. Venkatesh, B.; Cohen, J. Why the adjunctive corticosteroid treatment in critically Ill patients with septic shock (ADRENAL) trial did not show a difference in mortality. *Crit. Care Med.* **2019**, *47*, 1785–1788. [CrossRef] [PubMed]

12. Annane, D. Why my steroid trials in septic shock were "Positive". *Crit. Care Med.* **2019**, *47*, 1789–1793. [CrossRef] [PubMed]
13. Antcliffe, D.B.; Burnham, K.L.; Al-Beidh, F.; Santhakumaran, S.; Brett, S.J.; Hinds, C.J.; Ashby, D.; Knight, J.C.; Gordon, A.C. Transcriptomic signatures in sepsis and a differential response to steroids. from the VANISH randomized trial. *Am. J. Respir. Crit. Care Med.* **2019**, *199*, 980–986. [CrossRef]
14. Wilson, J.X. Mechanism of action of vitamin C in sepsis: Ascorbate modulates redox signaling in endothelium. *Biofactors* **2009**, *35*, 5–13. [CrossRef]
15. May, J.M.; Harrison, F.E. Role of vitamin C in the function of the vascular endothelium. *Antioxid. Redox Signal.* **2013**, *19*, 2068–2083. [CrossRef]
16. Okamoto, K.; Tanaka, H.; Makino, Y.; Makino, I. Restoration of the glucocorticoid receptor function by the phosphodiester compound of vitamins C and E, EPC-K1 (L-ascorbic acid 2-[3,4-dihydro-2,5,7,8-tetramethyl-2-(4,8,12-trimethyltridecyl)-2H-1-benzopyran-6-yl hydrogen phosphate] potassium salt), via a redox-dependent mechanism. *Biochem. Pharmacol.* **1998**, *56*, 79–86.
17. Fujita, I.; Hirano, J.; Itoh, N.; Nakanishi, T.; Tanaka, K. Dexamethasone induces sodium-dependant vitamin C transporter in a mouse osteoblastic cell line MC3T3-E1. *Br. J. Nutr.* **2001**, *86*, 145–149. [CrossRef]
18. De Andrade, J.A.A.; Gayer, C.R.M.; Nogueira, N.P.A.; Paes, M.C.; Bastos, V.; Neto, J.; Alves, S.C., Jr.; Coelho, R.M.; da Cunha, M.G.A.T.; Gomes, R.N. The effect of thiamine deficiency on inflammation, oxidative stress and cellular migration in an experimental model of sepsis. *J. Inflamm.* **2014**, *11*, 11. [CrossRef]
19. Woolum, J.A.; Abner, E.L.; Kelly, A.; Thompson Bastin, M.L.; Morris, P.E.; Flannery, A.H. Effect of Thiamine administration on lactate clearance and mortality in patients with septic shock. *Crit. Care Med.* **2018**, *46*, 1747–1752. [CrossRef]
20. Marik, P.E.; Khangoora, V.; Rivera, R.; Hooper, M.H.; Catravas, J. Hydrocortisone, vitamin c, and thiamine for the treatment of severe sepsis and septic shock: a retrospective before-after study. *Chest* **2017**, *151*, 1229–1238. [CrossRef]
21. Kim, W.Y.; Jo, E.J.; Eom, J.S.; Mok, J.; Kim, M.H.; Kim, K.U.; Park, H.K.; Lee, M.K.; Lee, K. Combined vitamin C, hydrocortisone, and thiamine therapy for patients with severe pneumonia who were admitted to the intensive care unit: Propensity score-based analysis of a before-after cohort study. *J. Crit. Care* **2018**, *47*, 211–218. [CrossRef] [PubMed]
22. Fowler, A.A., 3rd; Truwit, J.D.; Hite, R.D.; Morris, P.E.; DeWilde, C.; Priday, A.; Fisher, B.; Thacker, L.R., 2nd; Natarajan, R.; Brophy, D.F.; et al. Effect of vitamin C infusion on organ failure and biomarkers of inflammation and vascular injury in patients with sepsis and severe acute respiratory failure: the CITRIS-ALI randomized clinical trial. *JAMA* **2019**, *322*, 1261–1270. [CrossRef] [PubMed]
23. Vincent, J.L.; Moreno, R.; Takala, J.; Willatts, S.; De Mendonca, A.; Bruining, H.; Reinhart, C.K.; Suter, P.M.; Thijs, L.G. The SOFA (Sepsis-related Organ Failure Assessment) score to describe organ dysfunction/failure. On behalf of the working group on sepsis-related problems of the European society of intensive care medicine. *Intensive Care Med.* **1996**, *22*, 707–710. [CrossRef] [PubMed]
24. Rhodes, A.; Evans, L.E.; Alhazzani, W.; Levy, M.M.; Antonelli, M.; Ferrer, R.; Kumar, A.; Sevransky, J.E.; Sprung, C.L.; Nunnally, M.E.; et al. Surviving sepsis campaign: international guidelines for management of sepsis and septic shock: 2016. *Crit. Care Med.* **2017**, *45*, 486–552. [CrossRef] [PubMed]
25. Acute Respiratory Distress Syndrome Network; Brower, R.G.; Matthay, M.A.; Morris, A.; Schoenfeld, D.; Thompson, B.T.; Wheeler, A. Ventilation with lower tidal volumes as compared with traditional tidal volumes for acute lung injury and the acute respiratory distress syndrome. *N. Engl. J. Med.* **2000**, *342*, 1301–1308. [PubMed]
26. Knaus, W.A.; Draper, E.A.; Wagner, D.P.; Zimmerman, J.E. APACHE II: A severity of disease classification system. *Crit. Care Med.* **1985**, *13*, 818–829. [CrossRef]
27. Patel, B.M.; Chittock, D.R.; Russell, J.A.; Walley, K.R. Beneficial effects of short-term vasopressin infusion during severe septic shock. *Anesthesiology* **2002**, *96*, 576–582. [CrossRef]
28. Gaies, M.G.; Gurney, J.G.; Yen, A.H.; Napoli, M.L.; Gajarski, R.J.; Ohye, R.G.; Charpie, J.R.; Hirsch, J.C. Vasoactive-inotropic score as a predictor of morbidity and mortality in infants after cardiopulmonary bypass. *Pediatr. Crit. Care Med.* **2010**, *11*, 234–238. [CrossRef]
29. ARDS Definition Task Force; Ranieri, V.M.; Rubenfeld, G.D.; Thompson, B.T.; Ferguson, N.D.; Caldwell, E.; Fan, E.; Camporota, L.; Slutsky, A.S. Acute respiratory distress syndrome: The Berlin definition. *JAMA* **2012**, *307*, 2526–2533.

30. Griffee, M.J.; Merkel, M.J.; Wei, K.S. The role of echocardiography in hemodynamic assessment of septic shock. *Crit. Care Clin.* **2010**, *26*, 365–382. [CrossRef]
31. Kellum, J.A.; Lameire, N.; KDIGO AKI Guideline Work Group. Diagnosis, evaluation, and management of acute kidney injury: A KDIGO summary (Part 1). *Crit. Care* **2013**, *17*, 204. [CrossRef] [PubMed]
32. Oudemans-van Straaten, H.M.; Spoelstra-de Man, A.M.; de Waard, M.C. Vitamin C revisited. *Crit. Care* **2014**, *18*, 460. [CrossRef] [PubMed]
33. Dhar-Mascareno, M.; Carcamo, J.M.; Golde, D.W. Hypoxia-reoxygenation-induced mitochondrial damage and apoptosis in human endothelial cells are inhibited by vitamin C. *Free Radic. Biol. Med.* **2005**, *38*, 1311–1322. [CrossRef] [PubMed]
34. Carr, A.C.; Shaw, G.M.; Fowler, A.A.; Natarajan, R. Ascorbate-dependent vasopressor synthesis: A rationale for vitamin C administration in severe sepsis and septic shock? *Crit. Care* **2015**, *19*, 418. [CrossRef]
35. Busillo, J.M.; Cidlowski, J.A. The five Rs of glucocorticoid action during inflammation: Ready, reinforce, repress, resolve, and restore. *Trends Endocrinol. Metab.* **2013**, *24*, 109–119. [CrossRef]
36. Cain, D.W.; Cidlowski, J.A. Immune regulation by glucocorticoids. *Nat. Rev. Immunol.* **2017**, *17*, 233–247. [CrossRef]
37. Manzetti, S.; Zhang, J.; van der Spoel, D. Thiamin function, metabolism, uptake, and transport. *Biochemistry* **2014**, *53*, 821–835. [CrossRef]
38. Gibson, G.E.; Zhang, H. Interactions of oxidative stress with thiamine homeostasis promote neurodegeneration. *Neurochem. Int.* **2002**, *40*, 493–504. [CrossRef]
39. Krishnagopalan, S.; Kumar, A.; Parrillo, J.E.; Kumar, A. Myocardial dysfunction in the patient with sepsis. *Curr. Opin. Crit. Care* **2002**, *8*, 376–388. [CrossRef]
40. Hao, J.; Li, W.W.; Du, H.; Zhao, Z.F.; Liu, F.; Lu, J.C.; Yang, X.C.; Cui, W. Role of vitamin C in cardioprotection of ischemia/reperfusion injury by activation of mitochondrial KATP channel. *Chem. Pharm. Bull.* **2016**, *64*, 548–557. [CrossRef]
41. Rumbus, Z.; Matics, R.; Hegyi, P.; Zsiboras, C.; Szabo, I.; Illes, A.; Petervari, E.; Balasko, M.; Marta, K.; Miko, A.; et al. Fever Is Associated with Reduced, Hypothermia with increased mortality in septic patients: A meta-analysis of clinical trials. *PLoS ONE* **2017**, *12*, e0170152. [CrossRef] [PubMed]
42. Marik, P.E.; Zaloga, G.P. Hypothermia and cytokines in septic shock. Norasept II Study Investigators. North American study of the safety and efficacy of murine monoclonal antibody to tumor necrosis factor for the treatment of septic shock. *Intensive Care Med.* **2000**, *26*, 716–721. [CrossRef] [PubMed]
43. Wiewel, M.A.; Harmon, M.B.; van Vught, L.A.; Scicluna, B.P.; Hoogendijk, A.J.; Horn, J.; Zwinderman, A.H.; Cremer, O.L.; Bonten, M.J.; Schultz, M.J.; et al. Risk factors, host response and outcome of hypothermic sepsis. *Crit. Care* **2016**, *20*, 328. [CrossRef] [PubMed]
44. Hotchkiss, R.S.; Monneret, G.; Payen, D. Immunosuppression in sepsis: A novel understanding of the disorder and a new therapeutic approach. *Lancet Infect. Dis.* **2013**, *13*, 260–268. [CrossRef]
45. Bhavani, S.V.; Carey, K.A.; Gilbert, E.R.; Afshar, M.; Verhoef, P.A.; Churpek, M.M. Identifying novel sepsis subphenotypes using temperature trajectories. *Am. J. Respir. Crit. Care Med.* **2019**, *200*, 327–335. [CrossRef] [PubMed]
46. Sweeney, T.E.; Azad, T.D.; Donato, M.; Haynes, W.A.; Perumal, T.M.; Henao, R.; Bermejo-Martin, J.F.; Almansa, R.; Tamayo, E.; Howrylak, J.A.; et al. Unsupervised analysis of transcriptomics in bacterial sepsis across multiple datasets reveals three robust clusters. *Crit. Care Med.* **2018**, *46*, 915–925. [CrossRef]
47. Mira, J.C.; Gentile, L.F.; Mathias, B.J.; Efron, P.A.; Brakenridge, S.C.; Mohr, A.M.; Moore, F.A.; Moldawer, L.L. Sepsis pathophysiology, chronic critical illness, and Persistent Inflammation-Immunosuppression and Catabolism Syndrome. *Crit. Care Med.* **2017**, *45*, 253–262. [CrossRef]
48. Huijskens, M.J.; Walczak, M.; Sarkar, S.; Atrafi, F.; Senden-Gijsbers, B.L.; Tilanus, M.G.; Bos, G.M.; Wieten, L.; Germeraad, W.T. Ascorbic acid promotes proliferation of natural killer cell populations in culture systems applicable for natural killer cell therapy. *Cytotherapy* **2015**, *17*, 613–620. [CrossRef]
49. Manning, J.; Mitchell, B.; Appadurai, D.A.; Shakya, A.; Pierce, L.J.; Wang, H.; Nganga, V.; Swanson, P.C.; May, J.M.; Tantin, D.; et al. Vitamin C promotes maturation of T-cells. *Antioxid. Redox Signal.* **2013**, *19*, 2054–2067. [CrossRef]
50. Wilson, J.X. Evaluation of vitamin C for adjuvant sepsis therapy. *Antioxid. Redox Signal.* **2013**, *19*, 2129–2140. [CrossRef]

51. Keh, D.; Trips, E.; Marx, G.; Wirtz, S.P.; Abduljawwad, E.; Bercker, S.; Bogatsch, H.; Briegel, J.; Engel, C.; Gerlach, H.; et al. Effect of hydrocortisone on development of shock among patients with severe sepsis: The hypress randomized clinical trial. *JAMA* **2016**, *316*, 1775–1785. [CrossRef] [PubMed]
52. Naidu, K.A. Vitamin C in human health and disease is still a mystery? An overview. *Nutr. J.* **2003**, *2*, 7. [CrossRef] [PubMed]
53. Shin, T.G.; Kim, Y.J.; Ryoo, S.M.; Hwang, S.Y.; Jo, I.J.; Chung, S.P.; Choi, S.H.; Suh, G.J.; Kim, W.Y. Early vitamin C and thiamine administration to patients with septic shock in emergency departments: Propensity score-based analysis of a before-and-after cohort study. *J. Clin. Med.* **2019**, *8*, 102. [CrossRef] [PubMed]

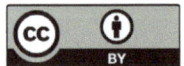

© 2019 by the authors. Licensee MDPI, Basel, Switzerland. This article is an open access article distributed under the terms and conditions of the Creative Commons Attribution (CC BY) license (http://creativecommons.org/licenses/by/4.0/).

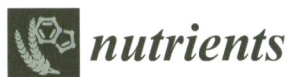

Editorial

The Emerging Role of Vitamin C in the Prevention and Treatment of COVID-19

Anitra C. Carr [1,*] and Sam Rowe [2,3]

1. Nutrition in Medicine Research Group, Department of Pathology & Biomedical Science, University of Otago, Christchurch 8011, New Zealand
2. Intensive Care Department, Newham University Hospital, Barts NHS Trust, London E13 8SL, UK; sam.rowe2@nhs.net
3. Clinical Sciences, Liverpool School of Tropical Medicine, Liverpool L3 5QA, UK
* Correspondence: anitra.carr@otago.ac.nz; Tel.: +64-3364-0649

Received: 15 October 2020; Accepted: 21 October 2020; Published: 27 October 2020

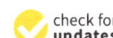

Abstract: Investigation into the role of vitamin C in the prevention and treatment of pneumonia and sepsis has been underway for many decades. This research has laid a strong foundation for translation of these findings into patients with severe coronavirus disease (COVID-19). Research has indicated that patients with pneumonia and sepsis have low vitamin C status and elevated oxidative stress. Administration of vitamin C to patients with pneumonia can decrease the severity and duration of the disease. Critically ill patients with sepsis require intravenous administration of gram amounts of the vitamin to normalize plasma levels, an intervention that some studies suggest reduces mortality. The vitamin has pleiotropic physiological functions, many of which are relevant to COVID-19. These include its antioxidant, anti-inflammatory, antithrombotic and immuno-modulatory functions. Preliminary observational studies indicate low vitamin C status in critically ill patients with COVID-19. There are currently a number of randomized controlled trials (RCTs) registered globally that are assessing intravenous vitamin C monotherapy in patients with COVID-19. Since hypovitaminosis C and deficiency are common in low–middle-income settings, and many of the risk factors for vitamin C deficiency overlap with COVID-19 risk factors, it is possible that trials carried out in populations with chronic hypovitaminosis C may show greater efficacy. This is particularly relevant for the global research effort since COVID-19 is disproportionately affecting low–middle-income countries and low-income groups globally. One small trial from China has finished early and the findings are currently under peer review. There was significantly decreased mortality in the more severely ill patients who received vitamin C intervention. The upcoming findings from the larger RCTs currently underway will provide more definitive evidence. Optimization of the intervention protocols in future trials, e.g., earlier and sustained administration, is warranted to potentially improve its efficacy. Due to the excellent safety profile, low cost, and potential for rapid upscaling of production, administration of vitamin C to patients with hypovitaminosis C and severe respiratory infections, e.g., COVID-19, appears warranted.

Keywords: vitamin C; ascorbate; ascorbic acid; COVID-19; pneumonia; sepsis; acute respiratory distress syndrome; randomized controlled trials; low-middle-income

---

For a quarter of a century, it has been known that critically ill patients, including those with sepsis and multiple organ failure, have very low vitamin C status [1–3]. It has also been demonstrated that these critically ill patients have higher requirements for vitamin C, with gram doses required to normalize their blood levels [4,5], 20–30 times more than is required for the general population. Despite these findings, critically ill patients with sepsis continue to be administered milligram amounts of vitamin C, which is insufficient to replete their vitamin C status [6]. In 2014, Dr Fowler and colleagues published the findings of a small clinical trial which indicated that intravenous administration of gram amounts of vitamin C to patients with sepsis could improve organ failure scores and decrease markers of inflammation (C-reactive protein) and tissue damage (thrombomodulin) [7]. In a larger randomized controlled trial (RCT) of septic patients with acute respiratory distress syndrome (ARDS), the CITRIS-ALI trial, intravenous administration of 200 mg/kg/d of vitamin C for 4 days resulted in a 28 day mortality of 30% relative to 46% in the placebo group ($p = 0.03$) and a hazard ratio (HR) of 0.55 (95% CI, 0.33–0.90, $p = 0.01$) [8]. The number of intensive care unit (ICU)- and hospital-free days was also significantly higher in the vitamin C group.

Administration of vitamin C late in the disease process, e.g., when ARDS has developed, likely attenuates its effectiveness. Earlier clinical trials have indicated that administration of vitamin C to patients with pneumonia can decrease the severity of the respiratory symptoms, particularly of the most severely ill patients, and the duration of hospital stay [9,10]. Thus, administration of vitamin C earlier in the respiratory infection process may prevent its progression to sepsis [11]. Survival data from the CITRIS-ALI trial has indicated that the effect of vitamin C on survival is most apparent during the 4 day infusion period [12]. Furthermore, pharmacokinetic research has indicated that upon cessation of vitamin C infusion, the vitamin C status of some patients returns to their low pre-infusion levels [5]. These findings call to sustained administration of the vitamin in the ICU. This will likely also improve the long-term outcomes of the patients, particularly if they continue to take the vitamin orally following discharge from ICU, due to its important roles in immunological function and in multiple organ systems [11].

Earlier this year, Dr Fowler and colleagues published a review on the emerging role of vitamin C as a treatment for sepsis [13]. In this review, they summarised the current state of knowledge around its pleiotropic physiological functions in sepsis. These include its roles as an antioxidant, a cofactor for the synthesis of vasopressors (norepinephrine and vasopressin), and roles in leukocyte and platelet functions, and endothelial and epithelial cell integrity. In the face of the current severe acute respiratory syndrome coronavirus (SARS-CoV-2) pandemic, this review has been very timely, with sepsis being a significant complication of severe coronavirus disease (COVID-19) [14].

Many of the functions of vitamin C appear relevant to COVID-19-related sepsis and ARDS. For example, recent research has uncovered a connection between SARS-CoV-2 infection and depleted levels of the antiviral cytokine interferon [15], and a negative association between interferon levels and disease severity [16,17]. Of note, vitamin C has been shown to augment interferon levels in animal models of viral infection [18,19]. Another characteristic of severe COVID-19 is elevated inflammatory markers and this can present as a 'cytokine storm' in some cases [14]. Vitamin C has anti-inflammatory and antioxidant activities which can potentially counteract this phenomenon [13]. Preliminary evidence from a small COVID-19 trial indicates that administration of intravenous vitamin C can significantly decrease IL-6 levels by day 7 of infusion [20].

Other common complications of COVID-19 are coagulopathy and microthrombi formation [14], which is likely a major component of COVID-19 lung pathology [21]. Early injection of vitamin C has been shown to prevent microthrombi formation and capillary plugging [22], and a case series has shown decreased D-dimer levels in COVID-19 patients who were administered intravenous vitamin C [23]. Neutrophil extracellular traps (NETs) have been implicated in COVID-19-related thrombotic complications [24,25]. Previous research has indicated that vitamin C administration can attenuate NETs in sepsis models [26], and post-hoc analysis of the CITRIS-ALI trial indicated decreased circulating cell-free DNA 48 h after administration of intravenous vitamin C [27]. Neutrophil-derived oxidative stress is believed to induce tissue damage in COVID-19 [28,29]. Patients with pneumonia and sepsis have significantly elevated oxidative stress markers relative to other critically ill patients [30,31], and early studies indicated that administration of vitamin C and other antioxidants to patients with septic shock and ARDS stabilized oxidative stress markers and improved cardiovascular parameters and survival [32,33].

In March, the World Health Organization published a coordinated global research roadmap for the 2019 novel coronavirus in which they identified a number of scientific knowledge gaps around determination of interventions that improve the clinical outcome of COVID-19-infected patients, including optimal selection of strategies for supportive care of seriously ill patients [34]. Of note, vitamin C was highlighted as an adjunctive intervention with biologic plausibility. Meta-analyses of relevant clinical trials have indicated that administration of vitamin C to critically ill patients can decrease the duration of mechanical ventilation and length of stay in ICU [35,36]. This is pertinent given global shortages of ICU capacity and may be particularly important for resource-limited settings such as those found in low–middle-income countries (LMICs) [37]. Of note, vitamin C production could be rapidly up-scaled globally, unlike many of the novel pharmacological treatments, some of which, e.g., remdesivir, have global shortages.

It is noteworthy that a majority of the top 10 countries with the highest COVID-19 case-loads are LMICs. In a recent review we highlighted the high prevalence of hypovitaminosis C and deficiency in LMICs (Figure 1) [38]. Furthermore, many of the risk factors for COVID-19 overlap with risk factors for vitamin C deficiency, such as poverty [39,40]. People who already have hypovitaminosis C are particularly susceptible to developing outright deficiency, and ergo more likely to respond to vitamin C administration. Therefore, the baseline vitamin C status of people with COVID-19 will likely affect their outcomes and their response to intervention [41,42].

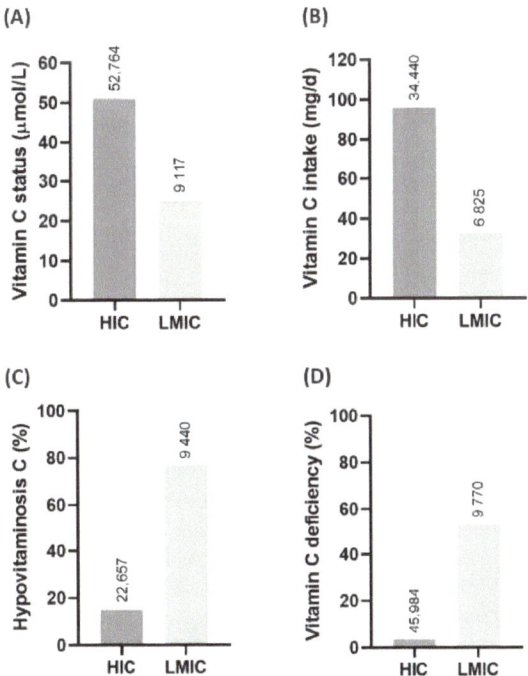

Figure 1. Summary of global vitamin C status (**A**) and intake (**B**) and prevalence of hypovitaminosis (**C**) and vitamin C deficiency (**D**). HIC—high-income countries; LMICs—low-middle-income countries. Hypovitaminosis C, <23 µmol/L; vitamin C deficiency, <11 µmol/L. Numbers above bars indicate the total number of individuals assessed. Data from [38].

As yet, there have been few publications reporting on the vitamin C status of patients with COVID-19. An observational study in the USA has indicated a mean vitamin C status of 22 ± 18 µmol/L in a cohort of 21 critically ill patients with COVID-19 [43], which is comparable to other studies of critically ill patients with sepsis [11]. An earlier case series from Spain indicated the absence of any detectable vitamin C in 17 of a cohort of 18 COVID-19 patients with ARDS [44]. However, the veracity of the methodology used to assess the vitamin C status of the patients was not clear, so the values could be artifactually low [45].

There are a number of clinical trials registered globally assessing intravenous vitamin C monotherapy in COVID-19 patients (Table 1). The first trial off the ground was in Hubei, China (NCT04264533) [46]. In this trial the investigators planned to treat 140 patients with a placebo control or intravenous vitamin C at a relatively high dose of 24 g/day for 7 days, and assess requirements for mechanical ventilation and vasopressor drugs, organ failure scores, ICU length of stay and mortality. A preprint of the findings of 54 patients from this trial is currently under peer review [15]. Although the investigators reported no differences between the treatment and placebo groups for the above outcomes, when a subgroup of the most severely ill patients (SOFA scores ≥ 3) was assessed, a significant decrease in ICU and hospital mortality was observed in the vitamin C group—18% vs. 50% in the placebo group (HR 0.2, 95% CI 0.1–0.9, $p = 0.03$). Unfortunately, the baseline vitamin C status of the patients was not reported.

The USA currently has the highest number of COVID-19 cases globally, however despite this, there are only a couple of small intravenous vitamin C monotherapy and COVID-19 trials registered in the USA (NCT04344184 and NCT04363216). A trial at the Cleveland Clinic is assessing oral vitamin C with and without zinc (NCT04342728). However, due to the pharmacokinetics of enteral and parenteral vitamin C differing dramatically, and the higher requirement for vitamin C during respiratory infections, oral vitamin C may not be as efficacious as intravenous vitamin C [42]. As such, future meta-analyses of vitamin C and COVID-19 clinical trials should include subgroup analyses of studies comprising intravenous vs. oral vitamin C. Furthermore, subgroup analysis of low vitamin C populations could also be carried out as RCT findings will likely vary depending on the country and hence the baseline vitamin C status of the population in which the study was carried out [47]. In populations with a high prevalence of chronic hypovitaminosis C, vitamin C intervention may show greater efficacy.

Overall, vitamin C exhibits plausible mechanisms of action that are of relevance to severe respiratory infection, including antioxidant, anti-inflammatory, antithrombotic, and immuno-modulatory functions. Based on the findings from clinical trials of patients with pneumonia and sepsis, and preliminary observational and interventional studies of COVID-19 patients, it is likely that vitamin C administration will improve outcomes in COVID-19. The upcoming findings from the larger RCTs currently underway (e.g., LOVIT-COVID), including introduction of intravenous vitamin C arms to large adaptive trials (e.g., REMAP-CAP; NCT02735707), will provide more definitive evidence. Some of these trials (e.g., LOVIT-COVID) are also examining the longer-term quality of life effects of short-term vitamin C administration. Optimization of the intervention protocols in future trials, e.g., earlier and sustained administration, is warranted to potentially improve its efficacy. Due to the excellent safety profile, low cost, and potential for rapid upscaling of production, administration of vitamin C to patients with hypovitaminosis C and severe respiratory infections, e.g., COVID-19, appears warranted.

Table 1. Summary of registered intravenous vitamin C (IVC) monotherapy and COVID-19 trials globally.

Country Study ID	Title	Participants	Intervention	Primary Outcome(s)
Canada NCT04401150	Lessening Organ Dysfunction with VITamin C—COVID-19 (LOVIT-COVID)	800 hospitalized patients with COVID-19	50 mg/kg/6 h IVC for 96 h vs. placebo	Death or persistent organ dysfunction
Italy NCT04323514	Use of Ascorbic Acid in Patients With COVID-19	500 patients with COVID-19 pneumonia	10 g/d IVC for 72 h uncontrolled	In-hospital mortality
USA NCT04344184	Early Infusion of Vitamin C for Treatment of Novel COVID-19 Acute Lung Injury (EVICT-CORONA-ALI)	200 patients with COVID-19 acute lung injury	100 mg/kg/8 h IVC for 96 h vs. placebo	Number of ventilator-free days
USA NCT04363216	Pharmacologic Ascorbic Acid as an Activator of Lymphocyte Signaling for COVID-19 Treatment	66 patients with COVID-19	0.3–0.9 g/kg/d IVC for 6 days vs. control	Clinical Improvement
China NCT04264533	Vitamin C Infusion for the Treatment of Severe 2019-nCoV Infected Pneumonia	140 patients with COVID-19 pneumonia	12 g/12 h IVC for 7 days vs. placebo	Ventilator-free days
China ChiCTR-2000032400	The efficacy and safety of high dose IVC in the treatment of novel coronavirus pneumonia (COVID-19)	120 patients with COVID-19 pneumonia	100 mg/kg/d IVC for up to 7 days vs. placebo	CRP, ESR, existence of SIRS
Iran IRCT2020-0411047025N1	Evaluation of effectiveness of IVC in Patients with COVID-19 Referred to Imam Khomeini Hospital	110 patients with COVID-19	1.5 g/6 h IVC for up to 5 days vs. control	Improvement of SPO_2
Iran IRCT2019-0917044805N2	Effects of High-dose Vitamin C on Treatment, Clinical Symptoms and Laboratory Signs of Iranian COVID-19 Patients	60 patients with COVID-19	12 g/d IVC for 4 days vs. placebo	Time to clinical improvement
Iran IRCT2020-0516047468N1	Interventional study of IVC in definitive patients with COVID-19 and its effect on changes in lung CT scan and clinical and laboratory symptoms of patients	50 patients with COVID-19	2 g/6 h IVC for 5 days vs. control	The amount of lung involvement in a CT scan

Author Contributions: Conceptualization, A.C.C.; writing—original draft preparation, A.C.C.; writing—review and editing, S.R. All authors have read and agreed to the published version of the manuscript.

Funding: This research received no external funding.

Acknowledgments: A.C.C. is the recipient of a Health Research Council of New Zealand Sir Charles Hercus Health Research Fellowship.

Conflicts of Interest: The authors declare no conflict of interest.

References

1. Schorah, C.J.; Downing, C.; Piripitsi, A.; Gallivan, L.; Al-Hazaa, A.H.; Sanderson, M.J.; Bodenham, A. Total vitamin C, ascorbic acid, and dehydroascorbic acid concentrations in plasma of critically ill patients. *Am. J. Clin. Nutr.* **1996**, *63*, 760–765. [CrossRef] [PubMed]
2. Galley, H.F.; Davies, M.J.; Webster, N.R. Ascorbyl radical formation in patients with sepsis: Effect of ascorbate loading. *Free Radic. Biol. Med.* **1996**, *20*, 139–143. [CrossRef]
3. Borrelli, E.; Roux-Lombard, P.; Grau, G.E.; Girardin, E.; Ricou, B.; Dayer, J.; Suter, P.M. Plasma concentrations of cytokines, their soluble receptors, and antioxidant vitamins can predict the development of multiple organ failure in patients at risk. *Crit. Care Med.* **1996**, *24*, 392–397. [CrossRef] [PubMed]
4. Long, C.L.; Maull, K.I.; Krishnan, R.S.; Laws, H.L.; Geiger, J.W.; Borghesi, L.; Franks, W.; Lawson, T.C.; Sauberlich, H.E. Ascorbic acid dynamics in the seriously ill and injured. *J. Surg. Res.* **2003**, *109*, 144–148. [CrossRef]
5. de Grooth, H.J.; Manubulu-Choo, W.P.; Zandvliet, A.S.; Spoelstra-de Man, A.M.E.; Girbes, A.R.; Swart, E.L.; Oudemans-van Straaten, H.M. Vitamin-C pharmacokinetics in critically ill patients: A randomized trial of four intravenous regimens. *Chest* **2018**, *153*, 1368–1377. [CrossRef] [PubMed]
6. Carr, A.C.; Rosengrave, P.C.; Bayer, S.; Chambers, S.; Mehrtens, J.; Shaw, G.M. Hypovitaminosis C and vitamin C deficiency in critically ill patients despite recommended enteral and parenteral intakes. *Crit. Care* **2017**, *21*, 300. [CrossRef]
7. Fowler, A.A.; Syed, A.A.; Knowlson, S.; Sculthorpe, R.; Farthing, D.; DeWilde, C.; Farthing, C.A.; Larus, T.L.; Martin, E.; Brophy, D.F.; et al. Phase I safety trial of intravenous ascorbic acid in patients with severe sepsis. *J. Transl. Med.* **2014**, *12*, 32. [CrossRef] [PubMed]
8. Fowler, A.A., 3rd; Truwit, J.D.; Hite, R.D.; Morris, P.E.; DeWilde, C.; Priday, A.; Fisher, B.; Thacker, L.R., 2nd; Natarajan, R.; Brophy, D.F.; et al. Effect of vitamin C infusion on organ failure and biomarkers of inflammation and vascular injury in patients with sepsis and severe acute respiratory failure: The CITRIS-ALI randomized clinical trial. *JAMA* **2019**, *322*, 1261–1270. [CrossRef]
9. Hunt, C.; Chakravorty, N.K.; Annan, G.; Habibzadeh, N.; Schorah, C.J. The clinical effects of vitamin C supplementation in elderly hospitalised patients with acute respiratory infections. *Int. J. Vitam. Nutr. Res.* **1994**, *64*, 212–219.
10. Mochalkin, N.I. Ascorbic acid in the complex therapy of acute pneumonia. (English translation: http://www.mv.helsinki.fi/home/hemila/T5.pdf). *Voen. Med. Zhurnal* **1970**, *9*, 17–21.
11. Carr, A.C. Vitamin C in pneumonia and sepsis. In *Vitamin C: New Biochemical and Functional Insights. Oxidative Stress and Disease*; Chen, Q., Vissers, M., Eds.; CRC Press/Taylor & Francis: Boca Raton, FL, USA, 2020; pp. 115–135.
12. Hemilä, H.; Chalker, E. Reanalysis of the effect of vitamin C on mortality in the CITRIS-ALI trial: Important findings dismissed in the trial report. *Front. Med.* **2020**, *7*, 590853. [CrossRef]
13. Kashiouris, M.G.; L'Heureux, M.; Cable, C.A.; Fisher, B.J.; Leichtle, S.W.; Fowler, A.A. The emerging role of vitamin C as a treatment for sepsis. *Nutrients* **2020**, *12*, 292. [CrossRef] [PubMed]
14. Wiersinga, W.J.; Rhodes, A.; Cheng, A.C.; Peacock, S.J.; Prescott, H.C. Pathophysiology, Transmission, Diagnosis, and Treatment of Coronavirus Disease 2019 (COVID-19): A Review. *JAMA* **2020**, *324*, 782–793. [CrossRef] [PubMed]
15. Blanco-Melo, D.; Nilsson-Payant, B.E.; Liu, W.C.; Uhl, S.; Hoagland, D.; Møller, R.; Jordan, T.X.; Oishi, K.; Panis, M.; Sachs, D.; et al. Imbalanced host response to SARS-CoV-2 drives development of COVID-19. *Cell* **2020**, *181*, 1036–1045. [CrossRef] [PubMed]
16. Zhang, Q.; Bastard, P.; Liu, Z.; Le Pen, J.; Moncada-Velez, M.; Chen, J.; Ogishi, M.; Sabli, I.K.D.; Hodeib, S.; Korol, C.; et al. Inborn errors of type I IFN immunity in patients with life-threatening COVID-19. *Science* **2020**, *370*, eabd4570. [CrossRef]

17. Bastard, P.; Rosen, L.B.; Zhang, Q.; Michailidis, E.; Hoffmann, H.H.; Zhang, Y.; Dorgham, K.; Philippot, Q.; Rosain, J.; Béziat, V.; et al. Auto-antibodies against type I IFNs in patients with life-threatening COVID-19. *Science* **2020**, *370*, eabd4585. [CrossRef]
18. Kim, Y.; Kim, H.; Bae, S.; Choi, J.; Lim, S.Y.; Lee, N.; Kong, J.M.; Hwang, Y.I.; Kang, J.S.; Lee, W.J. Vitamin C is an essential factor on the anti-viral immune responses through the production of interferon-α/β at the initial stage of influenza A virus (H3N2) infection. *Immune Netw.* **2013**, *13*, 70–74. [CrossRef]
19. Geber, W.F.; Lefkowitz, S.S.; Hung, C.Y. Effect of ascorbic acid, sodium salicylate, and caffeine on the serum interferon level in response to viral infection. *Pharmacology* **1975**, *13*, 228–233. [CrossRef]
20. Zhang, J.; Rao, X.; Li, Y.; Zhu, Y.; Liu, F.; Guo, G.; Luo, G.; Meng, Z.; De Backer, D.; Xiang, H.; et al. High-dose vitamin C infusion for the treatment of critically ill COVID-19. *Res. Sq.* **2020**. [CrossRef]
21. José, R.J.; Williams, A.; Manuel, A.; Brown, J.S.; Chambers, R.C. Targeting coagulation activation in severe COVID-19 pneumonia: Lessons from bacterial pneumonia and sepsis. *Eur. Respir. Rev.* **2020**, *29*, 200240. [CrossRef]
22. Tyml, K. Vitamin C and microvascular dysfunction in systemic inflammation. *Antioxidants* **2017**, *6*, 49. [CrossRef] [PubMed]
23. Hiedra, R.; Lo, K.B.; Elbashabsheh, M.; Gul, F.; Wright, R.M.; Albano, J.; Azmaiparashvili, Z.; Patarroyo Aponte, G. The use of IV vitamin C for patients with COVID-19: A case series. *Expert Rev. Anti Infect. Ther.* **2020**, 1–3. [CrossRef]
24. Middleton, E.A.; He, X.Y.; Denorme, F.; Campbell, R.A.; Ng, D.; Salvatore, S.P.; Mostyka, M.; Baxter-Stoltzfus, A.; Borczuk, A.C.; Loda, M.; et al. Neutrophil extracellular traps contribute to immunothrombosis in COVID-19 acute respiratory distress syndrome. *Blood* **2020**, *136*, 1169–1179. [CrossRef]
25. Skendros, P.; Mitsios, A.; Chrysanthopoulou, A.; Mastellos, D.C.; Metallidis, S.; Rafailidis, P.; Ntinopoulou, M.; Sertaridou, E.; Tsironidou, V.; Tsigalou, C.; et al. Complement and tissue factor-enriched neutrophil extracellular traps are key drivers in COVID-19 immunothrombosis. *J. Clin. Investig.* **2020**. [CrossRef]
26. Mohammed, B.M.; Fisher, B.J.; Kraskauskas, D.; Farkas, D.; Brophy, D.F.; Fowler, A.A.; Natarajan, R. Vitamin C: A novel regulator of neutrophil extracellular trap formation. *Nutrients* **2013**, *5*, 3131–3151. [CrossRef]
27. Qiao, X.; Fisher, B.; Kashiouris, M.G.; Truwit, J.D.; Hite, R.D.; Morris, P.E.; Martin, G.S.; Fowler, A.A. Effects of high dose intravenous vitamin C (IVC) on plasma cell-free DNA levels in patients with sepsis-associated ARDS. *Am. J. Respir. Crit. Care Med.* **2019**, *201*, A2100.
28. Schönrich, G.; Raftery, M.J.; Samstag, Y. Devilishly radical NETwork in COVID-19: Oxidative stress, neutrophil extracellular traps (NETs), and T cell suppression. *Adv. Biol. Regul.* **2020**, *77*, 100741. [CrossRef] [PubMed]
29. Laforge, M.; Elbim, C.; Frère, C.; Hémadi, M.; Massaad, C.; Nuss, P.; Benoliel, J.J.; Becker, C. Tissue damage from neutrophil-induced oxidative stress in COVID-19. *Nat. Rev. Immunol.* **2020**, *20*, 515–516. [CrossRef]
30. Carr, A.C.; Spencer, E.; Mackle, D.; Hunt, A.; Judd, H.; Mehrtens, J.; Parker, K.; Stockwell, Z.; Gale, C.; Beaumont, M.; et al. The effect of conservative oxygen therapy on systemic biomarkers of oxidative stress in critically ill patients. *Free Radic. Biol. Med.* **2020**. under consideration. [CrossRef] [PubMed]
31. Carr, A.C.; Spencer, E.; Dixon, L.; Chambers, S.T. Patients with community acquired pneumonia exhibit depleted vitamin C status and elevated oxidative stress. *Nutrients* **2020**, *12*, 1318. [CrossRef] [PubMed]
32. Galley, H.F.; Howdle, P.D.; Walker, B.E.; Webster, N.R. The effects of intravenous antioxidants in patients with septic shock. *Free Radic. Biol. Med.* **1997**, *23*, 768–774. [CrossRef]
33. Sawyer, M.A.J.; Mike, J.J.; Chavin, K.; Marino, P.L. Antioxidant therapy and survival in ARDS. *Crit. Care Med.* **1989**, *17*, S153.
34. World Health Organization. *A Coordinated Global Research Roadmap: 2019 Novel Coronavirus*; World Health Organization: Geneva, Switzerland, 2020.
35. Hemila, H.; Chalker, E. Vitamin C may reduce the duration of mechanical ventilation in critically ill patients: A meta-regression analysis. *J. Intensive Care* **2020**, *8*, 15. [CrossRef] [PubMed]
36. Hemila, H.; Chalker, E. Vitamin C can shorten the length of stay in the ICU: A meta-analysis. *Nutrients* **2019**, *11*, 708. [CrossRef] [PubMed]
37. Siow, W.T.; Liew, M.F.; Shrestha, B.R.; Muchtar, F.; See, K.C. Managing COVID-19 in resource-limited settings: Critical care considerations. *Crit. Care* **2020**, *24*, 167. [CrossRef]
38. Rowe, S.; Carr, A.C. Global vitamin C status and prevalence of deficiency: A cause for concern? *Nutrients* **2020**, *12*, 2008. [CrossRef] [PubMed]

39. Carr, A.C.; Rowe, S. Factors affecting vitamin C status and prevalence of deficiency: A global health perspective. *Nutrients* **2020**, *12*, 1963. [CrossRef]
40. Centres for Disease Control and Prevention. Assessing Risk Factors for Severe COVID-19 Illness 2020. Available online: https://www.cdc.gov/coronavirus/2019-ncov/covid-data/investigations-discovery/assessing-risk-factors.html (accessed on 5 September 2020).
41. Carr, A.C. Micronutrient status of COVID-19 patients: A critical consideration. *Crit. Care* **2020**, *24*, 349. [CrossRef] [PubMed]
42. Lykkesfeldt, J. On the effect of vitamin C intake on human health: How to (mis)interprete the clinical evidence. *Redox Biol.* **2020**, *34*, 101532. [CrossRef]
43. Arvinte, C.; Singh, M.; Marik, P.E. Serum levels of vitamin C and vitamin D in a cohort of critically ill COVID-19 patients of a north American community hospital intensive care unit in may 2020. A pilot study. *Med. Drug Discov.* **2020**, *8*, 100064. [CrossRef]
44. Chiscano-Camón, L.; Ruiz-Rodriguez, J.C.; Ruiz-Sanmartin, A.; Roca, O.; Ferrer, R. Vitamin C levels in patients with SARS-CoV-2-associated acute respiratory distress syndrome. *Crit. Care* **2020**, *24*, 522. [CrossRef] [PubMed]
45. Pullar, J.M.; Bayer, S.; Carr, A.C. Appropriate handling, processing and analysis of blood samples is essential to avoid oxidation of vitamin C to dehydroascorbic acid. *Antioxidants* **2018**, *7*, 29. [CrossRef] [PubMed]
46. Liu, F.; Zhu, Y.; Zhang, J.; Li, Y.; Peng, Z. Intravenous high-dose vitamin C for the treatment of severe COVID-19: Study protocol for a multicentre randomised controlled trial. *BMJ Open* **2020**, *10*, e039519. [CrossRef] [PubMed]
47. Hemilä, H.; Suonsyrjä, T. Vitamin C for preventing atrial fibrillation in high risk patients: A systematic review and meta-analysis. *BMC Cardiovasc. Disord.* **2017**, *17*, 49. [CrossRef]

Publisher's Note: MDPI stays neutral with regard to jurisdictional claims in published maps and institutional affiliations.

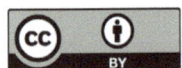

© 2020 by the authors. Licensee MDPI, Basel, Switzerland. This article is an open access article distributed under the terms and conditions of the Creative Commons Attribution (CC BY) license (http://creativecommons.org/licenses/by/4.0/).

MDPI
St. Alban-Anlage 66
4052 Basel
Switzerland
Tel. +41 61 683 77 34
Fax +41 61 302 89 18
www.mdpi.com

Nutrients Editorial Office
E-mail: nutrients@mdpi.com
www.mdpi.com/journal/nutrients

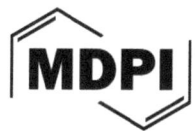

www.ingramcontent.com/pod-product-compliance
Lightning Source LLC
LaVergne TN
LVHW072344090526
838202LV00019B/2475